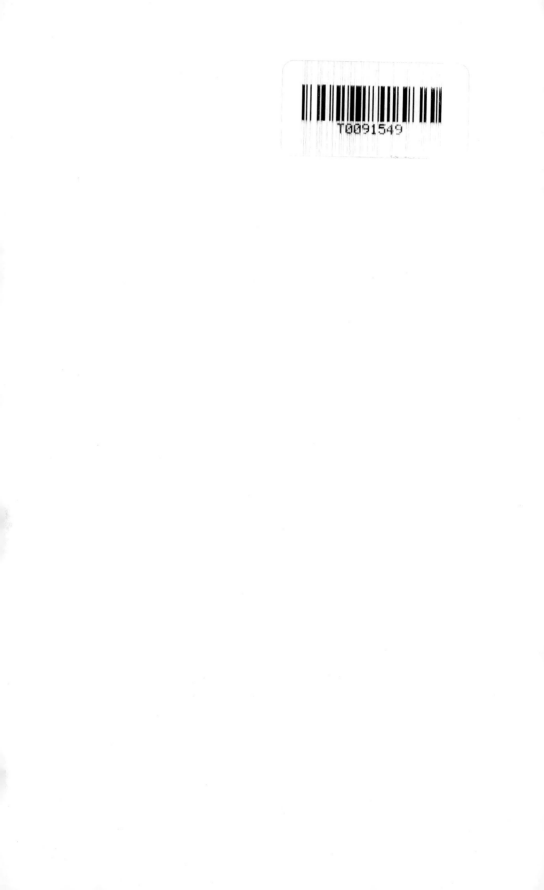

How to Write Better Medical Papers

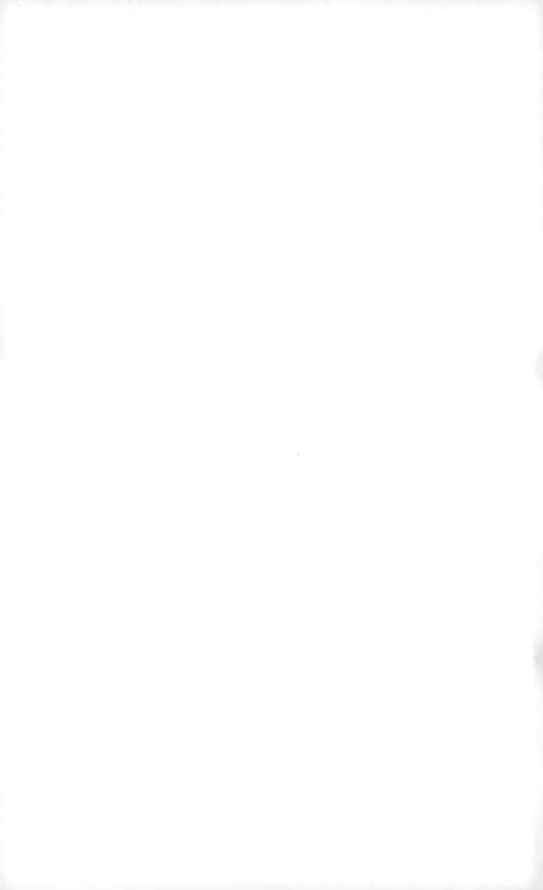

Michael Hanna

How to Write
Better Medical Papers

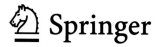 Springer

Michael Hanna
Mercury Medical Research & Writing
New York, NY
USA

ISBN 978-3-030-02954-8   ISBN 978-3-030-02955-5   (eBook)
https://doi.org/10.1007/978-3-030-02955-5

Library of Congress Control Number: 2018964919

This Springer imprint is published by the registered company Springer Nature Switzerland AG
The registered company address is: Gewerbestrasse 11, 6330 Cham, Switzerland

*Den Stil verbessern – das heisst
den Gedanken verbessern, und
gar Nichts weiter!*

– Friedrich Nietzsche
(Der Wanderer und sein Schatten, §131)

[Translation: Improving your writing style means
nothing other than improving your thinking.]

Contents

Part III   Drafting

Part IV   Special Types of Articles

Part V   Revising

Chapter 1
Introduction

Scientific journal papers are the predominant means of communicating new information and ideas in the fields of medicine, life sciences, and health sciences. They serve many important functions in society today. Physicians and healthcare professionals routinely consult journal papers to guide their decisions on patient care and learn about anything new since they left medical school. Researchers and companies rely heavily on journal papers in their work to gradually develop new medical treatments. Government agencies draw on the scientific literature to set health policies and provide proper healthcare and public health programs. Even some patients and their family members sometimes look at medical journal papers to learn about their health conditions and possible treatments. Over 1.1 million journal items were published in 2017 and indexed in PubMed by the US National Library of Medicine [1].

Unfortunately, the published journal literature of medicine, including the related life sciences and health sciences, is plagued with substantial errors, nonsensical statements, lethal omissions, illogical reasoning, false discoveries, and misleading conclusions. For example, the world-famous German pharmaceutical firm, Bayer, has tried to reproduce many promising preclinical studies published by other researchers, but Bayer reports that about two out of every three such studies were so irreproducible that the projects were canceled [2]. Similarly, the well-known American biotech firm, Amgen, has reported that they were only able to confirm the findings of 6 out of 53 "landmark" preclinical studies on cancer, even after conferring with the original investigators [3]. Thus the leaders of the National Institutes of Health (NIH) in the United States recognized that the irreproducibility of published studies and the frequent failure to publish studies at all are widespread problems in preclinical medical research, and they attributed these problems in large part to poor training of researchers and poor quality of research reporting [4]. Several other leaders in medical science have also discussed the extent and gravity of irreproducible preclinical research [5–8].

Clinical research also has its own laundry list of problems. Numerous reviews of the published literature have shown that papers frequently lack essential information about the methods and results [9–13], report their studies in self-contradicting ways

© Springer Nature Switzerland AG 2019
M. Hanna, *How to Write Better Medical Papers*,
https://doi.org/10.1007/978-3-030-02955-5_1

[14–17], and draw conclusions that are unsupported by their own results [18, 19]. Errors in statistical analysis, methodology, and reporting are so frequent and serious that one leading expert has described the medical literature as a "scandal" [20, 21]. Other experts have expressed similarly dismal viewpoints [22–25]. Subtle and non-so-subtle forms of bias are considered to be pervasive in the literature [26–30], as well as in the selection of what actually gets published at all [31–34]. And much of the published medical scientific literature is so badly written that even other native English-speaking researchers and clinicians struggle to understand what it even says [35–42]. Thus, it is no wonder that most medical doctors rarely bother to read anything more than the Abstracts, if even that much [43–45].

It must be emphasized that none of these problems refer to illicit deviations from the expectations of the medical community, such as falsified data or plagiarized articles, which are retracted from the literature when they are caught. Instead, all the problems described above refer to the "normal" state of affairs, regrettably. They can be found throughout the medical literature, even in the most prominent journals. Thus, much of the published medical scientific literature could be viewed as a waste [46]. Furthermore, over half the research studies that are completed are never published in a scientific journal at all [47–50], so virtually no one even knows what they found. In most cases, those studies remain unpublished because the researchers simply did not have all the capabilities and resources needed to write up a report that would meet even the current low standards of typical scientific journals.

But what is the root cause of all these deficiencies in the medical scientific literature that are decried by leaders in the medical research establishment? There are two closely related reasons for these deficiencies, one of which is discussed here, the other of which is discussed at the end of this book. The first part of the explanation is that universities, governments, and societies fail to provide sufficient education and training specifically for the performance and reporting of scientific research. The usual four-year medical school program is designed – rightly so – to train future physicians to take care of patients, not to conduct scientific research. Medical school provides excellent education about human health and diseases, the underlying biology, the available treatments, the clinical reasoning and medical skills needed to provide good healthcare, and so on. But medical school provides virtually no classwork in statistics or research methodology, and provides no training in how to write academic essays. Because most graduates of medical school will dedicate their lives to patient care instead of scientific research, there is little or no reason why the medical curriculum should change. Unfortunately, the opportunities after medical school to retrain for scientific research are mostly haphazard and unappealing. The need for better training of medical researchers has been widely recognized by leaders in the scientific community [4, 20, 51–58], but actual changes to the education and training system have been sparse.

Consequently, most people involved in performing and reporting medical research have insufficient education and training in the specific skills that are needed to be doing that research work, such as ethics, methodology, statistics, logic, and writing. They have only subject knowledge about the disease or treatment they studied. Some medical doctors fill this training gap by pursuing an additional university degree, such as a Master of Public Health (MPH); others fill this gap by just working together closely with life scientists and/or health scientists who have spent years learning these subjects and skills (instead of clinical subjects and patient care). But in most cases, medical doctors simply perform and report their research as best they can, on the basis of their expert subject knowledge, despite insufficient formal education and training in the subjects and skills needed specifically to perform and report scientific research. Even in the life sciences and social sciences – where the doctoral degree programs are geared toward producing scientific researchers – education and training in the specific skills needed to write scientific papers is often less than adequate, (and thus is supplemented by years of post-doctoral training). At bottom, the blame here lies entirely with the educational system and society for failing to provide medical researchers with sufficient education and training to do that work as well as everyone says it should be.

The consequence of these shortcomings in the education system is that most medical researchers struggle to write their journals papers and struggle to get them published – understandably so. They spend substantial amounts of time and energy trying to figure out what to write and how, and then trying to find a journal that will agree to publish their paper after further extensive revisions. Even after the papers are published, they are often still full of problems, as described above, that will be critiqued in later review papers or subsequent research publications. And unfortunately, less than half of all completed research studies are ever published in a scientific journal at all [47–50]. Undoubtedly this reflects the real difficulty of writing and publishing a journal paper [59, 60].

Researchers whose native language is not English but who strive to publish their work in English anyway have the added challenge of trying to write in a non-native language. It seems reasonable to estimate that more than half the co-authors of medical journal papers published in English today are not native speakers of English, so this is important to address here. Unfortunately, the difficulty for non-native speakers to write in English often hides the fact that these researchers (just like most native English speaking researchers) have many other difficulties with scientific writing that have no relation to using English as a second language. In other words, non-native speakers often believe – quite mistakenly – that if someone would just correct the English grammar of their manuscript, it would be perfect for publication. Unfortunately, that is rarely the case. Most of the problems that lead journals to reject manuscripts (besides the scientific contents) are more substantial than mere problems with just the English language itself. These problems are frequently encountered among native English speaking researchers too. Thus when peer reviewers recommend that non-native researchers have someone correct "the English" of their manuscript, the peer reviewers are usually pointing to larger problems of composition and logic that go far beyond mere issues of English grammar. When peer reviewers encounter such problems in manuscripts by native speakers of English, instead of recommending that the authors find someone to correct "the English", the peer reviewers simply say that the manuscript is poorly written and difficult to comprehend and should be rewritten. So both native and non-native speakers of English have mostly the same needs for improvement of their scientific writing – most of which is not simply an issue of the English language itself. Most non-native speakers may need some additional support in English as a second language. But honestly, many native English speaking medical researchers also have bad English grammar in need of improvement. At least non-native speakers are conscious of their need to achieve good English grammar; whereas, most native English speakers remain oblivious to their poor written English.

This book serves as an initial "self-teaching" book that guides researchers through the main phases of writing better research papers: preparing, analyzing, drafting, revising, and publishing. It aims to enable medical researchers (including also life scientists and health scientists) to get their papers published with less struggle and fewer rejections – precisely by improving the quality of their papers. No one book can substitute for years of university teaching and training in the subjects mentioned above – ethics, methodology, statistics, logic, writing. But hopefully this book will be worth your time to read and reread, by reducing the amount of time needed to get your papers written and published, while simultaneously improving their quality. This book provides explanations and justifications for its recommendations – it does not simply tell you what to do, but also why, so you can use your own mind to decided if the advice is any good. This book also strives, whenever possible, to guide readers to the vast but poorly known literature on various aspects of medical scientific communication, so you will know where to find further guidance whenever needed. (In this regards, this book may be one of the first on this topic that consciously strives to go beyond mere "expert opinion" and develop a scholarly account of the subject of medical scientific writing, grounded in the relevant literature. And hopefully, the annotated bibliography will serve as a valuable resource.)

Books and articles about scientific writing often think about "good writing" mainly in terms of English grammar and style. They equate "good" scientific writing with texts that would be pleasing to a secondary school English teacher. They then proceed to instruct researchers about the rules of good grammar, simple syntax, clear word choices, proper punctuation, etc. Good English grammar and a clear writing style are important, and they are often sorely lacking in the medical scientific literature. So this book provides some guidance on these issues in part V, "Revising". However, these issues of grammar, word choices, syntax, and so on are a rather limited notion of "writing". These aspects are really just the *craft* of writing, or more precisely, the craft of editing. The craft of editing is important, to ensure that your paper communicates clearly. Otherwise, people will not understand what you are telling them, regardless of how brilliant your research findings might be. But these aspects of good English grammar are not specific to medical science and are not sufficient to ensure high-quality medical scientific papers. Beautifully written sentences will still be terrible scientific writing, if the content is irrelevant, illogical, erroneous, muddled, incomplete, inconsistent, biased, scatter-brained, etc. Better scientific writing requires eliminating these kinds of problems from the thoughts being expressed. Editing for good English grammar is then just further fine polishing.

Excellent scientific writing requires excellent scientific thinking. In fact, the process of writing up a scientific paper is equivalent to thinking scientifically about what you want to say, why, and how. The majority of published scientific papers are poorly written, not mainly because the authors have bad English grammar that got past the journal Editors, (though that happens frequently too). Instead, most medical scientific papers are poorly written because the authors really were not sure what exactly their research was really about: which results to present, why, how, what to say about them, and many other such substantial scientific issues of the contents and presentation. These kinds of issues are beyond the capabilities of any English language copy-editor to fix for you. Clear scientific writing is a reflection of clear scientific thinking, which can only come from scientists themselves.

The writing process is not a mere supplemental task to do after the research is done. Instead, writing is an essential continuation of the scientific research, whereby the researchers think through their data and what they mean. In some sense, the write-up phase (not the data collection phase) is the true core of science because this is when a nebulous amount of private thoughts from a long period of time must finally crystallize into a permanent public record. The writing phase is when researchers must make final fixed decisions about what they really did, what they found, and what it all really means. For example, do you discuss the high economic costs of the current standard treatment for disease X as part of the rationale for why you performed this study on a potential new form of treatment? How much detail should you provide to explain how you recruited and selected patients to participate in the study? Do you compare each study group's clinical score at baseline versus follow-up and report the p-values for each group's change across time, or do you calculate the median and 95% confidence interval of the difference between the two groups' clinical scores at baseline and at follow-up, or do you report on a multivariable linear regression analysis with the change in clinical score from baseline to follow-up as the outcome variable and the study group as one of several predictor variables? Do you conclude that your study shows that treatment X is safe for use in adolescents or do you instead focus on the 6% loss-to-follow up as a puzzling study limitation? These are examples of some of the kinds of choices you will make during the writing phase of your research. Writing forces you to put your thinking into final form. (And again, neither a copy-editor nor your secondary school English teacher can provide you any guidance about how to write better papers in regards to these kinds of substantial aspects of scientific thinking/writing.)

A written text is also the social transmission of your thoughts from your mind over to the minds of the readers. In order to transmit your thoughts clearly to someone else, you must first clarify to yourself exactly what you are thinking. Muddled writing reflects muddled research and muddled thinking. Learning to write better scientific papers goes hand in hand with doing better research and thinking more scientifically. Indeed, learning to communicate clearly is an essential prerequisite to becoming a fully qualified scientist. Otherwise, no one will know what you are doing or why it matters, and no one will support your research work.

The goal of this book is to improve the quality of the scientific medical literature, by improving your capabilities to write better scientific medical papers. This book does not accept the notion that getting a paper published is "good enough", because the published medical journal literature, including the life sciences and health sciences, is plagued with substantial errors, nonsensical statements, lethal omissions, illogical reasoning, false discoveries, and misleading conclusions. We can and should do better. So this book assumes that even if you are writing your very first paper, you will need to exceed the current level of quality in the published literature. If you have already published journal papers, your forthcoming papers should get better and contribute to quality improvement of the literature. That is what is meant by "scientific progress": every year, we learn more and reach new higher standards. This book will help you write better papers and contribute to scientific progress. Better quality medical research publications will lead to better health for humanity.

References

1. US National Library of Medicine. PubMed. Accessed on 22 April 2018 (with a publication data range filter for 2017, and use of the "Results by year" graph and further examining of the search results) at: https://www.ncbi.nlm.nih.gov/pubmed
2. Prinz F, Schlange T, Asadullah K. Believe it or not: how much can we rely on published data on potential drug targets? Nat Rev Drug Discov. 2011; 10: 712.
3. Begley CG, Ellis LM. Raise standards for preclinical cancer research. Nature. 2012; 483: 531-533.
4. Collins FS, Tabak LA. NIH plans to enhance reproducibility. Nature. 2014; 505: 612-613.
5. Landis SC, Amara SG, Asadullah K, Austin CP, Blumenstein R, Bradley EW, Crystal RG, Darnell RB, Ferrante RJ, Fillit H, Finkelstein R, Fisher M, Gendelman HE, Golub RM, Goudreau JL, Gross RA, Gubitz AK, Hesterlee SE, Howells DW, Huguenard J, Kelner K, Koroshetz W, Krainc D, Lazic SE, Levine MS, Macleod MR, McGall JM, Moxlex RT III, Narasimhan K, Noble LJ, Perrin S, Porter JD, Steward O, Unger E, Utz U, Silberberg SD. A call for transparent reporting to optimize the predictive value of preclinical research. Nature. 2012; 490: 187-191.
6. Drug targets slip-sliding away. Nature. 2011; 17: 1155.
7. The long road to reproducibility. Nat Cell Biol. 2015; 17: 1513-1514.
8. Marcus E. Credibility and Reproducibility. Cell. 2014; 159: 965-966.
9. Berwanger O, Ribeiro RA, Finkelsztejn A, Watanabe M, Suzumura EA, Duncan BB, Devereaux PJ, Cook D. The quality of reporting of trial abstracts is suboptimal: survey of major general medical journals. J Clin Epidemiol. 2009; 62: 387-392.
10. Junker CA. Adherence to Published Standards of Reporting: A Comparison of Placebo-Controlled Trials Published in English or German. JAMA. 1998; 280: 247-249.
11. Bernal-Delgado E, Fisher ES. Abstracts in high profile journals often fail to report harm. BMC Med Res Methodol. 2008; 8: 14.
12. Pitrou I, Boutron I, Ahmad N, Ravaud P. Reporting of Safety Results in Published Reports of Randomized Controlled Trials. Arch Intern Med. 2009; 169: 1756-1761.
13. Golder S, Loke YK, Wright K, Norman G. Reporting of Adverse Events in Published and Unpublished Studies of Health Care: A Systematic Review. PLoS Med. 2016; 13: e1002127.
14. Altwairgi AK, Booth CM, Hopman WM, Baetz TD. Discordance Between Conclusions Stated in the Abstract and Conclusions in the Article: Analysis of Published Randomized Controlled Trials of Systemic Therapy in Lung Cancer. J Clin Oncol. 2012; 30: 3552-3557.
15. Estrada CA, Bloch RM, Antonacci D, Basnight LL, Patel SR, Patel SC, Wiese W. Reporting and Concordance of Methodologic Criteria Between Abstracts and Articles in Diagnostic Test Studies. J Gen Intern Med. 2000; 15: 183-187.
16. Pitkin RM, Branagan MA, Burmeister LF. Accuracy of Data in Abstracts of Published Research Articles. JAMA. 1999; 281: 1110-1111.

17. Pitkin RM, Branagan MA. Can the accuracy of abstracts be improved by providing specific instructions? A randomized controlled trial. JAMA. 1998; 280: 267-269.
18. Jonville-Béra AP, Giraudeau B, Autret-Leca E. Reporting of Drug Tolerance in Randomized Clinical Trials: When Data Conflict with Authors' Conclusions. Ann Intern Med. 2006; 144: 306-307.
19. Mathieu S, Giraudeau B, Soubrier M, Ravaud P. Misleading abstract conclusions in randomized controlled trials in rheumatology: comparison of the abstract conclusions and the results section. Joint Bone Spine. 2012; 79: 262-267.
20. Altman DG. The scandal of poor medical research. BMJ. 1994; 308: 283-284.
21. Jones R, Scouller J, Grainger F, Lachlan M, Evans S, Torrance N. The scandal of poor medical research: Sloppy use of literature often to blame. BMJ. 1994; 308: 591.
22. Bailar JC III. Science, Statistics, and Deception. Ann Intern Med. 1986; 104: 259-260.
23. Smith GD, Ebrahim S. Data dredging, bias, or confounding: They can all get you into the BMJ and the Friday papers. BMJ. 2002; 325: 1437-1438.
24. Marušić M, Marušić A. Good Editorial Practice: Editors as Educators. Croat Med J. 2001; 42: 113-120.
25. Ioannidis JPA. Why Most Published Research Findings Are False. PLoS Med. 2005; 2: e124.
26. The *PLoS Medicine* Editors. An Unbiased Scientific Record Should Be Everyone's Agenda. PLoS Med. 2009; 6: 0119-0121.
27. Chiu K, Grundy Q, Bero L. 'Spin' in published biomedical literature: A methodological systematic review. PLoS Biol. 2017; 15: e2002173.
28. Lazarus C, Haneef R, Ravaud P, Boutron I. Classification and prevalence of spin in abstracts of non-randomized studies evaluating an intervention. BMC Med Res Methodol. 2015; 15: 85.
29. Young SN. Bias in the research literature and conflict of interest: an issue for publishers, editors, reviewers and authors, and it is not just about the money. J Psychiatry Neurosci. 2009; 34: 412-417.
30. Gross RA. Style, spin, and science. Neurology. 2015; 85: 10-11.
31. Chalmers TC, Frank CS, Reitman D. Minimizing the Three Stages of Publication Bias. JAMA. 1990; 263: 1392-1395.
32. Guyatt GH, Oxman AD, Montori V, Vist G, Kunz R, Brozek J, Alonso-Coello P, Djulbegovic B, Atkins D, Falck-Ytter Y, Williams JW Jr., Meerpohl J, Norris SL, Akl EA, Schünemann HJ. GRADE guidelines: 5. Rating the quality of evidence—publication bias. J Clin Epidemiol. 2011; 64: 1277-1282.
33. Kicinski M, Springate DA, Kontopantelis E. Publication bias in meta-analysis from the Cochrane Database of Systematic Reviews. Stat Med. 2015; 34: 2781-2795.
34. Landewé RBM. How Publication Bias May Harm Treatment Guidelines. Arthritis Rheumatol. 2014; 66: 2661-2663.
35. Asher R. Why are medical journals so dull? BMJ. 1958; 2 (5094): 502-503.
36. Davis AJ. Readers don't have to come from overseas to benefit from plain English. BMJ. 1997; 314: 753.
37. How experts communicate. Nat Neurosci. 2000; 3: 97.
38. In pursuit of comprehension. Nature. 1996; 384: 497.
39. Plain English. J Coll Gen Pract. 1958; 1: 311-313.
40. Ronai PM. A Bad Case of Medical Jargon. AJR Am J Roentgenol. 1993; 161: 592.
41. O'Donnell M. Evidence-based illiteracy: time to rescue "the literature". Lancet. 2000; 355: 489-491.
42. Knight J. Clear as mud. Nature. 2003; 423: 376-378.
43. Howie JW. How I read. BMJ. 1976; 2 (6044): 1113-1114.
44. Groves T, Abbasi K. Screening research papers by reading abstracts. BMJ. 2004; 329: 470-471.
45. Smith R. Doctors are not scientists. BMJ. 2004; 328 (7454): 0-h.
46. Chalmers I, Glasziou P. Avoidable waste in the production and reporting of research evidence. Lancet. 2009; 374: 86-89.

47. von Elm E, Costanza MC, Walder B, Tramèr MR. More insight into the fate of biomedical meeting abstracts: a systematic review. BMC Med Res Methodol. 2003; 3: 12.
48. Weber EJ, Callaham ML, Wears RL, Barton C, Young G. Unpublished Research from a Medical Specialty Meeting: Why Investigators Fail to Publish. JAMA. 1998; 280: 257-259.
49. Sprague S, Bhandari M, Devereaux PJ, Swiontkowski MF, Tornetta P III, Cook DJ, Dirschl D, Schemitsch EH, Guyatt GH. Barriers to Full-Text Publication Following Presentation of Abstracts at Annual Orthopaedic Meetings. J Bone Joint Surg Am. 2003; 85-A: 158-163.
50. Smith MA, Barry HC, Williamson J, Keefe CW, Anderson WA. Factors Related to Publication Success Among Faculty Development Fellowship Graduates. Fam Med. 2009; 41: 120-125.
51. Moher D, Altman DG. Four Proposals to Help Improve the Medical Research Literature. PLoS Med. 2015; 12: e1001864.
52. Doctors and medical statistics. Lancet. 2007; 370: 910.
53. Masterson GR, Ashcroft GS. Better libraries and more journal clubs would help. BMJ. 1994; 308: 592-593.
54. Miedzinski LJ, Davis P, Al-Shurafa H, Morrison JC. A Canadian faculty of medicine and dentistry's survey of career development needs. Med Educ. 2001; 35: 890-900.
55. Marušić A, Marušić M. Teaching Students How to Read and Write Science: A Mandatory Course on Scientific Research and Communication in Medicine. Acad Med. 2003; 78: 1235-1239.
56. Bland CJ, Schmitz CC. Characteristics of the Successful Researcher and Implications for Faculty Development. J Med Educ. 1986; 61: 22-31.
57. Putnam W. Funding protected time for research: New opportunities from the Canadian Institutes of Health Research. Can Fam Physician. 2003; 49: 632-633.
58. North American Primary Care Research Group Committee on Building Research Capacity, The Academic Family Medicine Organizations Research Subcommittee. What Does It Mean to Build Research Capacity? Fam Med. 2002; 34: 678-684.
59. DeMaria AN. Of Abstracts and Manuscripts. J Am Coll Cardiol. 2006; 47: 1224-1225.
60. Erren TC. The Long and Thorny Road to Publication in Quality Journals. PLoS Comput Bio. 2007; 3: e251.

Chapter 2
The Ethical Foundations of Medical Scientific Writing

Introduction

Striving to be a better person, who lives more ethically today than you did yesterday, is the first and most essential step for writing better scientific papers. If you give only superficial thought and lip-service to the ethics of scientific research – i.e. if you simply think "yeah, yeah, yeah, I already know all this ethics stuff; let's move along to the 'real' science" – then you will not know the *right* way to conduct and report medical research. And if you do not know the right way to conduct and report medical research, you will do it in ways that are wrong. Conducting and reporting research involves making dozens, or even hundreds, of little choices per day – most of them without much conscious realization that another little choice is actually being made. Even if one does stop to notice them, most of these choices seem to be only technical choices about methods or grammar or whatever else, but they are not only that. Viewed in another light, they are also moral choices about what to do and say, or not do and say, why, and how. If you do not recognize this deeper moral dimension of scientific research, or if you fail to respond to it appropriately, then you risk making choices that will seem appropriate for reaching your practical goals, but which may often run counter to the greater purposes of scientific medical research. When you spend time reading the ethical guidelines and earnestly reflecting on how they apply to your research, the quality of your research and reporting will improve. You will find yourself making subtle but important changes in your work. And you will find yourself prepared to make better decisions going forward.

Unfortunately, following all the ethical guidelines and expectations for scientific research and writing does not in any way guarantee that you will publish good scientific papers. You might lack access to interesting and strong data; you might lack enough practice writing and rewriting; you might simply be a mediocre scientist; you might just have bad luck. But if you do not make conscience efforts to always follow all the ethical guidelines and expectations, then you will be stuck circulating

© Springer Nature Switzerland AG 2019
M. Hanna, *How to Write Better Medical Papers*,
https://doi.org/10.1007/978-3-030-02955-5_2

lousy manuscripts not worth reading. Indeed, there would even be a real risk that you would write junk science worthy of retraction if it ever did get published. If you lack the proper moral motivation and ethical guidance, your scientific work and writing will stagger off track at every step, without your awareness, like a drunk trying to walk home in the dark. And like most drunks, you will probably deny there is any shortcoming or fault in what you are doing. If you want to perform and publish high-quality research, the first and most essential step is to improve the ethical foundation of your work, so you will be able to run fast in a straight line.

Discussions of the ethical aspects of specific stages of the research, analysis, writing, and publishing are provided in later chapters of this book. Chapter 3 in the part "Preparing" briefly summarizes the main ethical aspects relevant to conducting the research, including ethical approval of the study protocol, registration of clinical trials, written informed consent of the human subjects or animal welfare, and following ethical guidelines. Chapter 11 in the part "Analyzing" discusses the major misconduct issues of fabricating data or results and falsifying data or results, as well as the need to archive raw data. Chapter 21 in the part "Drafting" discusses the ethical issues that arise mainly during the phase of writing up the research, above all plagiarism, but also preserving patient confidentiality, avoiding so-called "salami publication" (i.e. dividing the research into too many separate papers), and the obligation to actually write up and publish the research. Chapter 46 in the part "Publishing" discusses the ethical issues that arise during the publishing phase, including redundant publication, falsification of authorship lists, disclosing potential conflicts of interest, and reporting errors discovered after publication. This introductory chapter here addresses only the deeper ethical issues that serve as the foundation for excellent science across all phases of research, analysis, writing, and publishing.

Most unethical behavior arises when researchers are acting primarily for their own gain (advancing their careers, getting more money for themselves, etc.) If making more money or advancing your career are really your main goals, there are many other not disreputable fields where that is accepted or even expected, and where one has much higher chances of reaching those goals. The goal of medicine and science by contrast is to improve the health and knowledge of humanity. That can only be achieved if everyone contributing does so honestly and for the right humanitarian reasons. Most ethical rules in scientific publishing revolve around honest communication, because dishonest communication winds up wasting other people's time and resources and demoralizes them. Adhering to high ethical standards also improves the scientific quality of research and reporting and puts authors in a stronger moral position to defend their work.

Moral Vices and Virtues

Although there are many different kinds of ethical violations in research and reporting, they can all be explained, at bottom, by just three root causes: ignorance, laziness, and/or greed. Of these three, ignorance is surely the most widespread and forgivable cause of unethical conduct in research and reporting. Many people contributing to medical research and reporting are either relatively new and inexperienced in this field (i.e. junior researchers and trainees) or are only sporadically or tangentially involved in the work (e.g. healthcare professionals not working primarily in research). Such people often have inadequate education and training specifically about the ethics of research and scientific reporting. Because they are not thoroughly familiar with the ethical guidelines and expectations, they sometimes violate them, unknowingly. In other words, ignorance can result in unethical conduct. Second, somewhat less forgivable but still not quite reprehensible in most cases is laziness. Sometime people know or sense that what they are doing is not really the right way that research or reporting should be done, but doing things the right way would require more time and effort (often unpaid). Because they do not want to expend more time and effort to do things the right way, some people simply try to slip by with the work done in ways they know are not right or at least have been told are not right. In some cases one might be able to argue that the root problem is not simply laziness but instead that the researchers have not been provided sufficient resources to do the work any better. In most cases though, authors of papers know that they could correct or improve something in their paper that is not right ethically (or not right scientifically and therefore also ethically), but they simply do not want to be bothered. In other words, laziness is the bottom line explanation for the ethical problems, not merely insufficient resources. Finally, and most reprehensibly, many ethics problems – including nearly all of the most unbelievable scandals – can be explained entirely by the greed of the researchers for more money, either directly or indirectly. Greed for money also usually explains most misconduct of people who are well-established in research and know (or surely should know) how unethical their misconduct really is. Whenever someone is caught falsifying their data or reports, or stealing other people's work (through plagiarism or otherwise), or even "merely" falsifying authorship lists, the explanation almost always is that the culprits expected to obtain more money than they otherwise would have, through commercial profits, obtaining research grants, increased clinical activity through "fame" of research, advancing their career, etc. So greed for money and other personal gains is almost always the root cause of the worst ethical violations in medical research in the current era. The explanation is not something else.

Thus almost all ethical problems in research and reporting have the root causes of ignorance, laziness, or greed. In other words, unethical conduct in medical research is ultimately due to character flaws or vices of the researchers themselves (and not really to some other external or systemic factors).

It is important for all medical researchers to realize that these vices – ignorance, laziness, and greed – are the root causes of nearly all unethical misconduct in medical research, because that realization points the way toward better prevention of unethical misconduct. Because these vices are the root causes of unethical misconduct, researchers must make efforts to cultivate the opposite moral virtues, in order to reduce their own risk of acting unethically. And because the vices are specifically ignorance, laziness, and greed, the specific virtues that researchers should make efforts to cultivate are their opposites: ethical knowledge, "extra-mile" diligence (or "extra-kilometer" diligence), and disinterest of money and personal/career gains. Gaining ethical knowledge is the first and easiest virtue to cultivate. It starts by reading the relevant ethical guidelines. Most of them are only a page or two in length, so it is odd that they are not all routinely read and discussed by the medical research community. Because they are so brief, it is helpful to reread them at the start of every new study and paper and reflect on how they apply to your ongoing work. Cultivating the virtue of diligence is a bit more elusive. But most people who gain some experience in research and reporting will quickly notice that many little situations arise, where they know (or have been told) that something they are doing is not really right (ethically, or scientifically and therefore also ethically), but they do not want to bother doing more work to fix it, because "extra" work seems tedious and time-consuming. Cases where this would be financially difficult (e.g. additional data collection is needed) are different, but in most cases, the only barrier is the researcher's willingness to expend more time and effort doing the work. The amount of extra work required is often not much (a few hours to a couple days), especially considering the bigger picture of how much work a person can do in a year, but strangely many people still put up quite a fuss at the thought of having to do even a small amount of "extra" work. People often rationalize their laziness with phrases such as "it's good enough", "no one will notice", "it doesn't really matter", and so on. When researchers find themselves in those situations, where a choice must be made between either leaving things as they are, despite knowing that something is wrong or suboptimal, or being *diligent* and going the extra mile to do things the right way, researchers should make that choice of going the extra mile, for the mere sake of doing better quality work and being a better researcher. Finally, researchers should cultivate disinterest in financial or personal/career gains. Of course most everyone in medical research will say that they do not give much thought to money and that it does not affect their decisions in their research and reporting. To a large degree, that is indeed true. But it is quite rare that this is completely true. Most people in medical research still hope to obtain better positions, more salary, more research funding, more fame and recognition, more everything. Understandably so. But not really. It is very rare to find anyone who comprehends that money is actually a noxious system of artificial rewards (like food pellets for lab rats) that can distort their judgments and behaviors and therefore is better to avoid and give away than to want and pursue. True scientific curiosity, objectivity, and judgment begins just a little bit beyond the point where all interest in money, praise, and career advancement truly ends. So researchers must make a choice. Just ask Dr. Faust.

Responding to Ethical Misconduct

Regrettably, there is one more major reason why you need to know all the ethical guidelines and expectations really well. One might assume that people working in medical research have above average moral character and high ethical standards.

And most of them do. But unethical conduct, especially in minor forms, is also not uncommon in the world of medical research [1]. A metaanalysis of 18 surveys found that 12.3% of respondents had observed data fabrication or falsification by their colleagues, an unweighted median of about 40% of respondents from a sub-sample of 10 studies knew of cases of fraudulent reporting more broadly defined, and overall "misconduct was reported more frequently by medical/pharmacological researchers than others" [2]. These were conservative estimates that excluded pla-giarism and several other forms of misconduct unrelated to changing study results. So if you spend at least a year in medical research, there is a substantial likelihood that you will notice at least some minor forms of unethical conduct. Indeed, you might even find yourself being negatively affected by that misconduct. Therefore, you need to thoroughly learn the research ethics ahead of time, so you are able to clearly identify misconduct as such when you encounter it, and so you are ready to report it, if it is not simply an unintended mistake. Fortunately, most unethical mis-conduct in medical research is unintentional and is quickly corrected by the people involved when someone else makes them aware of it.

But if you observe unethical misconduct that appears conscious/deliberate or that does not get fully corrected when pointed out, you have an ethical obligation to report it [3], even if it seems that doing so will have negative repercussions for you. Start by documenting everything (including conversations) very well. People who knowingly engage in misconduct may also destroy evidence, and they will certainly deny or reframe anything that lacks undeniable evidence. Next, contact lawyers to discuss the situation and get their advice. Always follow your lawyer's advice; if you are not satisfied with your lawyer's advice, find a new lawyer, and follow his or her advice. Never report cases of research misconduct to the institution where it is occurring, (unless your lawyer advises you do to so). Regardless of whether the institution is a university, a company, a government agency, or whatever else, it is not an independent and neutral institution of justice, and you should not expect neutrality or justice from them [3, 4]. Instead, these institutions all have their own self-interests [5]. Any internal committees they have set up to field such complaints about misconduct exist primarily to protect the self-interests of the institution, not to administer justice and promote ethics. The one and only goal of institutions is to protect themselves from lawsuits and/or bad press, because those consume their finances and damage their reputation (and thus their future revenues). Cases of mis-conduct will only receive a fair and objective review from courts of law or other external commissions with absolute nothing to lose by reaching a guilty verdict and proclaiming it publicly in full detail.

So never make a report or complain to your university or other institution, nei-ther in writing nor orally, unless your lawyer advises you to do so and writes it for you. Anything you report to your institution will be used by their legal team to protect the institution and possibly to attack you. Do not be fooled by their pre-tenses to neutrality, whistleblower policies, and so on. If there is a problem, let your law firm handle it for you. Because of the potential legal issues, no university ethics board will ever provide feedback on anything you tell them, unless the university's legal team has assured themselves that there is no basis for your claims and wants you to stop complaining. If you bring research misconduct to light, it is probably a good idea to start looking for another job elsewhere. Even if you are entirely innocent, the institution will probably try to get rid of you, because your complaints are potentially damaging to their reputation. Moreover, it is usually easier for them to shoot the messenger than to address any real problems reported to them. Finally, whatever the situation is or however much it is harming you, do not take it personally or get too upset. Just follow your lawyer's advice and move forward. There is always some other better research paper you could be writing somewhere else instead.

Conclusion

The purpose of medical scientific research is to improve the health of humanity, by increasing our collective knowledge on how best to prevent, identify, and treat illnesses. People who want to do better medical research should commit themselves to serving that deeper purpose of medical research. Ethical guidelines on the performing and reporting of research (discussed in subsequent chapters) serve as an initial explanation of how researchers are expected to behave. Ethical guidelines tell researchers what they should and should not do, but the guidelines are generally unable to provide guidance about why. Although researchers should always follow the explicitly recommended behaviors of the ethical guidelines, it is even more important to recognize the underlying, unspoken moral foundation of the guidelines, and then adopt that spirit in everything you do. Primarily that means recognizing that the only purpose of medical scientific research is to improve the health of humanity, by increasing our collective knowledge on how best to prevent, identify, and treat illnesses. Researchers who dedicate themselves to this intrinsic purpose of medical research will find that it goes a long way toward ensuring ethical conduct more reliably and robustly, right down into little detail choices that ethical guidelines often fail to consider. Dedication to this purpose of medical research has a further advantage besides ensuring better ethical conduct. People dedicated to this deeper intrinsic purpose of medical research will also find that it leads them toward accomplishing research with greater relevance and impact. Without this proper deeper moral orientation, researchers inevitably drift down toward narrow technical studies on obscure topics. Their work then achieves their petty practical goals of career advancement and so on, but it has limited real impact on human health and knowledge. You should of course always read and follow the ethical guidelines (which are discussed in subsequent chapters). Yet ideally you should also honestly assess your motivations for doing medical research (rather than clinical care, non-medical research, or whatever else). And you should assess how well your motivations are aligned with the deeper inherent purpose of medical research – to improve the health of humanity, by increasing our collective knowledge on how best to prevent, identify, and treat illnesses.

References

1. The *PLoS Medicine* Editors. Getting Closer to a Fully Correctable and Connected Research Literature. PLoS Med. 2013; 10: e1001408.
2. Fanelli D. How Many Scientists Fabricate and Falsify Research? A Systematic Review and Meta-Analysis of Survey Data. PLoS One. 2009; 4: e5738.
3. Sigma Xi. Honor in Science. Research Triangle Park, NC, USA: Sigma Xi; 2000.
4. Van Der Weyden MB. Managing allegations of scientific misconduct and fraud: lessons from the "Hall affair". MJA. 2004; 180: 149-151.
5. Gillman MA. Checking for plagiarism, duplicate publication, and text recycling. Lancet. 2011; 377: 1403.

Part I
Preparing

Chapter 3
Ethics of Conducting Research

Introduction

Medical research must be conducted ethically. That requires preparation before beginning to collect any data. It is the one most important matter to attend to *before* starting the research, because it is the one aspect that cannot be corrected later during the writing phase. Moreover, laying a solid ethical foundation for the research before it ever starts will substantially improve the scientific quality of the research as well. This book is not about how to conduct research, nor about the ethics of research, so these topics will not be discussed in much depth here. But they must be presented briefly, because the quality of the papers depends fundamentally on these matters and because the Methods section of any paper must mention the ethical aspects of the research. There are four main elements for ethical research: ethics committee approval, study registration, written informed consent or animal welfare, and following ethical guidelines.

Ethics Committee Approval

First, the study protocol should be approved by a Research Ethics Committee (often referred to as an "Institutional Review Board" (IRB), regrettably [1]) – *before* the research begins [2, 3]. The ethics committee is a panel of people responsible for ensuring that research studies have been designed to be sufficiently safe, sensible, and fair to the subjects who will be participating [4–6]. If your institution does not have an ethics committee or if your research is being conducted outside of any such institution, you must still find some other independent ethics committee that can review the study protocol [7, 8]. Although some research ethics committees require extensive paperwork and/or revisions to the study protocol, nearly all submissions will eventually be approved [9], unless the risks to the participants clearly outweigh the possible benefits of the research or there are irresolvable concerns about the participants' rights. The process of having the study protocol reviewed by the ethics committee and revising for their concerns and questions usually leads to substantial

© Springer Nature Switzerland AG 2019
M. Hanna, *How to Write Better Medical Papers*,
https://doi.org/10.1007/978-3-030-02955-5_3

quality improvements in the research methods. If you are conducting a retrospective study, you still need to obtain approval from an ethics committee – before you begin extracting data from the medical records into a study database. Some other types of human research that are not actually medical are exempt from the requirement for approval by an ethics committee, but it is strongly advisable to ask an ethics committee (or a lawyer) to confirm that exemption in writing, even though this is legally superfluous if the research is indeed exempt. If a research study should have obtained approval from an ethics committee but did not, it will be virtually impossible to publish it in any scientific journal.

Study Registration

Second, if you are conducting a clinical trial, you must register it in a registry of clinical trials, *before* recruiting any subjects, (but after obtaining approval by an ethics committee) [2, 3, 10, 11]. A "clinical trial" is defined by the International Committee of Medical Journal Editors (ICMJE) in this context as essentially any prospective study of any health intervention on people [3]; only retrospective studies, observational studies, or studies without human subjects or samples would fall outside that definition of a "clinical trial". Registration is not currently required for research that is not a clinical trial, but registration of such non-trial research is still encouraged [3]. Inadequate registration of clinical trials makes it difficult for the scientific community to estimate the degree to which the available scientific literature provides an incomplete and distorted body of evidence, due to publication bias in favor of positive findings [10–14]. If you do not register your study *before* starting data collection, the best journals will refuse to even review your manuscripts about that clinical trial [3, 10], and many reviewers at standard journals will cite that as a reason to reject your manuscript. A list of clinical trial registries can be found on the website of the World Health Organization. The registration must contain adequate information for all trial registration items [3]; there is little point in registration with blank or vague entries.

Written Informed Consent and Animal Welfare

Third, "written informed consent" must be obtained from each of the subjects participating in the research, if your research is a prospective study on humans (or on samples collected from humans) [2, 15–17, 18 (pp. 20–21)]. The study purpose and risks must be clearly explained to them, and they must have the opportunity to ask any questions. The subjects must be able to freely choose to participate or not [2, 15]. They must sign a written statement that they agree to participate in scientific research, which should document real understanding and willingness, rather than being an empty bureaucratic formality [16, 19–22]. This written informed consent to participate in research is distinctly different from whatever consent documents they must sign to receive medical treatment.

Furthermore, the subjects should clearly understand that they are participating in scientific research, and therefore any drugs, devices, or interventions that they are receiving may be inadequately understood and/or not necessarily in their personal best interest [23–25]. People who are not clearly able to provide written informed consent (e.g. minors or people with substantial mental health problems) may still participate in research if they provide assent and their legal guardian provides consent [2, 15, 17]. The ethics committee reviewing your protocol can provide further guidance on such scenarios. Written informed consent is not necessary for retrospective studies of data that were already collected for routine patient care. And written informed consent is of course not applicable to studies that do not involve human subjects (or human samples). Because animals cannot provide informed consent (and surely would not if they could), researchers are instead expected to uphold high standards of animal welfare, to minimize the suffering and distress of the animals involved.

Use of animal models plays an important and well-established role in basic scientific research. However, there is obviously something about animal research that is ethically fragile. It is beyond the scope of this book to discuss the ethical aspects of animal research, much less to take a position on it. But as stated in the previous chapter, the first and most essential step to improving the quality of your research and your papers is to make efforts to act more ethically today than you did yesterday. (Further improvement is always possible for anything we do.) Many scientists may legitimately reach the conclusion that the use of animals is a necessary and ethical part of their research, and this book does not debate that. But what must be said here is that any scientist who does not seriously reflect on the ethical issues of conducting research on animals will be missing a major opportunity to improve the quality of his or her research and journal papers. Reflecting on the ethical issues of animal research forces you to reflect also on important methodological and epistemological aspects of your research that otherwise remain hidden from view. It may lead you to methodological improvements or innovations that are not only better for the animals but also for the scientific knowledge gained. Above all, researchers should think seriously about how to apply "the 3 Rs" – replacement, reduction, and refinement – to their research plans potentially involving animals [26–28]. Because written informed consent is not applicable to research on animals, best practice would instead involve documenting (e.g. in the study protocol) the variety of measures taken to minimize or eliminate harm (pain, stress, disability, etc.) to the animals.

Following Ethical Guidelines

Fourth, the research must be conducted in accordance with the Declaration of Helsinki [2], any applicable laws, and any relevant guidelines. Every researcher should devote some time to reading the relevant guidelines, applicable laws, and ethical literature, and understanding how they apply to his or her research projects. As mentioned before, making efforts to live more ethically today than you did yesterday, is the first and most essential step for writing better papers. Part of those efforts is rereading the relevant ethical guidelines yet again every time you start a new study. It is not sufficient that you read them a couple years ago, unless you also memorized them. Whenever you reread ethics guidelines, you will be reminded of important details you had forgotten. Always check that you have the most recent version; guidelines are often updated for recent advances in science, law, ethical reasoning, societal concerns, public consensus, and so on.

Conclusion

The four ethics elements discussed in this chapter should be fulfilled before the research even begins, for three reasons. First, the scientific community will hold researchers accountable for their ethical conduct. Journals will reject (or retract) manuscripts that are based on unethical research, at which point it is too late to correct the problem. Second, the process of ensuring that research is ethical improves the quality of the research. The researcher is obliged to review all the details of his or her research plan and to obtain approval from other people who are unfamiliar with the topic. Aside from ethical issues, this communication and review process always leads to identifying methodological points in the research plan that could be done better some other way or otherwise need refinement. Third, these three ethics elements should be fulfilled simply because it is the right thing to do. Presumably, we all want to live in a fair and just world [29], so we all have to make the extra effort to live in a fair and just way. If you yourself do not make that effort, do not be surprised to find yourself living in a world where no one else does either [30].

References

1. Emanuel EJ. Institutional Review Board Reform. NEJM. 2002; 347: 1285-1286.
2. World Medical Association. Declaration of Helsinki – Ethical Principles for Medical Research Involving Human Subjects. Accessed on 10 January 2018 at: https://www.wma.net/policies-post/wma-declaration-of-helsinki-ethical-principles-for-medical-research-involving-human-subjects/
3. International Committee of Medical Journal Editors. Recommendations for the Conduct, Reporting, Editing, and Publication of Scholarly Work in Medical Journals. Philadelphia: American College of Physicians; 1978, 2017. Accessed on 12 January 2018 at: www.icmje.org/icmje-recommendations.pdf
4. Enfield KB, Truwit JD. The Purpose, Composition, and Function of an Institutional Review Board: Balancing Priorities. Respir Care. 2008; 53: 1330-1336.
5. Schwenzer KJ. Practical Tips for Working Effectively With Your Institutional Review Board. Respir Care. 2008; 53: 1354-1361.
6. Colt HG, Mulnard RA. Writing an Application for a Human Subjects Institutional Review Board. Chest. 2006; 130: 1605-1607.
7. Rice TW. How to Do Human-Subjects Research If You Do Not Have an Institutional Review Board. Respir Care. 2008; 53: 1362-1367.
8. Lemaire F. Do All Types of Human Research Need Ethics Committee Approval? Am J Respir Crit Care Med. 2006; 174: 363-364.
9. Boyce M. Observational study of 353 applications to London multicentre research ethics committee 1997-2000. BMJ. 2002; 325: 1081.

10. DeAngelis C, Drazen JM, Frizelle FA, Haug C, Hoey J, Horton R, Kotzin S, Laine C, Marušić A, Overbeke AJPM, Schroeder TV, Sox HC, Van Der Weyden MB. Clinical Trial Registration: A Statement from the International Committee of Medical Journal Editors. NEJM. 2004; 351: 1250-1251.
11. Weber WEJ, Merino JG, Loder E. Trial registration 10 years on: The single most valuable tool we have to ensure unbiased reporting of research studies. BMJ. 2015; 351: h3572.
12. Chalmers I, Glasziou P. Avoidable waste in the production and reporting of research evidence. Lancet. 2009; 374: 86-89.
13. Guyatt GH, Oxman AD, Montori V, Vist G, Kunz R, Brozek J, Alonso-Coello P, Djulbegovic B, Atkins D, Falck-Ytter Y, Williams JW Jr., Meerpohl J, Norris SL, Akl EA, Schünemann HJ. GRADE guidelines: 5. Rating the quality of evidence—publication bias. J Clin Epidemiol. 2011; 64: 1277-1282.
14. Rosenthal R. The "File Drawer Problem" and Tolerance for Null Results. Psychol Bull. 1979; 86: 638-641.
15. United Nations Educational, Scientific and Cultural Organization (UNESCO). Universal Declaration on Bioethics and Human Rights. Paris: UNESCO; 2006.
16. Neff MJ. Informed Consent: What Is It? Who Can Give It? How Do We Improve It? Respir Care. 2008; 53: 1337-1341.
17. del Carmen MG, Joffe S. Informed Consent for Medical Treatment and Research: A Review. Oncologist. 2005; 10: 636-641.
18. Bland M. An Introduction to Medical Statistics, 4th ed. Oxford: Oxford University Press; 2015.
19. Bramstedt KA. A guide to informed consent for clinician-investigators. Cleve Clin J Med. 2004; 71: 907-910.
20. Lentz J, Kennett M, Perlutter J, Forrest A. Paving the way to a more effective informed consent process: Recommendations from the Clinical Trials Transformation Initiative. Contemp Clin Trials. 2016; 49: 65-69.
21. Cressey D. Informed consent on trial. Nature. 2012; 482: 16.
22. Rossel M, Burnier M, Stupp R. Informed Consent: True Information or Institutional Review Board–Approved Disinformation? J Clin Oncol. 2007; 25: 5835-5836.
23. Appelbaum PS, Roth LH, Lidz C. The Therapeutic Misconception: Informed Consent in Psychiatric Research. Int J Law Psychiatry. 1982; 5: 319-329.
24. Appelbaum PS, Roth LH, Lidz CW, Benson P, Winslade W. False Hopes and Best Data: Consent to Research and the Therapeutic Misconception. Hastings Cent Rep. 1987; 17: 20-24.
25. Lidz CW, Appelbaum PS. The Therapeutic Misconception: Problems and Solutions. Med Care. 2002; 40: V55-V63.
26. Council for International Organizations of Medical Sciences, International Council for Laboratory Animal Science. International Guiding Principles for Biomedical Research Involving Animals, December 2012. Accessed on 7 January 2018 at: iclas.org/wp-content/uploads/2013/03/CIOMS-ICLAS-Principles-Final.pdf
27. Guidelines for the treatment of animals in behavioral research and teaching. Animal Behavior. 2012; 83: 301-309.
28. Smith R. Animal research: the need for a middle ground. BMJ. 2001; 322: 248-249.
29. Rawls J. A Theory of Justice. Cambridge, MA, USA: Belknap Press; 1971.
30. Kant I. Grundlegung zur Metaphysik der Sitten. Leipzig: Verlag von Felix Meiner; 1785, 1792, 1947.

Chapter 4
Foresight

Some medical researchers spend a substantial amount of time and resources performing and writing up a study only to discover in the end that it is impossible (or very difficult) to publish their manuscript, because of some specific problem with the study. Most journals are quite selective about which manuscripts they will publish, and passing peer review is a necessary (but not sufficient) prerequisite for journals to accept a manuscript, (as discussed in more detail in part VI, "Publishing"). Most of the critical feedback from peer reviewers can be overcome by rewriting the manuscript and revising the data analysis if necessary. But there are many problems that are embedded so fundamentally into a study that no amount of rewriting or additional analysis can correct them. Most of these shortcomings of study design or methodology will not preclude publication at some good journal somewhere, if they are adequately addressed in the limitations section of the Discussion. But some of these problems of study design and methodology are so serious that they will lead to complete rejection of the manuscript at every journal to which it is sent. These kinds of problems are sometimes called "fatal flaws". Regrettably, many authors are quite oblivious to the existence of a fatal flaw in their manuscript until they receive several rejection letters in a row, at which point it is far too late to salvage all their work.

So the purpose of this chapter is to make you aware of these potential fatal flaws, which cannot be revised during the journal submission phase, and which make it difficult or even impossible to publish the manuscript in any respectable journal. If you consider them from the very outset, most of these fatal flaws can be completely avoided with just a little effort. Sometimes, some of these fatal flaws cannot be solved. In such cases, it is best to know that from the start, before wasting time and energy naively pursuing a particular study that has little or no chance of ever being published. Foresight about potential fatal flaws will help ensure that you channel your time and efforts into work that has reasonable chances of being published in an appropriate journal. This chapter presents ten fatal flaws, roughly in the order in which they should be considered and resolved.

© Springer Nature Switzerland AG 2019
M. Hanna, *How to Write Better Medical Papers*,
https://doi.org/10.1007/978-3-030-02955-5_4

First, you should always conduct a thorough literature review on your precise study topic, to ensure that the study question is relevant but has not already been answered sufficiently. Most medical researchers substantially overestimate their own familiarity with the scientific literature that is available on their topic [1, 2]. Many manuscripts are rejected from journals because they address questions that have already been answered sufficiently in previous publications, and therefore the new manuscript would not add anything much to the existing literature [3, 4]. Even when a topic does need more research, reviewing the literature often leads to important refinements of the study question and methods. Further discussion about reviewing the literature is provided mainly in chapters 6 ("Reading") and 7 ("Searching the Literature"). Failure to conduct a thorough literature review before performing a study will not preclude publication, but it will lead to multiple weaknesses of the study that are difficult or impossible to remedy during the publication phase and that push the paper toward much lower quality journals. If a literature review is done well enough, it could even serve as its own publication.

Second, you should give careful consideration to your study design and/or consult with a methodologist about it. The overall study design is fundamental for determining the study's level of evidence [5–8] and for grading the quality of the evidence [9–11]. In particular, prospective studies are generally much stronger than retrospective studies. Choices about the details of the study design will have a major influence on the quality of the evidence collected and therefore of the responses of the journals. Indeed, one study suggests that poor study design may be the leading cause of outright rejection of most manuscripts [12]. Furthermore, there is very little that can be done during the publishing phase to try to correct problems related to study design [13]. Consequently, problems with study design will push a manuscript toward lower quality journals, and if the problems are serious enough, they may lead even low-quality journals to reject the manuscript as invalid. Study design is a vast topic, just outside the scope of this book on medical writing, so it will not be discussed much further here. Readers are advised to read the relevant literature on study design, and/or to consult with methodologists. Researchers should take all reasonable steps to strength their study design from the outset, and they should avoid investing their time in studies with inherently weak designs. Improving the study design as much as possible prior to ever starting the study will greatly improve the quality of the research and the chances of publication.

Third, you should always use a valid comparison and/or control group whenever sensible. Preliminary research – such as pilot studies, case series, or retrospective analyses – can normally be published just fine without any kind of comparison or control group. But research that aims to provide more definitive answers – such as prospective clinical trials – can be difficult to interpret without a valid comparison and/or control group. In particular, placebo control groups are really only acceptable if there is no other available treatment in routine practice. Otherwise, the comparison group should always receive the current standard of medical care. Matched case-control studies should be carefully matched for the variables that other researchers will consider most relevant. Cross-over studies should have sufficient wash-out time and random assignment to the sequencing, to ensure that each subject is reliably serving as his or her own control. Experimental studies should have both positive and negative control groups. Failure to use an appropriate comparison group will not preclude publication, but it will normally push a manuscript toward lower quality journals, because the results become difficult to interpret without a valid comparison group. Using a valid comparison group more than doubles what you can do in the statistical analysis. Further information on appropriate comparison groups can be found by reading the relevant literature on research methodology or even simply by consulting any experienced researcher in your field.

Fourth, always use validated methods to collect data, and use the best such methods whenever possible. Above all, this point refers to any questionnaires being used in the research. Many researchers have a strange tendency to reinvent the wheel and make up their own questionnaires for their research studies. Except in surveys, this is always a very bad idea, unless it can be rigorously documented that no other relevant questionnaires have already been developed – something which is rarely the case anymore for anything you might want to assess. Data that is collected with questionnaires that have never been validated will generally be viewed as invalid data. Manuscripts that contain invalid data are essentially worthless and unpublishable. Furthermore, for many commonplace patient outcomes (such as depression, quality-of-life, patient satisfaction, etc.), there are many different questionnaires available. But some of them are better quality than others, and some of them may be better suited than others to your specific research topic or study population. So you should not simply use the first questionnaire that comes to mind or the one that seems easiest to use. Instead, you should find out what all the possible questionnaires are and then carefully choose the ones that will be viewed as most appropriate for your study. Otherwise, peer reviewers will assert that the questionnaires you used were not so good, and therefore neither are your data. Using validated questionnaires also ensures that there will be a body of literature you can draw upon to interpret your results. If you cannot find relevant questionnaires or you are not sure which questionnaires are most suitable for your study, consult a social scientist, psychometrician, or other appropriate expert.

Fifth, always calculate how large your study needs to be, before you actually start it. Many research studies – even those that are published – are too small to provide reliable answers to the questions they address [14, 15]. So whenever the results are not statistically significant, it is difficult to know if this is because the results would always be negative or simply because the study was too small to obtain statistically significant results. These issues of statistical power and adequate sample size are discussed further in chapters 14 ("Statistics: Common Mistakes"), 23 ("The Methods"), and 24 ("The Results"). If you are conducting a pilot study or other preliminary research, the sample size may be determined mainly by practical issues, especially if you are not intending to publish it. Otherwise, a power analysis should always be performed – before starting the research – to determine how large a sample size is needed to answer the study question [14, 16]. It is advisable to ask a statistician to perform the sample size estimate for you. You should also seriously consider how to minimize loss to follow-up and other causes of missing or invalid data [17]. These issues of sample size, missing data, and statistical power are generally not themselves reasons that journals give for rejecting a manuscript (though sometimes they are). Instead, excessive missing data and/or insufficient statistical power will lead to results that are inconclusive, vague, non-significant, and unreliable. That will disappoint and bewilder you, and it will make it difficult to publish the manuscript. Giving thought from the outset to these issues of sample size and missing data will help ensure that your database can provide useful results.

Sixth, if your research involves human or animal subjects, or even just biological samples from them, then you must obtain approval of an ethics committee – before you start the research, (or before you start the data extraction and analysis, in the case of retrospective studies). Most researchers know this, but attempts to publish manuscripts lacking approval from an ethics committee are not unknown. The topic of obtaining approval by an ethics committee was discussed in the previous chapter, "Ethics of Conducting Research". Failure to obtain the necessary approval of an ethics committee prior to starting the research will make it virtually impossible to publish the research anywhere. Seeking and obtaining approval of an ethics committee almost always leads to at least some improvement of the study, because it forces the researchers to explicitly articulate what they intend to do and why, and sometimes leads to feedback from other experts (the ethics committee).

Seventh, if your research is a clinical trial, you must register your trial in a trial registry prior to starting data collection. The topic of trial registration was discussed in the previous chapter, "Ethics of Conducting Research". Failure to register a trial will make it impossible to publish the paper in top-tier journals and will be viewed by peer reviewers and Editors at all other journals as a sufficiently good reason to reject your manuscript, if they feel a need to provide a reason. Registering a trial completely and correctly will improve your research by making you explicitly consider many methodological issues that might otherwise remain vague or overlooked.

Eighth, if your research was prospective and involved human subjects (or samples from them), then you must obtain written informed consent from them – to participate in a research study. If your research was prospective and involved animals, then you must follow all applicable guidelines to ensure animal welfare. These issues of written informed consent and animal welfare were discussed in the previous chapter, "Ethics of Conducting Research". Failure to obtain written informed consent from human subjects will make it virtually impossible to publish the research anywhere. Failure to implement appropriate animal welfare measures will make it much more difficult to publish your research, proportional to how much your research deviated from what would have been expected if you had implemented appropriate animal welfare measures. Obtaining written informed consent and following all possible measures of animal welfare will help ensure that your research subjects are cooperative willing partners, rather than being stressed-out resisting objects of undesired investigation.

Ninth, you should meet with all your co-researchers to assess their intended involvement in the project and their expectations of what they will receive in return. In fact, best practices involve writing up an informal agreement or formal contract among everyone involved, detailing who will do what, what they will get in return, how decisions will be made, and who will be the co-authors on the publications [18–23]. Miscommunication and/or misunderstandings about such matters are regrettably uncommon, and often lead to bitter disputes [24–27]. Failure to properly assess everyone's intended contributions has caused many research projects to fall apart before they are even completed [18, 28–30]. Disputes during the write-up and publication stage have also led to many manuscripts remaining unpublished and/or people losing credit for the work they did [21, 25, 31–35]. The best way to prevent these kinds of problems is to solve them from the outset before they even occur, by getting everyone involved to make a written agreement. Such a written agreement ensures everyone is committed to the research and will be contributing as much as expected.

Tenth, you should estimate the time and effort that are needed to carry out all the research work and honestly assess whether sufficient finances and other resources are available to complete the research, including getting it published. Data collection is often started but never completed, due to lack of resources or other unanticipated but foreseeable difficulties [28, 36]. About half of all studies that are presented at conferences are never published in journals [29, 30, 37]. The main explanation given by the authors of such unpublished studies is lack of time [29, 30, 36], which is another way of saying that there was a lack of funding to pay people to spend their time doing the write-up. Research that is started but never published is essentially a waste of time and resources [4]. So it is prudent to realistically assess whether or not you have sufficient time and resources to actually finish and publish the research – before you actually start it, not a year after the whole project is obviously dead in the water. If everything takes twice as long as you think it should, will you still be able to finish and publish the research? If not, you should probably acquire more funding first, or plan a more modest research study, or just direct your time and energy to some other activity. In particular, early career-phase researchers should seek and heed advice from disinterested experienced colleagues about the amount of time and effort really needed to collect new data of publishable quality. Although prospective studies are generally stronger than retrospective studies, it is far better to finish and publish a retrospective study than to undertake a prospective study that never reaches completion and publication. Realistically assessing the research workload and available resources will ensure that you channel your life toward fruitful undertakings.

These ten fatal flaws relate mostly to research methodology, research ethics, and the socioeconomic practicalities of carrying out research. Any of these ten fatal flaws can make it difficult or even impossible to publish manuscripts from that research. During the publication phase, there is almost never any way to resolve these kinds of problems by rewriting the manuscript, or even redoing the data analysis. So the only way to avoid such heartbreaking rejections is to consider and avoid all these fatal flaws from the very outset. Whenever you start to think about a research study or paper, you should consider these ten fatal flaws. If you cannot adequately resolve all ten, then it is probably better to not proceed with that study at all, because it may be difficult or impossible to publish it. At the very least, these problems will push the paper toward much lower quality journals (and make presentation at conferences less likely). In such cases, it is better to just direct your time and resources into some other research study or some other activity. The best proof that someone is a master of the game of chess is that he or she recognizes a checkmate scenario many moves before it happens, and either takes steps to avoid it, or gracefully admits defeat and stops the game. By contrast, inexperienced or lousy players of chess walk right into checkmate, and even then sometimes do not recognize it, until someone else carefully explains it to them. Foresight has a similar role in scientific research and publication.

References

1. Smith AJ, Goodman NW. The hypertensive response to intubation. Do researchers acknowledge previous work? Can J Anaesth. 1997; 44: 9-13.
2. Chalmers TC, Frank CS, Reitman D. Minimizing the Three Stages of Publication Bias. JAMA. 1990; 263: 1392-1395.
3. Jones R, Scouller J, Grainger F, Lachlan M, Evans S, Torrance N. The scandal of poor medical research: Sloppy use of literature often to blame. BMJ. 1994; 308: 591.
4. Chalmers I, Glasziou P. Avoidable waste in the production and reporting of research evidence. Lancet. 2009; 374: 86-89.
5. Oxford Centre for Evidence-Based Medicine, Levels of Evidence Working Group. Oxford Centre for Evidence-Based Medicine 2011 Levels of Evidence. Accessed on 18 February 2018 at: https://www.cebm.net/wp-content/uploads/2014/06/CEBM-Levels-of-Evidence-2.1.pdf
6. Howick J, Chalmers I, Glasziou P, Greenhalgh T, Henghan C, Liberati A, Moschetti I, Phillips B, Thornton H. The 2011 Oxford CEBM Levels of Evidence: Introductory Document. Accessed on 18 February 2018 at: https://www.cebm.net/wp-content/uploads/2014/06/CEBM-Levels-of-Evidence-Introduction-2.1.pdf
7. Gross RA, Johnston KC. Levels of evidence. Neurology. 2009; 72: 8-10.
8. Wright JG, Swiontkowski MF, Heckman JD. Introducing Levels of Evidence to *The Journal*. J Bone Joint Surg Am. 2003; 85-A: 1-3.
9. GRADE Working Group. Grading quality of evidence and strength of recommendations. BMJ. 2004; 328: 1490.
10. Guyatt G, Oxman AD, Akl EA, Kunz R, Vist G, Brozek J, Norris S, Falck-Ytter Y, Glasziou P, deBeer H, Jaeschke R, Rind D, Meerpohl J, Dahm P, Schünemann HJ. GRADE guidelines: 1. Introduction—GRADE evidence profiles and summary of findings tables. J Clin Epidemiol. 2011; 64: 383-394.
11. Balshem H, Helfand M, Schünemann HJ, Oxman AD, Kunz R, Brozek J, Vist GE, Falck-Ytter Y, Meerpohl J, Norris S, Guyatt GH. GRADE guidelines: 3. Rating the quality of evidence. J Clin Epidemiol. 2011; 64: 401-406.
12. Byrne DW. Common Reasons for Rejecting Manuscripts at Medical Journals: A Survey of Editors and Peer Reviewers. Sci Ed. 2000; 23 (2): 39-44.
13. Pierson DJ. The Top 10 Reasons Why Manuscripts Are Not Accepted for Publication. Respir Care. 2004; 49: 1246-1252.
14. Altman DG, Bland JM. Absence of evidence is not evidence of absence. BMJ. 1995; 311: 485.
15. Detsky AS, Sackett DL. When Was a 'Negative Clinical Trial Big Enough? How Many Patients You Needed Depends on What You Found. Arch Intern Med. 1985; 145: 709-712.
16. Sprent P. Statistics in medical research. Swiss Med Wkly. 2003; 133: 522-529.
17. Little RJ, D'Agostino R, Cohen ML, Dickersin K, Emerson SS, Farrar JT, Frangakis C, Hogan JW, Molenberghs G, Murphy SA, Neaton JD, Rotnitzky A, Scharfstein D, Shih WJ, Siegel JP, Stern H. The Prevention and Treatment of Missing Data in Clinical Trials. NEJM. 2012; 367: 1355-1360.
18. Primack RB, Cigliano JA, Parsons ECM. Coauthors gone bad; how to avoid publishing conflict and a proposed agreement for co-author teams. Biol Conserv. 2014; 176: 277-280.

19. Cals JWL, Kotz D. Effective writing and publishing scientific papers, part IX: authorship. J Clin Epidemiol. 2013; 66: 1319.
20. Albert T, Wager E. How to handle authorship disputes: a guide for new researchers. In: Committee on Publication Ethics. The COPE Report 2003. Norfolk, England: Committee on Publication Ethics; 2003, pp. 32-34.
21. Chakravarty K. Excluding authors may be impossible. BMJ. 1997; 315: 748.
22. Riesenberg D, Lundberg GD. The Order of Authorship: Who's on First? JAMA. 1990; 264: 1857.
23. Scientific Integrity Committee of the Swiss Academies of Arts and Sciences. Authorship in scientific publications: analysis and recommendations. Swiss Med Wkly. 2015; 145: w14108.
24. Wilcox LJ. Authorship: The Coin of the Realm, The Source of Complaints. JAMA. 1998; 280: 216-217.
25. Ezsias A. Authorship is influenced by power and departmental politics. BMJ. 1997; 315: 746.
26. Jain SH. Negotiating Authorship. J Gen Intern Med. 2011; 26: 1513-1514.
27. Jia J-D. Fierce disputes about order of authors sometimes occur in China. BMJ. 1997; 315: 746.
28. Mireles-Cabodevila E, Stoller JK. Research During Fellowship. Chest. 2009; 135: 1395-1399.
29. Weber EJ, Callaham ML, Wears RL, Barton C, Young G. Unpublished Research from a Medical Specialty Meeting: Why Investigators Fail to Publish. JAMA. 1998; 280: 257-259.
30. Sprague S, Bhandari M, Devereaux PJ, Swiontkowski MF, Tornetta P III, Cook DJ, Dirschl D, Schemitsch EH, Guyatt GH. Barriers to Full-Text Publication Following Presentation of Abstracts at Annual Orthopaedic Meetings. J Bone Joint Surg Am. 2003; 85-A: 158-163.
31. Currie C. Author saw fraud, misconduct, and unfairness to more junior staff. BMJ. 1997; 315: 747-748.
32. Boerma T. New authorship practices are needed in developing countries. BMJ. 1997; 315: 745-746.
33. Lawrence PA. Rank injustice. Nature. 2002; 415: 835-836.
34. Kwok LS. The White Bull effect: abusive coauthorship and publication parasitism. J Med Ethics. 2005; 31: 554-556.
35. Wagena EJ. The scandal of unfair behaviour of senior faculty. J Med Ethics. 2005; 31: 308.
36. Smith MA, Barry HC, Williamson J, Keefe CW, Anderson WA. Factors Related to Publication Success Among Faculty Development Fellowship Graduates. Fam Med. 2009; 41: 120-125.
37. von Elm E, Costanza MC, Walder B, Tramèr MR. More insight into the fate of biomedical meeting abstracts: a systematic review. BMC Med Res Methodol. 2003; 3: 12.

Chapter 5
Time

Writing a paper does not take much time, but writing a paper that a scientific journal Editor will offer to publish does require a substantial amount of time. A paper that is written quickly and carelessly will simply be rejected from the journals. So the first step for writing up a good scientific journal paper is to plan when and how you are going to dedicate the necessary time from your life to do all the work involved in writing a publishable paper. Several scientific studies have reported that "lack of time" is the leading explanation that researchers give for why they have not published their work as journal papers [1–3]. So if you cannot find the time to do the writing, then your paper will also never get written and published, regardless of whatever else this book or anyone else teaches you about writing a journal paper. *Time* is the fundamental prerequisite for writing. And taking *more* time is the essential prerequisite for writing a *better* paper that will be published in a better journal.

So how much time does it really take to write a paper? Most researchers underestimate this substantially, partly because they do not have much experience with being the lead author [4], partly because they never keep precise track of what they do with their time. Furthermore, the time spent working on a paper is often spread out over weeks or months, with various people contributing to various parts of the work. Consequently, it is easy to lose sight of everything that is actually involved in the whole process, from the day data collection is completed to the day the final paper appears in the journal. But many different time-consuming tasks are involved in writing a journal paper: searching and reading the literature, preparing the database, discussing the intended paper and outline with the co-authors, performing statistical analysis, making figures and tables, drafting the manuscript, revising the contents of the manuscript, revising for co-author feedback, revising for good English composition, writing up legends and references, selecting potential target journals, formatting for the journal, writing a cover letter, submitting the manuscript to the journals, revising for peer review feedback, resubmitting to the journal (or reformatting and submitting to a new journal), correcting the printer's proofs, etc. Altogether this easily adds up to about 100–200 hours of work, depending on the type of paper, the complexity of the data, the extensiveness of the relevant literature,

© Springer Nature Switzerland AG 2019
M. Hanna, *How to Write Better Medical Papers*,
https://doi.org/10.1007/978-3-030-02955-5_5

the quality standards of the target journal, the contributions of the co-authors, etc. That is about 2–4 weeks of full-time work. If you are inexperienced (i.e. if you have not already written five or more published papers as the lead author), it will take you even longer. If you are writing in a language that is not your native language, the writing and editing will take you longer. If neither you nor anyone else on your team has a strong command of statistical analysis, the process will take you longer (and yield a weaker paper). But if you put in all the time required, you can write and publish a good journal paper.

So you need to plan when you are going to put in that time to do all that work [5]. If you simply try to do it whenever you find some time between seeing patients or doing lab duties or during lunch breaks without actually scheduling dedicated writing sessions on your calendar, then you can be certain that the work will never actually get done. So if you want to write a paper, start by blocking off 100 hours of work time on your calendar to do the writing and related work on the paper. It is best that you schedule *blocks* of a few hours or more, rather than many short periods, so you can really sink into the work. Although there are some tasks that can be done with an hour here and an hour there (such as writing legends or formatting the manuscript for the journal), the core activities of analyzing your data and drafting the paper require longer periods of sustained thinking and working. If you try to work just an hour per day, it is inefficient, because you stop thinking and working each time just as you are getting started. So start by trying to schedule, for example, 25 sessions of 4 hours each. If you block off 2 afternoons per week, with 4 hours each session, then within about 3 months, you should have completed about 100 hours of work on your paper. Hopefully a good quality first draft will be ready to circulate to your co-authors by then. By scheduling time each week to focus on doing the work, you will ensure that the paper actually gets done. If you cannot schedule the time, (or if you schedule time but then do not actually do the writing during the scheduled time), then the paper will not get written.

Each time one of your scheduled writing sessions arrives, you need to be mentally focused on the writing work that you are doing. In this busy and noisy day and age, you need to take measures to secure your concentration, in order to ensure that you will remain mentally focused on that work. First, disappear someplace quiet – such as the top floor of the library or an unused exam room in another wing of the hospital – where other people cannot find you and nothing else can distract you. If you sit in your usual office, other people will knock on your door and bother you about other nonsense, or you will fiddle with other paperwork, etc. Furthermore, turn off all your communication gadgets – mobile phones, beepers, internet, fax machines, smart watches, google glasses, etc. – so no one can interrupt your concentration and work. Otherwise, people, robots, and other machines will interrupt you constantly to discuss some other pointless nonsense, and your scientific paper will never get written. As the solitude and calm quiet settles in around you, you will be amazed to rediscover that you have a thinking human mind with something so important to say that it is actually worth writing down and publishing.

Of course, writing a scientific paper is usually not a solitary undertaking but instead a team project. The work to write-up the paper might be distributed to some degree among the various co-authors, but the team altogether still needs to put in the time to do the work. Most often, the first author takes the lead to write the first draft [6], while other co-authors make more limited contributions (oftentimes too limited). The team should decide from the outset who will do what to produce the paper and how they will be credited [7–10]. If you are the lead author, you can expect that you will probably put in at least one-third of the total time, regardless of how many other co-authors there might be. If you expect other co-authors to make specific contributions to the paper, make sure that you get them to schedule the corresponding amount of time on their calendar to do that work. Otherwise, that work will not get done. Indeed, it is a good idea to schedule a weekly team meeting to make sure that everyone is making appropriate progress on the work that each person agreed to do.

Writing a scientific paper requires sufficient "protected time" to actually do that work. "Protected time" is the specific paid hours during the work week, when your supervisor and employer will expect you to be working on writing up the paper and not be giving you other work responsibilities to do instead [11–13]. As discussed above, writing a publishable journal paper can require about 100–200 hours of work from the time data collection is complete until the time the journal actually publishes the paper, and you must deliberately schedule that volume of time onto your calendar (or your co-authors' calendars). If your supervisor or employer disrupts that work with other assignments and responsibilities – taking care of patients, doing lab experiments, filling out paperwork, or whatever else – then the paper will not get written. Moreover, writing up a scientific paper is indeed work being done for your employer, just like any other work; it is often enjoyable, but no one is doing it merely for their own amusement. There is no reason why you should be volunteering to do unpaid overtime work on the evenings and weekends in order to write up the research and publish it. You could be visiting your friends and family instead. If you are spending time writing up research, you should be paid for that work time. Do not fool yourself into thinking that writing several papers will lead to better work opportunities later, because most often that is not really the case. If no one is willing to pay you to write the paper you are currently working on, then no one is going to pay you later to write the follow-up paper either. So if your supervisor or employer wants you to write up papers for publication, then your supervisor or employer must provide you with paid protected hours to actually do that work [14, 15]. If they do not provide you with protected time, then the work will not get done [16]. Regrettably, your supervisors and employers will probably never tell you that. They will just pretend that writing a paper does not take much time, and they will implicitly expect you to put in unpaid overtime, evenings and weekends, to do that writing, for the great honor of being named as a co-author. So you need to discuss all this with them clearly from the outset – do they expect you to work on the write-up of papers? If so, how many papers as lead author, how many as a mere co-author? And when exactly during the work week would they like to schedule the protected time for you to do that writing work? If they are not willing to schedule at least 100–200 hours per paper as lead author and 20–40 hours per paper as co-author, then you are in an unrealistic and/or exploitative work situation. As mentioned already, several scientific studies have reported that "lack of time" is the leading explanation that researchers give for why they have not published their work as journal papers [1–3]. So if your supervisor or institute is not giving you protected time to write your papers, then your papers will probably also never get written and published. Protected time is the necessary prerequisite for writing scientific papers.

So far, for simplicity and ease of understanding, I have been making statements such as, "writing requires a substantial amount of time" and "time is the prerequisite for writing". But even these formulations are superficial and make time seem less essential and more external to writing that it actually is. In reality, writing is essentially nothing more than the process of converting some amount of your finite time alive on earth into a printed document that you hope will be read by other people and maybe even outlive you. The thinking of the human mind is more invisible than air and more immaterial than light. Writing is like the sedimentation of human thoughts from a period of time into the durable visible record of a publication. So the final paper will always reveal how much time and thought was actually put into it.

References

1. Weber EJ, Callaham ML, Wears RL, Barton C, Young G. Unpublished Research from a Medical Specialty Meeting: Why Investigators Fail to Publish. JAMA. 1998; 280: 257-259.
2. Sprague S, Bhandari M, Devereaux PJ, Swiontkowski MF, Tornetta P III, Cook DJ, Dirschl D, Schemitsch EH, Guyatt GH. Barriers to Full-Text Publication Following Presentation of Abstracts at Annual Orthopaedic Meetings. J Bone Joint Surg Am. 2003; 85-A: 158-163.
3. Smith MA, Barry HC, Williamson J, Keefe CW, Anderson WA. Factors Related to Publication Success Among Faculty Development Fellowship Graduates. Fam Med. 2009; 41: 120-125.
4. Asher R. Six Honest Serving Men for Medical Writers. JAMA. 1969; 208: 83-87.
5. MacDonald NE, Ford-Jones L, Friedman JN, Hall J. Preparing a manuscript for publication: A user-friendly guide. Paediatr Child Health. 2006; 11: 339-342.
6. Riesenberg D, Lundberg GD. The Order of Authorship: Who's on First? JAMA. 1990; 264: 1857.
7. Primack RB, Cigliano JA, Parsons ECM. Coauthors gone bad; how to avoid publishing conflict and a proposed agreement for co-author teams. Biol Conserv. 2014; 176: 277-280.
8. Wilcox LJ. Authorship: The Coin of the Realm, The Source of Complaints. JAMA. 1998; 280: 216-217.
9. Albert T, Wager E. How to handle authorship disputes: a guide for new researchers. In: Committee on Publication Ethics. The COPE Report 2003. Norfolk, England: Committee on Publication Ethics; 2003, pp. 32-34.
10. Scientific Integrity Committee of the Swiss Academies of Arts and Sciences. Authorship in scientific publications: analysis and recommendations. Swiss Med Wkly. 2015; 145: w14108.
11. Barnard JA. Protected Time: A Vital Ingredient for Research Career Development. J Pediatr Gastroenterol Nutr. 2015; 60: 292-293.
12. Smythe WR. Protected time. Surgery. 2004; 135: 232-234.
13. Bogdonoff MD. The Need for Faculty Protected Time. Arch Intern Med. 1972; 129: 363-365.
14. North American Primary Care Research Group Committee on Building Research Capacity, The Academic Family Medicine Organizations Research Subcommittee. What Does It Mean to Build Research Capacity? Fam Med. 2002; 34: 678-684.
15. Bland CJ, Schmitz CC. Characteristics of the Successful Researcher and Implications for Faculty Development. J Med Educ. 1986; 61: 22-31.
16. Young RA, DeHaven MJ, Passmore C, Baumer JG. Research Participation, Protected Time, and Research Output by Family Physicians in Family Medicine Residencies. Fam Med. 2006; 38: 341-348.

Chapter 6
Reading

If you want to write a good paper, you must read good papers [1–3]. You must read dozens of good papers. You must read the entire paper, closely, not only parts of it. By reading the literature, you will know which issues really interest the medical community and why. You will discover important details about "the facts" and what is known. You will notice important variations in the methods to take into account. You will find alternate theories and explanations that you have not yet considered. You will become up-to-date on the latest scientific findings and thinking on the subject. All great writers have done a lot of reading. Reading trains the mind to think better like other great writers.

One mistake many medical researchers make is that they read only the Abstracts of other papers. Medical researchers usually have many other responsibilities and not much time. They think that one way to get more done faster is to simply skim the Abstract, maybe glance at the figures and conclusions, and skip the rest of the paper. But if you do not read the full paper, then you have not really read the scientific literature. You will not know what other researchers really did in detail, and you will not know all the subtleties of what they are thinking. Reading the literature thoroughly is an integral part of doing the research.

You will gain two main benefits from reading the scientific literature. First, reading the literature will equip you with ideas and facts that you will use later to write a paper with rich content. Not reading the literature is like showing up an hour late for a meeting, and saying, "I'm not sure what exactly you all have been talking about or what was already said before I arrived, but I'd like you all to listen now to my opinions anyway." So reading the literature will give you a better sense of what might be worth saying versus what has already been discredited. Second, reading the literature provides you with examples of good writing, (or at least "not bad" writing). Medical scientific writing has a certain style, which is different from other kinds of writing. By reading the literature, you will become familiar with how medical papers should be written. But there is one caveat: many journal papers today are not written well, especially in run-of-the-mill journals. Fortunately, the papers in top-tier journals are usually very well written, so they are the preferred source for your readings.

© Springer Nature Switzerland AG 2019
M. Hanna, *How to Write Better Medical Papers*,
https://doi.org/10.1007/978-3-030-02955-5_6

Over one million journal papers are published every year, and it is impossible for anyone to read all the papers that might be relevant to their work. So researchers often wonder how to select the best papers to read, aside from just looking at the Abstract and deciding whether the paper seems relevant to their needs. Here are eight informal criteria to help steer you toward the more worthwhile readings. 1) Books are usually at least as reliable as journals, but their contents are often broader and less specialized. They serve as a good foundation but are generally insufficient as a basis for writing journal papers. 2) Papers in top tier journals are almost always of much better quality – regarding both the research and the writing – than papers in standard specialty journals. They should be a part of every research-er's reading diet. 3) If you need a broad overview, review papers and metaanalyses are generally much more useful than primary research papers. 4) Editorials are usu-ally very good to stimulate your thinking, and they are comparatively quick and easy to read. 5) Case reports and letters are anecdotal and therefore low priority options, unless they address something specific with direct relevance to your own work. 6) Conference abstracts, academic theses, and other gray literature are usually prelimi-nary, unreliable, and low quality; they should be avoided unless there are no journal papers on the topic. Webpages are almost always garbage because there is usually no quality control at all; you should avoid reading them even if you have all the time in the world. 7) Medicine and science are constantly progressing, so papers that are too old will probably have outdated information based on less valid methods. How old is "too old" depends greatly on the topic, but if a paper was published more than 10 or 20 years ago, you should ask yourself whether people still use the same medi-cal or scientific methods now as they did then. 8) The author(s) of the paper and the institution(s) where they work are misleading indicators of the paper's value. You should generally avoid selecting your reading based on who wrote it or where.

There are two ways to read a paper: a poor passive way and an enriching active way. In the poor passive way, the reader simply takes in the words and numbers, page after page, without pause, and without much reaction, just to see what it says and get to the end of it. That is fine if you are reading a Sunday newspaper to relax. But that is an inappropriate way to read scientific literature. Do not read scientific papers like a sponge absorbing water. Scientific literature must be read thoughtfully, critically, and reactively, in order for it to be enriching and useful. Actively reflect on the papers you are reading. Does the context and aim of the study really make sense? Has each step of the research been designed appropriately, or would you have done it differ-ently? Do the results really say what the authors claim, or would you interpret them some other way? Are their arguments and conclusions logical, relevant, and convinc-ing, or do you view the matter differently? Is the paper rigorous and insightful or dull and dubious? In your mind, dialogue further with the authors: argue back if they seem wrong, reflect further if they say something enlightening. When you get to the end of the paper, don't rush off to your next task; stop and think some about what you just read. Discuss the paper with your colleagues.

Part of the scientific process is that every researcher must assess the scientific merit of previous publications. If the evidence and thinking is good, researchers cannot simply ignore it. If the evidence or thinking is not good, they must reject it.

If researchers do not read and critically assess the papers they cite, then they do not contribute to creating true scientific knowledge. Instead, they only report their own tinkering and contribute to unfounded rumors ("So-and-so said that Goldberg et al. found that …"). Science depends centrally on this process of critically assessing the existing scientific literature and building further upon it. Reading the literature critically is fundamental to the scientific enterprise.

References

1. Jones R, Scouller J, Grainger F, Lachlan M, Evans S, Torrance N. The scandal of poor medical research: sloppy use of literature often to blame. BMJ. 1994; 308: 591.
2. Bourne PE. Ten Simple Rules for Getting Published. PLoS Comput Biol. 2005; 1: e57.
3. Marušić A, Marušić M. Teaching Students How to Read and Write Science: A Mandatory Course on Scientific Research and Communication in Medicine. Acad Med. 2003; 78: 1235-1239.

Chapter 7
Searching the Literature

So how do you find relevant papers to read and cite? There are three main ways, which should be sufficient, unless you are writing a literature review or cannot find references on some specific point.

First, choose half a dozen or more journals in your field and flip through the table of contents every time a new issue comes out. This will help ensure that you are familiar with the latest research findings, as well as the topics that currently interest journal Editors.

Second, look at the reference lists of the papers you read. Whenever someone writes something interesting followed by some endnote numbers, flip to the end of the paper, and look at what those references are. Often they will be uninteresting or outdated, but sometimes they will be worth tracking down and reading.

Third, and most importantly, use online search engines, such as PubMed (or other NCBI databases), Google Scholar, Europe PMC, PubPsych, and so on, to locate all the articles you would never have known about otherwise [1–5]. Whenever you write a paper, you should start by running multiple literature searches on different aspects of your paper (e.g. the patient population, the pathology, the treatment studied, the methods you used, etc.), to obtain some relevant literature on all aspects of your paper. Most search engines have various filters, so you can restrict your search in various ways to reduce the number of articles to a manageable list. You can then read the Abstracts to determine which papers will or will not be useful for you. But if a paper does seem useful, you should always retrieve and read the full article; do not rely only on the Abstract. The full paper will have much richer information and reflections, which is what you need, in order to write better papers.

Whenever you start to work on a new study or paper, you should run a thorough literature search on your study question and try to find the answer in the literature that has already been published [3, 6–8]. That is much easier than running a whole new research study, merely to confirm something that was already well-known to other people. If answers to your study questions have already been provided sufficiently in previous papers, then there is no need for you to conduct yet another study on that specific issue, (except perhaps a metaanalysis or systematic review of the

© Springer Nature Switzerland AG 2019
M. Hanna, *How to Write Better Medical Papers*,
https://doi.org/10.1007/978-3-030-02955-5_7

literature). This is particularly important for animal studies [9], because they are more likely to be small and reported only in poorly known gray literature (e.g. conference presentations, academic theses, etc.), and because there is an ethical need to reduce the use of animals in research [10]. So always start by running a thorough search, to find out whether you are really addressing questions that have not yet been answered adequately. When your research is completed and you are ready to start writing your paper, you should thoroughly search the literature again, to catch anything that you overlooked before or anything that was published after your initial literature search for your research design.

As a rough rule of thumb, you should read at least 2 papers and cite 1, for every 100 words of your paper's total word count. So if you're writing a 3000 word paper, you should read at least 60 papers, and cite 30; for a 500 word letter, read at least 10 and cite 5.

More importantly, every claim you make in a paper should be supported by citations (if not based on your own data). So for example, if your paper starts by saying, "Lower respiratory infections are the leading cause of death worldwide," go to a major search engine such as PubMed, run a search on the epidemiology of lower respiratory infections and/or the leading causes of death, and find papers to support that claim [11]. Maybe whatever you asserted is not really true, or at least not the exact way you formulated it. (For example, lower respiratory infections are the leading *infectious* cause of death worldwide [12, 13] or the leading cause of death *in children under five* worldwide [13; personal communication from AH Mokdad on 23 March 2018] or the *fifth* leading cause of death worldwide [12] or the *third* leading cause of *years of life lost to early mortality* worldwide [13]; whereas, "the leading cause of death worldwide" is actually ischemic heart disease [13]. Notice also how it is important to carefully verify that the assertion in your manuscript corresponds to what the references actually say. It is counterproductive, or even deceptive, to provide citations that do not actually support the statements to which they are attached.) Even if whatever you asserted is true and correctly formulated, readers will often want to know how you know that. If you fail to provide citations, readers may doubt what you say or be unable to obtain more information to improve their understanding. For example, if your manuscript says, "Road injury is among the top 10 causes of early mortality worldwide", but you do not provide any citations, then readers might wonder whether or not that statement is really true. So you should look at each sentence in your manuscript and reflect on whether it needs supporting citations. If you already have references to back up an assertion, it is often nonetheless helpful to run a quick literature search on that point anyway. More recent or better quality references might assert something somewhat different, in which case you will want to update your manuscript accordingly.

Similarly, if you use a particular questionnaire in your study, such as the CES-D, run a literature search on that instrument. Identify, read, and cite a few of the key papers on that instrument, so you are familiar with its measurement properties and applications. This will also enable other people to learn more about it if they are unfamiliar. This is especially important when using questionnaires that are new or not well known.

By searching, reading, and citing the scientific literature, you will embed your research and thinking within the investigations and debates of the broader scientific community. Science is scientific because it is based upon the conversation that the scientific community is publishing in the scientific literature.

References

1. Falagas ME, Pitsouni EI, Malietzis GA, Pappas G. Comparison of PubMed, Scopus, Web of Science, and Google Scholar: strengths and weaknesses. FASEB J. 2008; 22: 338-342.
2. Giglia E. Beyond PubMed: Other free-access biomedical databases. Eura Medicophys. 2007; 43: 563-569.
3. Cals JWL, Kotz D. Literature review in biomedical research: useful search engines beyond PubMed. J Clin Epidemiol. 2016; 71: 115-116.
4. Giustini D, Barsky E. A look at Google Scholar, PubMed, and Scirus: comparisons and recommendations. JCHLA / JABSC. 2005; 26: 85-89.
5. Doyle DJ. Search engines for scholarly research: a brief update for clinicians. Can J Anesth. 2007; 54: 336-341.
6. Chalmers I, Glasziou P. Avoidable waste in the production and reporting of research evidence. Lancet. 2009; 374: 86-89.
7. Chalmers TC, Frank CS, Reitman D. Minimizing the Three Stages of Publication Bias. JAMA. 1990; 263: 1392-1395.
8. Smith AJ, Goodman NW. The hypertensive response to intubation. Do researchers acknowledge previous work? Can J Anaesth. 1997; 44: 9-13.
9. Pound P, Ebrahim S, Sandercock P, Bracken MB, Roberts I; for Reviewing Animal Trials Systematically (RATS) Group. Where is the evidence that animal research benefits humans? BMJ. 2004; 328: 517-517.
10. Smith R. Animal research: the need for a middle ground. BMJ. 2001; 322: 248-249.
11. Jones R, Scouller J, Grainger F, Lachlan M, Evans S, Torrance N. The scandal of poor medical research: sloppy use of literature often to blame. BMJ. 1994; 308: 591.
12. GBD 2015 LRI Collaborators. Estimates of the global, regional, and national morbidity, mortality, and aetiologies of lower respiratory tract infections in 195 countries: a systematic analysis for the Global Burden of Disease Study 2015. Lancet Infect Dis. 2017; 17: 1133-1161.
13. GBD 2016 Causes of Death Collaborators. Global, regional, and national age-sex specific mortality for 264 causes of death, 1980-2016: a systematic analysis for the Global Burden of Disease Study 2016. Lancet. 2017; 390: 1151-1210.

Chapter 8
The Elevator Speech

Most researchers spend so much time deeply sunk into the details of their research that they lose sight of what they are doing or why. They can talk for hours about their research, but they cannot really sum it all up in one minute or less. Moreover, they simply assume that everyone else understands what they are talking about. But that is rarely the case. Scientific research today usually involves the study of unusual questions that very few people ever think about and no one already knows what the answer to them might be. It uses specialized terminology and unfamiliar concepts and methods. The consequence is that whenever researchers talk or write about their work, they often only spew out a long ramble of technobabble that remains incomprehensible to most everyone else.

So before you start drafting your paper, try to compose an "elevator speech": summarize your research in one minute or less, in such a way that any university student could understand what you are saying [1–3]. Your elevator speech should include the general problem that you are trying to address and a basic description of the study you are conducting. If the research is not yet completed, you should summarize your study aims and why it matters. If your research is already completed, you should summarize your main finding, and why it matters. Do not whip up a sloppy summary in ten minutes. Put some time and effort into it, reflecting on what exactly you are doing and why. Think about how best to communicate it clearly in one minute or less, as if all your research funding for the next year depended on this; (in fact, it might).

Then review this elevator speech with all your co-authors, and see if they agree with you that it is the clearest and most accurate summary possible of your research (or that specific paper) [4]. You will be surprised how often your own co-authors would summarize the work differently or put the focus on other aspects. If you reach consensus about the elevator speech before starting work on the paper, the rest of the write-up will go more smoothly.

If anyone else asks you about your research, you can deliver this elevator speech to tell them what you are doing and why they should care. Even if people do not ask you about it, stop anyone you see at work, and give them your elevator speech. It

© Springer Nature Switzerland AG 2019
M. Hanna, *How to Write Better Medical Papers*,
https://doi.org/10.1007/978-3-030-02955-5_8

does not matter who they are: your co-workers, your friends, the secretary, the Dean of the College, the cleaning lady, a visiting Professor from another field, the delivery man, the wisecracking teenage intern down the hall, the narcoleptic security agent at the building entrance, and so on. Give them your elevator speech, and then ask them: "Does that make sense to you?" If they respond, "Umm, well, uhhh…", then you and your co-authors need to revise your elevator speech before doing anything else.

If you cannot summarize what you did, why, what you found, and how it matters in a one-minute nutshell, they your paper lacks sufficiently sharp focus or your thinking is muddled. Similarly, if you cannot explain your research in a way that any university student (or patient) can understand, then either your research is too obscure and irrelevant or you yourself do not really understand clearly what you are doing. In either case, no one else will understand it either, including other experts in your field.

Do not skip the step of composing a good elevator speech; skipping it will only make the rest of the process of writing the paper much more difficult. When you have composed an elevator speech that other people understand and all your co-authors support, then you are ready to start writing the outline of your paper.

References

1. Annesley TM. The Abstract and the Elevator Talk: A Tale of Two Summaries. Clin Chem. 2010; 56: 521-524.
2. Griscom NT. Your research: How to get it on paper and in print. Pediatr Radiol. 1999; 29: 81-86.
3. Dubé CE, Lapane KL. Lay Abstracts and Summaries: Writing Advice for Scientists. J Cancer Educ. 2014; 29: 577-579.
4. Berk RN. Preparation of Manuscripts for Radiology Journals: Advice to First-Time Authors. AJR. 1992; 158: 203-208.

Chapter 9
The Outline

When you are ready to start writing, the first step is to write an outline of the paper. The outline of a paper is equivalent to the blueprint of a building. No one would try to build a real building these days without first creating a blueprint. The same principle applies to writing: never try to write a paper directly without first writing an outline.

So what does an outline look like and how do you write one? This is what the beginning of an outline might look like for a fictitious paper about a new treatment for children with "Kazil" disease who are not cured by conventional treatment.

Introduction
  A. General Background (Kazil disease)
      1. what is Kazil disease
      2. how many people have Kazil disease
      3. what its effects are on people who have it
      4. the current standard treatment options
  B. Specific Problem (children who become refractory)
      1. some children become refractory to treatment
      2. clinical description of what happens
      3. speculation on why this happens
      4. recent laboratory study in *Nature* that may be relevant to this
      5. suggested alternative treatment for these refractory children
  C. This Study
      1. general description of this research study
      2. the two treatment regimens that were compared
      3. the aim of this particular paper

© Springer Nature Switzerland AG 2019
M. Hanna, *How to Write Better Medical Papers*,
https://doi.org/10.1007/978-3-030-02955-5_9

Methods
    A. Ethics
        1. IRB approval
        2. study registration
        3. written informed consent from the patients' parents
        4. laws and guidelines followed
    B. Patient Population
        1. recruitment setting and timeframe
        2. inclusion criteria
        3. exclusion criteria
[etc.]

As you can see, the outline has three levels. The first level simply presents the major sections of the paper (for example, "Introduction, Methods, Results, Discussion" in a standard research paper). The second level (A, B, C, etc.) presents either the subsections (when using subsections, such as in the Methods) or the topics of the paragraphs (when there are no subsections, such as in the Introduction). The third level (1, 2, 3, etc.) then presents all the main points that you want to cover in that paragraph or subsection. Generally, three levels are sufficient for the outline of a journal paper.

So now that you see what an outline looks like, how do you go about writing an outline for a paper? You do not write an outline from start to finish, top to bottom, line by line, like the final outline will appear. Instead, you start by writing just the first level. Then you go back and expand out each section with just the second level (A, B, C, etc.) Then you go back again and expand out each of those sections with the third level (1, 2, 3, etc.) So start by writing just the major sections; for example:

Introduction
Methods
Results
Discussion

That first level is normally already determined by the type of paper you are writing and the format of your target journal. You do not have much choice about it, so that first level of the outline is very easy to write.

Next, go back and write briefly what each subsection or paragraph will be about; for example:

Introduction
    A. General Background (Kazil disease)
    B. Specific Problem (children who become refractory)
    C. This Study

Methods
>   A. Ethics
>   B. Patient Population
>   C. Study Design
>   D. Treatments
>   E. Outcome Measures
>   F. Statistical Analysis

[etc.]

That second level (A, B, C, etc.) depends some on the contents of your paper but also loosely follows some conventions. Later chapters of this book will provide more guidance about which subsections or paragraphs commonly make up the Introduction, Methods, Results, and Discussion. You can also look at recent papers in your target journal as model examples. When you are done writing the second level, stop, look it over, and make sure it seems complete, accurate, in the right order, and otherwise correct. Revise it as needed before proceeding.

Then go back through the outline and expand each subsection or paragraph by adding the specific points that each subsection or paragraph will cover. For example:

Introduction
>   A. General Background (Kazil disease)
>   1. what is Kazil disease
>   2. how many people have Kazil disease
>   3. what its effects are on people who have it
>   4. the current standard treatment options
>   B. Specific Problem (children who become refractory)
>   1. some children become refractory to treatment
>   2. clinical description of what happens
>   3. speculation on why this happens
>   4. recent laboratory study in *Nature* that may be relevant to this
>   5. suggested alternative treatment for these refractory children
>   C. This Study
>   1. general description of this research study
>   2. the two treatment regimens that were compared
>   3. the aim of this particular paper

The contents of this third level (1, 2, 3, etc.) depends mostly on the contents of your specific paper – i.e. what you want to say. Whatever you write here, you should try to write it simply in a "bullet-point" or "key idea" summary form, like you see above; do not try to write out full sentences. Writing full sentences is more difficult, and you will get caught up in the process of writing your paper rather than creating an outline. Also, using only "bullet-point" or "key idea" summary form will enable you and your co-authors to see the underlying logical skeleton of your paper, rather than looking at the "flesh" of how everything will be said.

Creating an outline enables you to plan ahead what you will write and make changes now before you begin writing. Don't worry about wording everything exactly right. This is only an outline. Just try to create a clear plan of what you will write later, on another day. When you are done, spend some time looking at your blueprint and reflecting on whether this is really the house you want to build, or did you want to say something else instead? Are you saying everything you need to say, but nothing more? Are you saying it all in the right order, or would it make more sense to readers if you switched around some sentences or sections?

After you are done drafting the detailed outline of your paper, you should also compare it to current reporting guidelines for your type of paper. Reporting guidelines for many different kinds of papers can be found online from the EQUATOR Network [1, 2]. Review your outline to check whether it contains all the essential elements in the applicable reporting guidelines. There may sometimes be good scientific reasons to not report every element recommended in some guidelines, but failure to review the guidelines is not one of those good reasons. Nonetheless, the reporting guidelines should be checked only after you have drafted a detailed outline yourself; otherwise your paper may become a mere "fill in the blanks" exercise that fails to communicate anything beyond the standardized basic information of the guidelines checklist.

You should ask all your co-authors to carefully read the outline and make revisions. Everyone should agree on a final outline before you start writing the actual paper. Even if you worked together closely on the actual research, they may think that the paper will present or discuss something in a different way. So it is important to agree upon the outline before you spend many hours writing a manuscript that they will not support. Once everyone agrees on the outline, it is relatively easy to convert this detailed outline into an actual paper.

Now you can see why it is so important to always write an outline first. It provides you with a clear blueprint for your building. It serves as the logical skeleton that you will "flesh out" into a full written paper. There would be two negative consequences if you did not write this outline first but instead tried to simply dive right into writing the paper directly without an outline. First, it would probably be much more difficult for you to find the words to say anything you find satisfying, because you would not have a clear plan of what the paper should say. You would spend more time staring at the computer not writing, or writing something you find unsatisfactory and then changing it again and again. Second, because you would not have a clear overview, you might start your paper in the wrong way (for example, with sentence #3 above – the effects of Kazil disease). Not sure what to say next, you might write about how expensive it is to treat Kazil disease. Then you might summarize a couple clinical studies you recently read. Soon the paper would be a disorganized mess. But after writing several pages of text, it would be more difficult to see why the paper was not coming out the way you hoped. So always always always write an outline first. Ultimately, it will save you a lot of time and lead to a much better paper.

References

1. Simera I, Altman DG. Writing a research article that is "fit for purpose": EQUATOR Network and reporting guidelines. Ann Intern Med. 2009; 151: JC2-2 to JC2-3.
2. Simera I, Moher D, Hoey J, Schulz KF, Altman DG. A catalog of reporting guidelines for health research. Eur J Clin Invest. 2010; 40: 35-53.

Chapter 10
Envision Your Readers

The purpose of a scientific paper is to communicate the work, findings, and thoughts of the authors to other people. If such communication was not the goal of the authors, there would be no need to write the paper. Yet writing is mostly a solitary activity done almost entirely in isolation from any readers. Authors generally do not see their readers or ever hear any feedback from them. The regrettable consequence is that many scientific papers are written in ways that show a lack of awareness of who the readers really are and what they will or will not understand in a paper. Insofar as a scientific paper is not understood by its readers, it does not succeed in fulfilling the purpose of a scientific paper.

Authors of scientific papers should repeatedly give thought to who their readership will probably be. This includes both the primary intended audience and the variety of other plausible types of readers. The primary intended audience is the set of people with whom the authors are trying to communicate. Authors should consider who exactly is the primary intended audience: other researchers vs. practicing clinicians, medical doctors vs. other healthcare professionals, specialists in a single field vs. a broader audience. Authors should also consider what other types of people might be reading the paper (besides the types just mentioned): medical students, patients, administrators, policy makers, other healthcare professionals, and so on. Generally speaking, technical research papers intended for specialists are not read by people outside that field, but major clinical studies, literature reviews, or viewpoint articles might indeed reach a broad and heterogeneous audience. Whomever the readership is, the authors should clearly envision those readers.

You should then write your paper with your primary intended audience always clearly in mind. Consider what they already know or do not know. If you are writing for a narrow audience of other specialists in your subfield, there is no need to belabor points that are already common knowledge in your field. If you are writing for a broad multidisciplinary audience, you may need to explain and justify many basic points that you otherwise just take for granted. For medical scientific papers, it is especially important to keep in mind how much knowledge the readers already have about the precise topic of your research and also how well they understand any

© Springer Nature Switzerland AG 2019
M. Hanna, *How to Write Better Medical Papers*,
https://doi.org/10.1007/978-3-030-02955-5_10

forms of statistical analysis you are reporting. If something might be unfamiliar to them, explain it (without being pedantic). You should always write in a way that is comprehensible to your primary intended audience. If you can make your paper accessible to other possible types of secondary readers without boring your primary readers, then do so.

The one and only legitimate goal of every medical scientific paper is to increase the knowledge of the readers. So whenever you have a choice between two different ways of writing something, choose the version that will be more effective at reaching that goal. There are many rules, recommendations, tips, and so on about how to write well. For medical scientific texts, all those rule and tips are ultimately subservient to this one general underlying principle: maximize the knowledge gained by the readers.

Part II
Analyzing

Chapter 11
Ethics of Data Analysis

Introduction

Research is the process of methodically gathering and analyzing new information on a topic, in order to generate more reliable knowledge about the world. The data that is gathered in research is often not accessible to other people reading the final reports and is only rarely reviewed by anyone else even when it is available. Because most readers of research reports do not have the time or even access to review the raw data from the research themselves, they place their trust in the authors of the report that the results refer to accurate data from research that truly took place as described. Thus the knowledge gained and shared from research depends critically on a system of social trust in the veracity of the data and results. So the ethics of data analysis concerns two major forms of research misconduct – fabrication of data or results and falsification of data or results – as well as the minor practical issue of preserving the data for future reexamination.

No Fabrication

"Fabrication" means making up numbers, in the database or reported results, without ever doing the research to which those numbers supposedly refer. It seems absurd that scientific researchers would ever need to be told, "Do not make up your data or results." Fabrication of the raw data or the results is so blatantly contradictory to the inherent purpose of scientific research that it is difficult to imagine who would ever do that. But it does happen. Although data fabrication is not commonplace, it is also not a very rare anomaly [1, 2]. After all, doing research and collecting real data requires time, effort, and funding, and then often fails to prove the conclusions that the researcher already had in mind from the outset anyway. So perhaps it is not so surprising that some people decide to simply skip all the work of research and create their data from their imagination instead.

© Springer Nature Switzerland AG 2019
M. Hanna, *How to Write Better Medical Papers*,
https://doi.org/10.1007/978-3-030-02955-5_11

Never fabricate your data. (Of course you would never do that, but it has to be said anyway for the record.)

Although you yourself will never fabricate data, you should remain aware that maybe one of your co-authors, or non-co-author research assistants charged with data collection, might sometimes fabricate data [3–6]. It does not happen very often, but when it does, it is a deadly problem, precisely because it is so antithetical to the essence of scientific research. If you co-author a paper using fabricated data, it may be difficult to absolve yourself of that research misconduct when it is discovered, even if someone else is guilty and you yourself honestly had no awareness of it at all [7]. So unless you were personally involved in all the data collection, you should always take a moment to mentally screen for this risk. Have you yourself seen the data collection and the original study records? If not, do the results seem "too good to be true"? Even if not, take a moment to skeptically suspect that some (but not all) of the data is fabricated. Can you somehow objectively disprove that doubt? If not, you should probably ask to see the original data records. If they are not forthcoming, you should probably remove yourself from the project.

No Falsification

Falsification of data or results is a related but different form of research misconduct. The difference here is that research is actually carried out and real data is collected, but then parts of the raw data and/or the reported results are altered ("falsified"), usually because they are not showing what the researcher wants to show. Regrettably, falsification of data or results is very easy to slip into and accordingly is not at all rare [1]. The most basic and crass form of falsification is simply changing numbers in the database to obtain different results or merely reporting different results than what was actually obtained. But falsification can take several other forms, which are not as obviously crass or blatant, and which may even seem to have a veneer of scientific rationale. Selective exclusion of data (e.g. removing some subjects from the database) is actually falsification, unless it is clearly reported, along with valid scientific justifications for the exclusion. Inappropriate editing or manipulation of images for figures is another form of falsification. (Chapter 19, "Figures: Photographs and Images", provides guidance on what is acceptable image editing and how to safeguard against suspicions of misconduct.) Not reporting known harms from a clinical study (or reporting them in a deliberately vague way) – a problem that is quite commonplace [8, 9] – is also actually a form of falsification of research results. Use of inappropriate statistical methods is equivalent to falsification of results, if it is done with awareness that the methods are (or may be) inappropriate and is nonetheless done for the purpose of obtaining results that are preferable for the researchers' wishes [10, 11, 12 (p. 453)]. Consciously misrepresenting or misinterpreting results to make unsupported statements may also be a borderline form of falsification, blending over into the problem of "spin" [13–15]. Of course, researchers who find themselves sliding into these various forms of falsification never admit to themselves that what they are doing is falsification.

Instead, they find various euphemisms, rationalizations, and doublespeak to make it all more palatable to themselves and others: "improving the presentation of the results", "focusing on the main message", "massaging the data", "enhancing the clarity of the figures", "database cleaning" (a term for legitimate procedures that is sometime misapplied to illegitimate procedures that should actually be termed "database cleansing"), etc.

It can be challenging to guard against falsification of data or results, because falsification takes so many forms, some of which are subtle and not far removed from legitimate preparation, analysis, and presentation of the data. Falsification usually arises when a researcher has a preferred conclusion in mind, and wants the data and results to support that conclusion. Falsification (or suppression) of data and results can also arise, inversely, when the researcher wants to avoid showing something from the research, (e.g. harms). In other words, when a researcher starts to feel pressure to make a certain conclusion that is not fully supported by the data, or to avoid a conclusion that is supported by the data, that mental pressure is usually what drives the falsification. But the moment a researcher starts to falsify (or suppress) data or results, the research is no longer scientific. Instead, the researcher drifts off into making statements that are not truly supported by empirical examination of reality. You must always keep in mind that drawing conclusions that are truly supported by accurate data and results is more important than maintaining any pet theory from your own mind, even if financial rewards depend on proving those pet theories. Falsification of data or results, however subtle, is an unscientific way of fooling yourself and others into believing something that is not true.

So always ask yourself: are you mentally ready to publish results that contradict your current beliefs or otherwise are inconsistent with your interests? If not, you may be experiencing the kind of mental pressure that puts people at risk for drifting off into subtle (or not so subtle) forms of falsification. One of the best safeguards against falsification of data or results is to work together with a statistician (or other methodologist) who has no personal preferences or interests for or against any particular conclusion on the research topic, but instead has only a strong professional interest in doing rigorously accurate data analysis, regardless of whatever it might show. It is also beneficial to document, report, and justify every step of your data preparation and analysis, especially any changes you make to the data or results, so it is all transparent to the readers. The line between legitimate and illegitimate preparation, analysis, and presentation of data is not always sharp and clear, so if you are anywhere in that gray zone, it is best to seek expert guidance from your colleagues and transparently document what you do. If you have other co-authors involved in the data preparation, analysis, and presentation, it is probably worth your time and efforts to reflect about whether they might have inadvertently drifted off into subtle forms of falsification without even realizing it [16]. Falsification of data or results can arise without deliberate malicious intent or conscious awareness. Indeed, that is part of the reason it occurs so easily and so often. And that is why you should scrutinize all your papers for it, rather than sleepily waiting for someone else to notice it and accuse you of misconduct.

Preservation of the Raw Data

The raw database, and all primary data collection forms, should be archived for a minimum of ten years after publication of the research [17], preferably in more than one location, so multiple back-up copies exist. In pure theory, destruction of the primary data is not by itself truly research misconduct. But if anyone ever asks to review the primary data later, the non-existence of the data would be viewed as strong circumstantial evidence that the published results and/or the data on which they were based were probably fabricated or falsified [18]. And even if no one ever questions the veracity of your results, destruction of raw data is very poor research practice and wasteful mismanagement of scientific resources, because it eliminates the possibility of further secondary data analysis studies or meta-analysis from combined primary data. For these ethical and scientific reasons, you should never delete the raw data or destroy the original study records, not even after publication of the paper. Instead, you should make adequate efforts to preserve multiple copies of them, in case there is ever any need later to review or audit the research or to reuse the data in further new analyses.

Conclusion

Ethical data analysis means honestly reporting appropriate analysis of accurate real data, and not "fudging" anything. Other people's research work and medical decisions will be influenced by the research they read. They must be able to trust that the results they read are a truthful and accurate report of real research. Research reports with fabricated or falsified data or results have direct negative consequences on readers who make use of those reports, but more importantly such reports also have a widespread corrosive effect on people's capacity to trust the veracity of research reports in general. To maintain that necessary system of social trust, researchers must themselves have the self-discipline to remain entirely truthful and transparent about their data and analysis.

References

1. Fanelli D. How Many Scientists Fabricate and Falsify Research? A Systematic Review and Meta-Analysis of Survey Data. PLoS One. 2009; 4: e5738.
2. Carlisle JB. Data fabrication and other reasons for non-random sampling in 5087 randomised, controlled trials in anaesthetic and general medical journals. Anaesthesia. 2017; 72: 944-952.
3. Kingori P, Gerrets R. Morals, morale and motivations in data fabrication: Medical research fieldworkers views and practices in two Sub-Saharan African contexts. Soc Sci Med. 2016; 166: 150-159.
4. Steen RG. Retractions in the scientific literature: do authors deliberately commit research fraud? J Med Ethics. 2011; 37: 113-117.
5. Baerlocher MO, O'Brien J, Newton M, Gautam T, Noble J. Data integrity, reliability and fraud in medical research. Eur J Intern Med. 2010; 21: 40-45.
6. Koshland DE Jr. Fraud in Science. Science. 1987; 235: 141.
7. Kennedy D. Multiple Authors, Multiple Problems. Science. 2003; 301: 733.

8. Golder S, Loke YK, Wright K, Norman G. Reporting of Adverse Events in Published and Unpublished Studies of Health Care: A Systematic Review. PLoS Med. 2016; 13: e1002127.

9. Haidich A-B, Birtsou C, Dardavessis T, Tirodimos I, Arvanitidou M. The quality of safety reporting in trials is still suboptimal: Survey of major general medical journals. J Clin Epidemiol. 2011; 64: 124-135.

10. Bailar JC III. Science, Statistics, and Deception. Ann Intern Med. 1986; 104: 259-260.

11. Sigma Xi. Honor in Science. Research Triangle Park, NC, USA: Sigma Xi; 2000.

12. Altman DG. Practical Statistics for Medical Research. Boca Raton, FL, USA: CRC Press; 1991, 1999.

13. Gross RA. Style, spin, and science. Neurology. 2015; 85: 10-11.

14. Lazarus C, Haneef R, Ravaud P, Boutron I. Classification and prevalence of spin in abstracts of non-randomized studies evaluating an intervention. BMC Med Res Methodol. 2015; 15: 85.

15. Chiu K, Grundy Q, Bero L. 'Spin' in published biomedical literature: A methodological systematic review. PLoS Biol. 2017; 15: e2002173.

16. A picture worth a thousand words (of explanation). Nat Methods. 2006; 3: 237.

17. International Committee of Medical Journal Editors. Recommendations for the Conduct, Reporting, Editing, and Publication of Scholarly Work in Medical Journals. Philadelphia: American College of Physicians; 1978, 2017. Accessed on 12 January 2018 at: www.icmje.org/icmje-recommendations.pdf

18. Organisation for Economic Co-Operation and Development, Global Science Forum. Best Practices for Ensuring Scientific Integrity and Preventing Misconduct. Accessed on 13 January 2018 at: www.oecd.org/science/inno/40188303.pdf

Chapter 12
Data Preparation

Most medical papers rely centrally on some kind of statistical analysis. Good statistical analysis starts with a good dataset: garbage in, garbage out; gold in, gold out. Yet it is amazing how many researchers try to generate a paper using a data spreadsheet that is a disorganized mess riddled with errors and useless numbers. Before you even begin any statistical analysis, you need to spend time: 1) organizing your database, 2) doing database cleaning, and 3) performing quality control of the dataset.

First, you need to organize your database. Researchers often collect more data in a study than they actually intend to use in the current paper they are writing. So the first step is to create a data file for the specific paper that you are writing. In that file, you should remove or separate out all the variables that you will not be using in the current paper. If you are not reporting on all the subjects for some reason, you should remove or separate out all the subjects that are being excluded. For example, if you are writing a paper on the subset of obese patients, create a column for BMI, delete the data on raw height and weight measurements, and eliminate all the subjects whose BMI is below your defined threshold of "obese". Further, you should arrange the variables in a logical order (e.g. the order you expect to present them). Also avoid using typographic formatting or other features that may be lost if the spreadsheet is imported into some other software program for statistical analysis, (except to temporarily mark data that needs further review). You should also write up a key to your data coding scheme and abbreviations, so anyone else who looks at the data spreadsheet can quickly understand it. Your spreadsheet should be well-organized and clear to read.

Second, you must spend time doing database cleaning. What this means is that you look through your database for missing or erroneous cells of data, or data that is poorly coded. Again, it is surprising how many researchers will run analyses on datasets that are missing data that they do in fact have in their records somewhere. So look at each and every cell in your spreadsheet. If there are any empty cells, go back to the original study records and see if the missing data is there. If not, see if the information is available in other patient records. If the data is still missing, you

© Springer Nature Switzerland AG 2019
M. Hanna, *How to Write Better Medical Papers*,
https://doi.org/10.1007/978-3-030-02955-5_12

should try to figure out why: what went wrong that the data is not there? You should also check for erroneous data. Typing numbers into a spreadsheet can be tedious, so people do make mistakes with it. The easiest and best way to check for errors is to have two different people type all the data into two original databases independently, and then compare the two files for discrepancies. It is unlikely that two people will both make the same error. You should also look through your entire database for implausible values. Numbers may have been recorded wrong on the original records, and they can skew your results. Finally, always make sure that each of your variables is coded in the most logical way. For example, if your database has a variable, "current smoker (Y/N)", do not code it as "1 = yes" and "2 = no". Instead, it should be coded as "0 = no" and "1 = yes", because zero represents the absence of something. Or if you asked your patients, "When you ride a bicycle, how often do you wear a helmet: always, usually, sometimes, never?", do not code the data as "1=always, 2=usually, 3=sometimes, 4=never". Instead, it should be coded as: "0=never, 1=sometimes, 2=usually, 3=always", because that order of the numbers corresponds more sensibly to the order of the words. Coding your variables in the most logical way will make it easier to perform, understand, and present your statistical analysis. This becomes particularly important for more complex analysis, such as multivariable regression. Scientifically correct data coding also depends critically on understanding the kinds of variables being coded; these issues related to data coding are discussed in chapter 14.

Third, you should perform quality control of your dataset. Take the original study records from say 10 random subjects, and compare those study records to your current dataset. If all the information matches correctly, you may proceed with some confidence that your dataset is correct. But if you find discrepancies in this random quality-control sample, then you should continue to compare the original study records to your database. This step is particularly important in retrospective studies on routine patient care, where both the original patient records and their subsequent entry into an electronic database may have been done with less diligence than they would be done in a carefully run prospective study.

Some people may feel that it is unnecessarily time-consuming to go through this triple process of database organization, database cleaning, and dataset quality-control, but there are several reasons why it should be done. First, this process ensures that your data and statistical analysis will be accurate. Second, it makes you more familiar with your raw dataset, which can lead to insights or a better understanding of your observations. It also helps you to organize and clarify the results that you will or will not be presenting in your paper. Third, "a stitch in time saves nine". If you do not go through this process, a peer-reviewer might question some "surprising" result in your paper, and you might then realize that this result was actually due to problems with your dataset. At that point you would have to redo your statistical analyses and figures and revise your paper accordingly. If you do careful good work from the outset, you will not be forced to waste more time and energy later cleaning up a mess. And last but not least, as mentioned in chapter 2, laziness is a vice that leads to scientifically and ethically dubious research; whereas, diligence is an ethical virtue that leads to better science.

Chapter 13
Statistics: General Principles

Most medical research papers rely upon at least some statistical analysis, so it is important to address this here. Yet, this is not a book of statistics, and it would not be fitting here to try to provide even a brief summary substitute for such a book. This book (about how to write medical papers) presupposes that you either already know how to do the statistical analysis for your paper or you are working together with someone else who does. In either case, there are many textbooks of statistics to guide you through that analysis with sufficiently full explanations and examples [1–3]. The journal literature also has numerous papers that either provide basic reviews of commonly used tests or discuss specific applications or advanced techniques. Search engines can point you toward any such papers you might need. On the other end, this is also not a book merely about how to properly type up your statistical results. So this book will not delve into all the tiny details of how exactly to present your statistics in your paper, as that has already been thoroughly covered elsewhere [4, 5].

This is a book about how to get your research written up and published. Getting your paper written and published requires making numerous substantial choices about which way to analyze your data and which way to present it. Most textbooks and classes about statistics do not really provide guidance on these issues. They will tell you which kinds of tests are appropriate for which kinds of data (e.g. to compare two independent groups for an ordinal variable, use a Mann-Whitney test). But they do not really provide any guidance about what is relevant or not (e.g. should you bother to calculate and report a Mann-Whitney U test at all, even if it is applicable to some selection of your data). So this chapter will briefly discuss how to conceptualize which statistical analyses will make a better paper. For any given scientific study, there are always many different legitimate ways to analyze the data and report the results. But some approaches to the analysis and presentation of statistics yield better papers than others. Moreover, there is never anywhere near enough space in a journal paper to report all the statistical analyses that could legitimately be performed. So the aim here is to improve the approach and quality of the statistical analysis that you report, so your paper will be published in a better journal with less revision.

© Springer Nature Switzerland AG 2019
M. Hanna, *How to Write Better Medical Papers*,
https://doi.org/10.1007/978-3-030-02955-5_13

The main challenge facing all medical researchers regarding statistics is envisioning the optimal way to analyze and present their data. This conundrum has two interrelated aspects: choosing which data to analyze and then choosing which statistical procedures to perform (from among those that are legitimately applicable for the data). All too often researchers run statistical analyses that are methodologically valid but nonetheless do not make much sense, in regards to the communicational goals of the paper. They also often choose the tests that they are most familiar with, not the ones that are most appropriate. And some researchers have an unfortunate tendency to present many statistical tests, simply because someone punched them out on a computer at some time in the past, even though those tests lack any clear relevance for their paper. In most medical studies, it is possible to do more statistical analysis than would ever possibly fit into the space limits of a journal paper. The selection of which statistical analyses to perform cannot be guided only by the principles of statistics and the data itself. The statistical analysis must also be guided by the line of thinking that the paper as a whole is developing, along with a sense of which analyses will advance the understanding of the readers.

The best way to prevent the analysis from becoming confusing and messy is to write out a *statistical plan* before doing any analysis on the data. A statistical plan is simply a list of all the statistical tests you are going to present in the paper, in the order you intend to present them, including which variables you will use for each test and how you intend to present the results (text, table, or figures, including which kinds exactly). This information might already be available in a general form in your study protocol, but usually more detail is needed. The statistical plan can also be seen as a technical elaboration on part of the outline you wrote for your paper. Writing out a statistical plan enables you and your co-authors to clearly see and discuss what you intend to do – and why and how – before you get caught up in the (often messy) process of actually doing the analysis. A further advantage of writing out a statistical plan before doing any data analysis is that your results will be, insofar as possible, preplanned instead of post hoc, and thus less susceptible to error and bias. Writing out a detailed statistical plan enables you to do the optimal analysis the first time (or close to it), and to spare yourself the time and effort of doing other pointless analyses that never make it into the final paper or that should not be in the paper.

So what might a statistical plan look like? For the sake of illustration, let us imagine a very simple study. Let us imagine that you have been using a new medication in an outpatient pain clinic, and it seems to be quite helpful among patients with co-morbid depression. So you want to publish a retrospective brief report on the clinical data you already have, as a basis for further work. Keeping it simple for the sake of illustration, a statistical plan for this study might be written as follows:

Sample Enrollment (text)
1. N of patients treated
2. n (%) of patients with follow-up data
3. qualitative comparison of baseline data of patients with versus without follow-up data

Sample Characteristics (text and table)
4. sex of patients: n (%) of majority group (text)
5. age of patients: median and range (text)
6. baseline pain score (0–100 VAS): min, 25th quartile, median, 75th quartile, max (table)
7. baseline depression score (0–60 CES-D): min, 25th quartile, median, 75th quartile, max (table)

Clinical Improvement (figure and text)
8. pain score: change scores from baseline to follow-up (histogram)
9. depression score: change scores from baseline to follow-up (histogram)
10. correlation coefficient of change in pain score and change in depression score (text) [Pearson's if both change scores are Normally distributed, Spearman's otherwise]

Analysis (text or table)
11. multivariable linear regression: do age, sex, and baseline depression predict change in pain score?
12. multivariable linear regression: do age, sex, and baseline pain predict change in depression score?

Do not worry too much here about the contents of such a study or whether this really would be the ideal approach to the statistical analysis. What is important to see here in this simple fictitious example is how you can write out a detailed plan (about how you intend to analyze and report the data), before you actually do that analysis. The statistical plan states clearly which variables you will analyze, using which tests or calculations, how you will present them, and in which order. The statistical plan can then be discussed with all the co-authors and/or statistical consultants, and improved accordingly, prior to spending time and effort actually doing that work. The statistical plan makes it easier for you to decide which analyses you are going to do, how, and why. It enables you to determine whether the statistical analysis you intend to perform is well matched to the precise points that the paper is supposed to address and also whether you have selected the optimal statistical procedures for each part of the analysis. The statistical plan also helps prevent you from falling into aimless data dredging.

So while you are developing your statistical plan, how do you decide which statistical procedures you should perform and report? Simple: look at the outline of the paper that you wrote and think about the questions you want to answer. You should choose statistical procedures that will enable you to discuss these questions with your readers in a sensible and comprehensible way. There should be a clear purpose behind each calculation that you perform and report. In other words, each test or calculation you report should correspond to a specific link in the chain of thinking you want to lead the readers through. Choose the tests that will advance your line of reasoning (not the tests yielding the smallest p-values or whatever else). When reviewing your statistical plan, weed out any statistical calculations that have no point for the further discussion and are not otherwise interesting for the readers.

Above all, avoid fishing around aimlessly for statistically significant findings or choosing which results to report based on the numbers themselves. Know ahead of time why you are running each analysis; if there is no strong reason for it, then just drop it. If there is a strong reason for it, then do it and report it, regardless of how it comes out. Here, a "strong reason" usually means "the readers need to know these numbers to understand our answers to the study questions".

When designing your statistical plan, it is important to keep in mind that nearly all research studies are performed only on a small sample from the entire population they represent [2 (pp. 26–31)]. If the study had been conducted in some other sample, the results would be different, perhaps even substantially so. This may seem self-evident, but researchers often lose sight of this point and start talking about their results (from their small study sample) as if they are identical with the results that would be found in everyone (in the larger population). The fact that research studies are conducted only on a small sample of the larger population has two important implications for the analysis and presentation that should be built into the statistical plan from the outset. First, it is important to thoroughly characterize the study sample, using descriptive statistics of their baseline characteristics [6, 7]. This enables readers to compare the study sample to their own patients, in order to form some sense of how applicable the study results might be to their sample of patients. Second, in addition to reporting the actual results of a study, it is important to calculate and report a confidence interval (CI) for those results whenever possible. For any result you report, that result is only for your study sample; the true result of the larger population, from which you drew your study sample, will be different. So the confidence interval is the possible range for the true result of the population from which your study sample was drawn [8–10]. More specifically, the 95% confidence interval is the range within which we are 95% confident that the true result from the larger population lies. Typically, researchers calculate the 95% CI, but other CIs such as 90% or 99% are also possible [1 (p. 163)]. The CI thus provides readers with an understanding of what the range of possible results might be in some other sample (such as their own patients) drawn from the same population [8–11]. When discussing the results, the range represented by the 95% CI is in some sense actually more important to report than the actual result itself, because the result only tells readers what was found in that particular study sample, while the CI tells them the range within which the real results in the larger population could possibly be. So a wide 95% CI leaves the research issue more indeterminate, while a narrow 95% CI provides a more definitive answer.

Although there are many different statistical tests, three broad types of statistical calculations will get you through most medical papers you might want to write: descriptive statistics, group comparisons, and regression analysis. Descriptive statistics (frequencies, percents, ranges, medians, quartiles, means, standard deviations, etc.) are the simplest form of statistical analysis [2 (pp. 41–53), 6]. They are used to report on the study sample itself (rather than to make inferences about the larger population from which the sample was drawn), primarily to characterize the sample at baseline. Their main graphic forms in medical research are histograms and box-and-whisker plots (see the chapters on figures) [2 (pp. 41–53), 6]. Strangely, descriptive statistics are somewhat underused, perhaps because researchers feel that their papers will not seem sophisticated if they rely too much on descriptive statistics [12]. But you can do a lot with simple descriptive statistics. Just tell us (or even show us): what did you find? How many patients reported whatever it is you studied? What was the distribution of values of the main variable you measured? Unless there are already many papers on the exact same topic, your simple data probably already contains novel knowledge, even without doing any more sophisticated analysis. If your sample size is small or your study is preliminary, it may be advisable to not go beyond descriptive statistics [13]. Descriptive statistics also have the major advantage that every reader quickly and clearly understands what they mean – something which is not often the case with most other types of statistical analysis. A clear presentation of descriptive statistics also provides a solid foundation for any further inferential statistics.

Group comparisons have become a standard workhorse in medicine. The tests most often used for this include paired and unpaired t-tests, Mann-Whitney U-test, Wilcoxon matched pairs test, Chi-squared test, and Fisher's exact test, depending on the type of variables, whether the groups are paired, and the distribution of the data [1 (pp. 179–181), 2 (pp. 214–216)]. In all these approaches, two groups are compared on some outcome variable (or two measurements for one group are compared). Generally, group comparisons are a simple and clear way to determine if one form of treatment is better than another. Since medical research does often involve comparing two kinds of treatments, group comparisons are often useful and easy to understand. Unfortunately, group comparisons are also widely overused. If your study was really designed to compare two groups – for example, a randomized trial comparing two kinds of treatment to decide which is more efficacious – then group comparisons are acceptable. Otherwise, there are probably better ways to analyze your data than to transform it into a football match of group A vs. group B; (e.g. comparing old patients vs. young patients). Unplanned comparisons of subgroups should also be avoided [1 (pp. 466–467), 2 (pp. 123–124), 14–19]. Furthermore, even if your study was designed well to compare two different groups, there is often a subtle mismatch between these statistical tests and the question you are really trying to answer. The real question that many clinical studies are trying to answer is not, "Was there a difference in outcome between group A and group B?" but instead, "Is treatment A more effective than treatment B?" The effectiveness of the treatment may depend on or be obscured by multiple other variables (e.g. age, sex, BMI, etc.), but simple group comparisons never account for these other factors, which are often imbalanced, even in randomized trials. Group comparisons in such situations are not invalid, but most researchers should be more reserved about their use and meaning.

Regression analysis is a powerful way to determine which variables had an influence on the outcomes [2 (pp. 159–167), 20–25]. For example, a multiple linear regression analysis can be used to determine how much influence age, sex, BMI, and smoking have on the patients' blood-pressure. The main forms of regression currently used in medical research are multivariable linear regression (for continuous outcome variables, such as blood pressure) and multivariable logistic regression (for dichotomous outcome variables, such as death). Unfortunately, regression analysis is not used nearly as often as it should be, probably because most medical researchers are not sufficiently familiar with this advanced technique. Regression analysis uses algebraic modeling to determine how much the value of the outcome variable (e.g. blood pressure) depends on the values of various predictor variables (e.g. age, sex, BMI, smoking, etc.) In the results, each predictor variable has a coefficient (for linear regressions) or an odds ratio (for logistic regression), which shows how much the outcome variable depends on that predictor variable. Each predictor variable also has a p-value, which tells how statistically significant that calculated relation is, or in other words how probable it would be to obtain that study's set of raw data (or more extreme data) if there was no such relation between that predictor variable and outcome variable in the larger population from which the study sample was drawn. Regression analyses also provide an overall "adjusted r^2" value for the entire model, which tells us how much of the total variance of the outcome variable is explained by the predictor variables in the regression model [1 (pp. 345–346)]. Since regression analysis can provide deeper insights in most clinical studies with a sufficient sample size, it should at least be considered for every report. So all medical researchers should become familiar enough with regression analysis to know how it could be used in their papers, even if they hand over the actual work to a statistician or someone else. (In fact, regression analysis should still be within the capabilities of most doctoral-level researchers to carry out themselves, though working together with a statistician is often advantageous.) Regression analysis enables researchers to disentangle the effects of a study intervention from other confounding factors, such as patient characteristics. It should be used more frequently. In particular, whenever the sample size is sufficiently large, multivariable regression is a better approach to statistical analysis than any kind of simple group comparison or correlation coefficient [1 (pp. 320–321), 2 (pp. 216, 227–228)].

Another set of statistical analyses called ANOVA (ANalysis Of VAriance) are closely related to regression analysis but with slightly different applications and output. They can be used when the main predictor variable is categorical, e.g. different study groups, and the outcome variable is continuous. However, ANOVA may only be used for experimental studies, not for observational studies, due to ANOVA's prerequisites about the data structure [1 (pp. 325–326, 336)]. So ANOVAs are used more frequently in the life sciences and behavioral sciences, but in clinical medicine, regression analysis is the right choice of method, not ANOVA.

Medical researchers should always consider working together with a statistician, especially when approaching the limits of their own capabilities [26–28]. Statistics is not a simple add-on to medical research that anyone can do after reading a few webpages or taking a quick tutorial on how to use some specific statistical software package. Statistics is its own complex field, in which people earn doctoral degrees. If your study involves more than some basic statistical analysis, it is sensible to at least consult a statistician or even hand over that part of the work to a statistician or other person with advanced training in statistics. Even if you know what you are doing, an expert in statistics can probably point out some better ways of doing the analysis or provide oversight that the approach is correct and optimal. At the same time, anyone planning to contribute to medical research for more than a few years ought to learn all the most commonly used techniques up through regression analysis, even if someone else is performing or supervising the actual analysis.

Finally, there is one last general principal that is crucial for good statistical analysis and write-up: keep your readers in mind. First, if you are doing any kind of statistical analysis that the majority of your readers will not immediately understand (i.e. anything much more than descriptive statistics and group comparisons), then you should try to explain your methods and results also in a simple non-technical way, so readers without a solid background in statistics will still be able to understand your findings. There is no point in presenting statistical analyses that are over the head of your readers, if you are not going to make it accessible to them. If your readers do not understand what you write, then you are talking only to yourself. Second, avoid doing anything so unusual that even people with a solid knowledge of statistics will not easily follow it. There is no need to be too clever for your own good. And medical research virtually never requires the use of statistical procedures that have not already become well-established and familiar through use in other neighboring fields first. So stick to the established approaches and explain them in a way that all healthcare providers should understand.

References

1. Altman DG. Practical Statistics for Medical Research. Boca Raton, FL, USA: CRC Press; 1991, 1999.
2. Bland M. An Introduction to Medical Statistics, 4th ed. Oxford: Oxford University Press; 2015.
3. Machin D, Campbell MJ, Walters SJ. Medical Statistics: A Textbook for the Health Sciences. West Sussex, England: John Wiley & Sons; 2007.
4. Lang TA, Secic Michelle. How to Report Statistics in Medicine, 2nd ed. Philadelphia: American College of Physicians; 2006.
5. Iverson C, Christianse S, Flanagin A, Fontanarosa PB, Glass RM, Gregoline B, Lurie SJ, Meyer HS, Winker MA, Young RK, eds. AMA Manual of Style: A Guide for Authors and Editors, 10th ed. Oxford: Oxford University Press; 2007.
6. Larson MG. Descriptive Statistics and Graphical Displays. Circulation. 2006; 114: 76-81.
7. Spriestersbach A, Röhrig B, du Prel J-B, Gerhold-Ay A, Blettner M. Deskriptive Statistik. Dtsch Arztebl Int. 2009; 106: 578-583.
8. Gardner MJ, Altman DG. Confidence intervals rather than P values: estimation rather than hypothesis testing. BMJ. 1986; 292: 746-750.
9. Braitman LE. Confidence Intervals Assess Both Clinical Significance and Statistical Significance. Ann Intern Med. 1991; 114: 515-517.
10. Guyatt G, Jaeschke R, Heddle N, Cook D, Shannon H, Walter S. Basic statistics for clinicians: 2. Interpreting study results: confidence intervals. CMAJ. 1995; 152: 169-173.
11. Cohen J. The Earth Is Round ($p < .05$). Am Psychol. 1994; 49: 997-1003.
12. Marincola FM. In support of descriptive studies; relevance to translational research. J Transl Med. 2007; 5: 1.
13. Young J. When should you use statistics? Swiss Med Wkly. 2005; 135: 337-338.
14. Guyatt GH, Oxman AD, Kunz R, Woodcock J, Brozek J, Helfand M, Alonso-Coello P, Glasziou P, Jaeschke R, Akl EA, Norris S, Vist G, Dahm P, Shukla VK, Higgins J, Falck-Ytter

Y, Schünemann HJ; GRADE Working Group. GRADE guidelines: 7. Rating the quality of evidence—inconsistency. J Clin Epidemiol. 2011; 64: 1294-1302.

15. Wang R, Lagakos SW, Ware JH, Huner DJ, Drazen JM. Statistics in Medicine—Reporting of Subgroup Analyses in Clinical Trials. NEJM. 2007; 357: 2189-2194.

16. Burke JF, Sussman JB, Kent DM, Hayward RA. Three simple rules to ensure reasonably credible subgroup analyses. BMJ. 2015; 351: h5651.

17. Moher D, Hopewell S, Schulz KF, Montori V, Gøtzsche PC, Devereaux PJ, Elbourne D, Egger M, Altman DG. CONSORT 2010 Explanation and Elaboration: updated guidelines for reporting parallel group randomised trials. BMJ. 2010; 340: c869.

18. Assmann SF, Pocock SJ, Enos LE, Kasten LE. Subgroup analysis and other (mis)uses of baseline data in clinical trials. Lancet. 2000; 355: 1064-1069.

19. Sterne JAC, Smith GD. Sifting the evidence–what's wrong with significance tests? BMJ. 2001; 322: 226-231.

20. Guyatt G, Walter S, Shannon H, Cook D, Jaeschke R, Heddle N. Basic statistics for clinicians: 4. Correlation and regression. CMAJ. 1995; 152: 497-504.

21. Lunt M. Introduction to statistical modelling: linear regression. Rheumatology. 2015; 54: 1137-1140.

22. Slinker BK, Glantz SA. Multiple Linear Regression: Accounting for Multiple Simultaneous Determinants of a Continuous Dependent Variable. Circulation. 2008; 117: 1732-1737.

23. LaValley MP. Logistic Regression. Circulation. 2008; 117: 2395-2399.

24. Bagley SC, White, H, Golomb BA. Logistic regression in the medical literature: Standards for use and reporting, with particular attention on one medical domain. J Clin Epidemiol. 2001; 54: 979-985.

25. McNamee R. Regression Modelling and Other Methods to Control Confounding. Occup Environ Med. 2005; 62: 500-506.

26. Elefteriades JA. Twelve Tips on Writing a Good Scientific Paper. Inter J Angiol. 2002; 11: 53-55.

27. Sprent P. Statistics in medical research. Swiss Med Wkly. 2003; 133: 522-529.

28. Tallis RC. Researchers forced to do boring research... BMJ. 1994; 308: 591.

Chapter 14
Statistics: Common Mistakes

Because most medical researchers do not have extensive training in statistics and fail to work together with someone who does, the published literature contains many mistakes in the analysis or presentation of data. These mistakes then become perpetuated, because new researchers see them and imitate them. Fortunately, these errors are often caught in the peer-review process, and manuscripts are sent back for revision. This chapter reviews some of the most commonplace errors, so you can avoid making them and improve the quality of your paper. Reading a textbook of statistics [1–3] will help you avoid making many other less common errors that are not covered here. Working together with a statistician (or someone with advanced training in statistics) and having him or her review the final manuscript is another good way to avoid making errors. (Nonetheless, it must be kept in mind that many statisticians have little sense about how to present statistical information for non-statisticians and/or in a medical scientific context, so care must be taken to not rely blindly on their approaches to reporting.)

First, the biggest and most common error medical researchers make when doing statistical analysis is that they rely on a computer to perform statistical analyses that they themselves do not adequately understand. A computer can crunch numbers a zillion times faster than you can, but it does not know what it is doing and it cannot correct any mistakes or outright foolishness of the user. So never rely on a computer to automatically spit out statistical analyses that you yourself do not really understand [1 (pp. 108–110), 2 (p. 2), 4]. Learn what you are doing before even turning on that machine – it is the most dangerous piece of equipment in your clinic or lab. Statistical software can spare you from learning mathematical formula and performing complex calculations. That is an enormous advantage, as anyone knows who has tried to calculate statistics with paper and pen, or even a calculator too. Many of the better statistical software programs will even provide you with some useful explanations and will block any attempts to perform entirely inappropriate analyses. But computer programs will not tell you which data to analyze, how, or why. They will not tell you what all the output really means, nor what you should report or not. So please, do not try to fly an airplane, without first going to flight school. Once you

© Springer Nature Switzerland AG 2019
M. Hanna, *How to Write Better Medical Papers*,
https://doi.org/10.1007/978-3-030-02955-5_14

have a solid understanding of which kinds of statistical analysis are appropriate and useful for which kinds of data and what all the output really means, then you can make use of the statistics software, to save yourself the Herculean labor of performing the mathematical calculations yourself. Indeed, although it can be helpful, you do not really need to learn all the mathematical formulas involved in statistics, as most old-school textbooks and courses still assume. The computer will do the math anyway [5]. But you do need to learn – conceptually – what is appropriate or not for which kinds of data, and what it really means. If you want to learn the math too, all the better; (doing the math yourself can be good exercise for your mind). Until you have thoroughly studied statistics, work together with someone else who has.

Second, recognize which kind of variables you have (continuous, ordinal, nominal, etc.) and analyze them accordingly. A continuous variable is one where all intermediate values are possible, such as weight. A categorical variable is one where intermediate values are not possible; they are further subclassified as follows. A dichotomous variable is one where there are only two possibilities, such as sex (M, F). A nominal variable is one where there are three or more possibilities, which have no inherent ordering, such as nationality (French, Belgian, Swiss, Italian, etc.) An ordinal variable is a categorical variable that has an inherent order, but intermediate values are not possible and the intervals between categories are not equivalent, such as rating the severity of a symptom as "0 – absent", "1 – mild", "2 – moderate" or "3 – severe". Researchers often make the error of converting a continuous variable (such as age, BMI, or visual analogue scale scores) into a categorical variable or the error of collapsing several categories of an ordinal variable together, usually so they can make a simple comparison of groups of subjects. That crude approach to statistical analysis has no justification and leads to a loss of information and statistical power [1 (pp. 12–13, 271–272), 6, 7]. So never convert continuous variables into dichotomous or ordinal variables; instead, analyze the continuous variable in its original form. For example, if you are thinking of creating two groups of patients (e.g. "normal" and "obese") to try to compare them, use regression analysis instead to examine the influence of the continuous variable (BMI) on the outcome. Similarly, do not collapse categories together for an ordinal variable (e.g. comparing "absent and mild" vs. "moderate and severe") [1 (p. 11)].

Third, the reverse error sometimes occurs quite unknowingly. Researchers often record some kind of ordinal variable and then code it numerically. For example, they might assess symptom severity as "absent, mild, moderate, severe" and then code this as 0–3, or they might ask a patient to rate symptom frequency as "never, rarely, sometimes, often, always" and code this as 0–4. That is entirely fine, but an error emerges if these numerical codings or groupings are then analyzed in the same way that a continuous variable such as BMI is analyzed. The problem is that the distance between ordinal categories cannot be assumed to be homogeneous. In other words, "moderate" (2) is not necessarily twice as bad as "mild" (1), and "always" (4) is not twice as often as "sometimes" (2). So ordinal variables cannot be analyzed in the same way as continuous variables are. For example, it does not make sense to calculate the means of an ordinal variable, because (using the examples above) it cannot be assumed that the difference between "moderate" symptoms (2) and "mild" symptoms (1) is the same magnitude as the difference between "mild" symptoms (1) and "no" symptoms (0). Instead, one can only report how many patients' symptoms were "mild", "moderate", etc.

Fourth, do not report means and standard deviations (SD) if your data is not "Normally distributed" (i.e. has a histogram with a "bell-shaped" curve). If your SD is greater than half the mean, then your data is definitely not Normally distributed. In that case, reporting the mean and SD will be very misleading for most readers and therefore is inappropriate, despite how frequently this basic misstep can be found in the literature. Instead, you should present the median and some kind of range, usually the interquartile range (the interquartile range is the 25th and 75th percentile datapoint, just as the median is the 50th percentile datapoint). Unlike the mean, it is never erroneous or misleading to present the median and interquartile range. Yet if the data is indeed Normally distributed, the mean and SD is more useful. But never report both the median and the mean for the same variable; that is pointless and tedious.

Fifth, many commonplace statistical calculations rest on the assumption that the data do represent a Normal distribution (aka "Gaussian distribution") [2 (pp. 86–93), 8, 9], so you should always determine whether or not your data are Normally distributed, if you might be using any such statistical calculations. There are many ways to test Normality, some better than others. Looking at a histogram of the data provides an initial sense but is not always reliable [1 (pp. 59–60), 2 (pp. 93–94), 8]. Currently, the best approach to determining whether data are Normally distributed seems to be a combination of: 1) a Normality plot (either a so-called "q-q plot" or a "p-p plot") and 2) the Shapiro-Wilk or Anderson-Darling tests of Normality [1 (pp. 132–142), 2 (pp. 93–96), 10]. Advanced researchers might also consider L-moments [10, 11]. If your data is Normally distributed, then you may use parametric statistical tests (e.g. t-tests or ANOVA). If your database is large enough (n>100), mild violations of the assumption of Normality sometimes may not matter much [1 (p. 223), 2 (pp. 141–142, 189–190), 12], but it is better to check with a statistician in such cases before using any methods with unconfirmed assumptions. If the data is not Normally distributed, textbooks of statistical analysis recommend transforming the data by taking the logarithm or other methods, in order to try to make it Normally distributed [1 (pp. 143–146), 2 (pp. 93, 138–141), 7, 8, 12, 13]. But in practice it seems rare to find that anyone actually did that, (probably because numbers on logarithmic scales are not intuitively comprehensible for most people). Using non-parametric tests (e.g. the Mann-Whitney U test or the Kruskal-Wallis test) is the much easier standard solution [2 (pp. 189–190), 9], albeit usually at the cost of a slight loss of statistical power [2 (p. 189), 12]. The problem of a non-Normal distribution of data seems to arise more often for small samples (where, moreover, it is more of a problem), so oftentimes the best solution would probably be to just go collect more data – especially if your study is underpowered. Space permitting, you should briefly state in the Methods how the assumption of a Normal distribution of data was confirmed (or simply that it was not), but the actual results of such checks should not be reported in journal papers, because those details are not relevant for most readers to review themselves.

Sixth, ensure that your study sample is large enough for each statistical test that you want to use. Many statistical tests may become unreliable or inapplicable if the sample size is too small. So if N<100, you should check whether the statistical tests you are using are still applicable [2 (pp. 142, 214, 215)]. If your sample size is too small for some test, statistical textbooks can always recommend an alternative test that is suitable for small samples. Using bootstrapping to calculate a 95% CI is also often a superior alternative approach. However, if your sample size is really small (say N<50), then the best solution these days is probably to just go back and collect more data, or to limit yourself to a brief report or case series type paper using only descriptive statistics. If a power analysis shows that your study is underpowered – i.e. is *too* small – then you should definitely go back and collect more data; (see the tenth point below for further explanations about power analyses). In today's era of *big data* and over a million new medical scientific papers being published each year, there is rarely any solid scientific justification for publishing clinical studies based on small samples. Experimental studies (especially with animals) or human studies on very rare conditions are probably the only situations where statistical tests designed for small samples are still defensible.

Seventh, many strange habits have become commonplace in the literature, because no one remembers anymore what p-values actually mean, above all the frequent habit of splitting results as "significant" or "not significant" around one arbitrary threshold of p=0.05 [14, 15]. Whenever a p-value is calculated, it always refers to a specific hypothesis (e.g. there is a difference between two groups), even if the researchers have never explicitly stated that hypothesis. The p-value is basically the probability that the results of that specific study sample could be obtained by random chance alone, if that hypothesis was not true in the larger population from which the study sample was drawn [1 (pp. 165–168, 170), 7, 16–18]. For example, a p-value of 0.35 means that there is a 35% probability (35 in 100) that the results are due to sampling chance if the hypothesis tested is not true; a p-value of 0.06 means that there is a 6% probability (6 in 100) that the results are due to chance alone; and a p-value of 0.003 means that there is a 0.3% probability (3 in 1000) that the results are due to chance alone if the hypothesis tested is not true. There is absolutely nothing magical about a p-value of 0.05. Traditionally, this was an arbitrary threshold for deciding whether or not the results were due to chance [18]. But as can be seen, there is hardly any difference in meaning between p=0.06 and p=0.04 [1 (p. 168), 2 (p. 117)]. In either case, the results are probably not due to sampling chance (but still might be); instead, the more likely explanation is that the hypothesis tested on the study sample is also true in the population from which the study sample was drawn. So instead of splitting your results into the black and white categories of "significant" or "non-significant", report the exact p-value and reflect more carefully about what it actually means – as a gray scale of probability [2 (p. 117), 14, 15].

Indeed, if p-values must be categorized at all, the threshold of p<0.05 is outdated and should be replaced. In the computer era, too much statistical testing is done to continue relying on p<0.05. At that threshold, 1 in 20 "statistically significant" findings are actually type I errors, i.e. false positives [1 (p. 170), 4, 14]. Furthermore, a single threshold is too dichotomous for such interpretations. A better approach for most clinical studies would be to consider that p≥0.1 is not statistically significant, 0.01<p<0.1 is inconclusive but strongly suggests that further research is warranted, and p≤0.01 is statistically significant [2 (p. 117), 14]. Why? Because at p≤0.01, a type I error (a false positive) is quite unlikely; at p≥0.1, a type II error (a false negative) is sufficiently unlikely; but with 0.1<p<0.01, neither possible error can be easily dismissed. In any case, you should decide your interpretive policy for p-values prior to doing the statistical analysis and state it clearly in the Methods section of your paper. And keep in mind that even very small p-values ("highly statistically significant" results) do not actually prove or disprove anything. The p-value is only the probability that the results from your sample were obtained by random chance and do not represent what would be found in the population from which your sample was drawn. Scientific "proof" is based on entirely different criteria, such as independent replication.

Eighth, many researchers report only p-values when presenting their results. That is insufficient. You should also report the actual results that you are analyzing and the 95% confidence interval [15, 19–23]. Your results are based on data from a sample of patients, not the entire population of people with that condition. The 95% CI is a statistical calculation that represents the range of values within which we have 95% confidence that the true results for the larger population lie, based on the data from your study sample. Thus a narrow 95% CI means that the true results must be quite close to the results that are reported; whereas, a wide 95% CI means that the true results may lie rather far from the reported results. Because the 95% CI is expressed as a range of the outcome variable, it simultaneously provides the necessary information about the statistical significance and the clinical relevance. It is therefore preferable to the p-value, which provides information only about statistical significance [15, 19–21]. The 95% CI is related to a p-value of 0.05 and is just as arbitrary. It is equally possible and sensible to calculate other CIs, such as a 90% CI or a 99% CI, though this remains quite uncommon so far [1 (p. 163)]. Whenever you want to report results with a p-value, try to calculate a 95% CI of your result and report that too. If your 95% CI is very narrow, you could calculate and report a 99% CI, though if it loses narrowness, it is not preferable. A 95% CI can also be calculated for results that do not have a p-value and sometimes it is sensible to calculate and report such 95% CIs. CIs can be calculated at any such width desired, for any statistical result you calculate, by using bootstrapping with 1000 or more iterations of the sample. This recent approach of using bootstrapping to generate CIs is currently still extremely rare to see but will surely become well-established and commonplace in the coming years. Making a graph (of the raw data and/or summary statistics of the results and confidence intervals) is another better approach to the statistical analysis than calculating p-values for hypothesis tests [24].

Ninth, many researchers make the blunder of emphasizing differences in out-comes while simultaneous conceding that these differences were not statistically significant. They are making double-talk that misleads the readers. They often use the phrase a "trend toward significance", but this shows a lack of comprehension of what statistical significance is all about. The lack of significance tells us that the difference observed in the study sample is probably due only to random chance of the sampling and thus does not represent a real difference in the larger popula-tion from which the study sample was drawn. There is no such thing as a "trend toward significance"; the p-value is exactly what the p-value is, no more, no less. A p-value of 0.08 means there is an 8% probability that the results are due to ran-dom chance. It does not mean that the results were moving toward a p-value less than 5% [25]. The expression "a trend toward significance" is simply nonsense written by biased researchers who refuse to admit that their own results do not meet their own standards for generalizability. It can be viewed as a commonplace form of "spin" [26, 27]. It is better to just report the results, the 95% CI, and the p-value, and avoid making any dichotomous judgments about the results being "statistically significant" or not. But if researchers are going to adopt thresholds for "statistical significance" (whether p<0.05 or p<0.01 or whatever other value), then they need to rigorously enforce those thresholds, not ignore them when a key result falls short. Yet keep in mind that the lack of statistical significance may be merely because the study was underpowered – i.e. too small to detect statistically significant findings. This is one reason why it is so important to always calculate and report a 95% confidence interval [15]. Oftentimes, when the p-value is between 0.05 and 0.1, most of the 95% CI will included values similar to the cal-culated results, thus reinforcing the interpretation that the effect observed proba-bly is real (but weak). In other cases, the 95% CI will be quite broad, including many values that do not have the same meaning or relevance as the result obtained, thus indicating that the results are imprecise, presumably because the study is indeed too small. So a 95% CI eliminates any perceived need to talk unscientifi-cally about "a trend toward significance" by showing instead the range of results that we are 95% confident would be found in the larger population from which the study sample was drawn.

Tenth, many studies are underpowered and lack awareness of this problem [28]. The consequence is that they make type II errors: they fail to find results that would be statistically significant and instead report false negatives. Researchers should always try to estimate how much data will be needed to address their main study aim before they actually start collecting data [7, 16, 29]. This is referred to as a "sample size estimate" or "power analysis". Very regrettably, only a minority of published studies ever actually do this, and among those that do, most fail to report this crucial information. If the main outcomes of the study are statistically signifi-cant, it probably does not matter so much. But if the main outcomes are not statisti-cally significant and the paper does not report this information about the study's power, then readers cannot be sure whether the main outcomes were not statistically significant because the results are indeed negative or only because the study was too small to find a reliable answer. This kind of power analysis or sample size estimate should always be performed prior to starting the research (even for retrospective analyses), so you know how large a sample you need and do not waste your time and resources conducting a study that is too hopelessly small to provide reliable results. (Generally speaking, power analyses are not highly complex to do, but they are so critical to study planning that they should be performed by a statistician or someone else with training and familiarity in doing them.) If your team performed a power analysis prior to collecting data (or for retrospective studies, prior to analyzing the data), then you should at least state that; if space permits, you should briefly summarize the most basic information for that calculation, as described further in the chapter on The Methods. If your main outcomes were not statistically significant, your 95% CI will provide the readers with some information about whether you might have missed a positive outcome [30]. Nonetheless, you should also perform a post hoc analysis of how much power your study actually had – using the results you actually obtained – and report that in the Results; that information enables readers to judge how much your results reflect the reality that would be found in the larger population from which your sample was drawn versus reflecting random chance of your study sampling [4, 16, 31].

Eleventh, "statistically significant" is not the same as "clinically meaningful" [2 (p. 119), 19, 20, 32]. As just discussed, "statistically significant" only means that the observed results are very probably not due to random chance. But the actual difference of the measurement between groups (or between timepoints or whatever is being analyzed) may not be very large. For example, if we conduct a clinical trial on a new weight-loss pill in a very large sample, we might find after ten weeks that the weight-loss pill group has lost a mean of 2 kg while the placebo group has lost a mean of 1 kg and that this difference is statistically significant (p=0.003). But the difference between losing 1 kg or 2 kg is not really relevant (and certainly would not justify any side-effects, risks, or costs). So it is not sufficient that your results are statistically significant. They must also be "clinically meaningful", i.e. the absolute difference between the two groups (or timepoints) for the outcome variable must be large enough to make a relevant difference for the patients' health. You must always make sure that your results are not only statistically significant but also clinically meaningful. As discussed above, it is better to avoid ever using the word "significant"; (just report the exact 95%CI and p-value instead, without making any dichotomizing judgments about them). But if you must use that word, always write "statistically significant", not merely "significant" [7, 22]. And then follow-up immediately with more information about whether that statistically significant finding was clinically meaningful or not. Many studies are available on the minimum clinically important differences for various measures. When such information is lacking, using sound clinical reasoning to comment is better than no such commentary at all. Finally, to avoid confusion, do not use the word "significant" if you do not mean "statistically significant"; use some other word, such as "substantial", "important", "meaningful", etc. depending on what you are trying to say.

There are of course many other mistakes that people make in their statistical analysis and presentation. But the errors listed above occur quite frequently, because these statistical procedures are performed often and because many researchers do not know better. If you can avoid all these common errors, your paper will get a much better start in the peer-review process. The best way to avoid these and other errors of statistical analysis is to study statistics (take a class, read a book, etc.) or to work together with someone who has.

References

1. Altman DG. Practical Statistics for Medical Research. Boca Raton, FL, USA: CRC Press; 1991, 1999.
2. Bland M. An Introduction to Medical Statistics, 4th ed. Oxford: Oxford University Press; 2015.
3. Machin D, Campbell MJ, Walters SJ. Medical Statistics: A Textbook for the Health Sciences. West Sussex, England: John Wiley & Sons; 2007.
4. Running the numbers. Nat Neurosci. 2005; 8: 123.
5. Efron B, Tibshirani R. Statistical Data Analysis in the Computer Age. Science. 1991; 253: 390-395.
6. Altman DG, Royston P. The cost of dichotomizing continuous variables. BMJ. 2006; 332: 1080.
7. Wright DB. Making friends with your data: Improving how statistics are conducted and reported. Brit J Educ Psychol. 2003; 73: 123-136.
8. Altman DG, Bland JM. The normal distribution. BMJ. 1995; 310: 298.
9. Maltenfort MG. Understanding a Normal Distribution of Data. J Spinal Disord Tech. 2015; 28: 377-378.
10. Henderson AR. Testing experimental data for univariate normality. Clin Chim Acta. 2006; 366: 112-129.
11. Hosking JRM. L-moments: Analysis and Estimation of Distributions using Linear Combinations of Order Statistics. J R Statist Soc B. 1990; 52: 105-124.
12. Lachenbruch PA. Proper metrics for clinical trials: transformations and other procedures to remove non-normality effects. Stat Med. 2003; 22: 3823-3842.
13. Maltenfort MG. Understanding a Normal Distribution of Data (Part 2). Clin Spine Surg. 2016; 29: 30.
14. Sterne JAC, Smith GD. Sifting the evidence–what's wrong with significance tests? BMJ. 2001; 322: 226-231.
15. Cohen J. The Earth Is Round ($p < .05$). Am Psychol. 1994; 49: 997-1003.
16. Detsky AS, Sackett DL. When Was a 'Negative Clinical Trial Big Enough? How Many Patients You Needed Depends on What You Found. Arch Intern Med. 1985; 145: 709-712.
17. Sprent P. Statistics in medical research. Swiss Med Wkly. 2003; 133: 522-529.
18. Guyatt G, Jaeschke R, Heddle N, Cook D, Shannon H, Walter S. Basic statistics for clinicians: 1. Hypothesis testing. CMAJ. 1995; 152: 27-32.
19. Gardner MJ, Altman DG. Confidence intervals rather than P values: estimation rather than hypothesis testing. BMJ. 1986; 292: 746-750.
20. Braitman LE. Confidence Intervals Assess Both Clinical Significance and Statistical Significance. Ann Intern Med. 1991; 114: 515-517.
21. Bahrami H. The Value of p-Value. Am J Gastroenterol. 2005; 100: 1427-1428.
22. Cummings P, Rivara FP. Reporting Statistical Information in Medical Journal Articles. Arch Pediatr Adolec Med. 2003; 157: 321-324.
23. Cals JWL, Kotz D. Effective writing and publishing scientific papers, part II: title and abstract. J Clin Epidemiol. 2013; 66: 585.
24. Loftus GR. A picture is worth a thousand p values: On the irrelevance of hypothesis testing in the microcomputer age. Behav Res Methods. 1993; 25: 250-256.

25. Lang TA, Secic M. How to Report Statistics in Medicine, 2nd ed. Philadelphia: American College of Physicians; 2006.
26. Chiu K, Grundy Q, Bero L. 'Spin' in published biomedical literature: A methodological systematic review. PLoS Biol. 2017; 15: e2002173.
27. Gross RA. Style, spin, and science. Neurology. 2015; 85: 10-11.
28. Altman DG, Bland JM. Absence of evidence is not evidence of absence. BMJ. 1995; 311: 485.
29. Whitley E, Ball J. Statistic review 4: Sample size calculations. Crit Care. 2002; 6: 335-341.
30. Guyatt G, Jaeschke R, Heddle N, Cook D, Shannon H, Walter S. Basic statistics for clinicians: 2. Interpreting study results: confidence intervals. CMAJ. 1995; 152: 169-173.
31. Bailar JC III. Science, Statistics, and Deception. Ann Intern Med. 1986; 104: 259-260.
32. Glatstein E. Restrictions of a Statistical Mind: Clinical Relevance versus P Values or When Less is More. Int J Radiation Oncology Biol Phys. 2007; 68: 322-323.

Chapter 15
Presentation: Figures versus Tables versus Text

There are three ways you can present your numerical results: in a figure, in a table, or in the text. Choose one place. *Never* present the same results in more than one way [1–3]. So how do you know which is the optimal form of presentation? There are two ways to think about this: a formal perspective and a functional perspective.

The formal perspective simply considers how your results will appear, and what the effects on the readers will be, in each of the three *forms*: figure vs. table vs. text. Figures and tables present your results in very different ways. A figure presents some overall pattern of your results, visually, within a spatial field. Thus the strength of a figure is that it enables your audience to quickly *see* some big picture of what your findings say. And that visual presentation usually captures readers' attention and makes a stronger impression on them than other forms of presentation would. The weakness of figures is that they almost never allow an exact numerical determination of the results or data (unless the results are superimposed in typed numbers), and even an approximate determination of the numbers by looking over at the axes can be a bit difficult and/or imprecise. A further limitation of figures is that some kinds of results do not lend themselves well, or at all, to graphing as figures, especially if you are trying to present unrelated kinds of results together at once. A table by contrast enables people to read many numbers, organized according to any two defined features of the results (in the rows and columns), without the interference of grammatical sentences. A table is capable of presenting results to any level of numerical precision, even far beyond what a figure could possibly achieve. Furthermore, while many results cannot be graphed easily or at all, tables should be capable of presenting any results you can possibly generate. The weakness of a table is that it is less engaging and interesting for readers, especially if it presents substantially more information than they really want to know. So use a figure if you want your readers to quickly *see* the big picture of what your results say or a pattern in your data. Use a table if you believe that your readers will want to scrutinize the exact numbers of your results or you believe it is important for them to know the exact numbers.

© Springer Nature Switzerland AG 2019
M. Hanna, *How to Write Better Medical Papers*,
https://doi.org/10.1007/978-3-030-02955-5_15

One other major capability of figures must be emphasized. Although figures are often used to simply present summary statistics (e.g. means, SD, range, etc.), they are also capable of presenting the raw data (e.g. in a scatter plot). Figures that plot raw data can have a powerful effect on the viewers. The human visual system has remarkable capabilities for processing complex visual information and patterns. So when used thoughtfully, figures that plot raw data can be highly engaging and highly informative [4 (pp. 13–14, 161–169), 5 (pp. 36–79), 6 (pp. 40, 221–222)]. In contrast, tables and text are generally incapable of presenting raw data, unless the sample size was very small. Thus if you believe that there are meaningful patterns in your raw data, you should try to plot that raw data, rather than generating summary statistics for a table or text.

If you present your results in a figure or table, it is acceptable to concisely summarize the main point in the one sentence of the text that refers to that figure or table, for example: "The treatment group recovered more quickly than the control group, but they had equivalent outcomes by the end of one year (figure X)" [where figure X shows the two groups' outcomes at several follow-up timepoints]. (Indeed, some such summary sentence will be necessary if you want to present that result in your paper's Abstract.) But you should not then repeat the results of the figure or table in further text. Even the one summary sentence referring to the table or figure should also not contain numbers that repeat the results in the table or figure.

From a formal viewpoint, text usually serves to present a small amount of numbers. Figures or tables that present very few numbers usually seem to be made by and for dimwits [4 (pp. 53, 79–81, 87, 136), 5 (pp. 33–35)]. So if you can replace all the results, data, and/or information of a table or figure with three sentences or less, you probably should. There is no need to make a pie chart to show us that 50% of the study sample were women (and wow, the other 50% were men!) Similarly, there is no need to make a pair of "dynamite plungers" (vertical bar charts with whiskers), if all you really want to report is the mean and SD for two groups with a p-value; that can be accomplished just fine in text, (e.g.: "The mean (SD) baseline heart-rate was statistically significantly higher in the hypochondriacs than in the controls (97 (4) vs. 82 (3) bpm, p=0.02"). So if there are not many numbers to actually present, it is usually best to present them in text [7]. How many is "not many" depends on the kind of information, but surely a half a dozen or fewer should always be presented in text. If a table or figure presents few numbers but relies critically upon organizing the information spatially in two directions, then there is somewhat greater justification for using a table or figure despite the low quantity of numbers represented.

On the other end of the spectrum, text is usually not capable of presenting a large amount of numbers without losing the readers' attention. A single sentence that contains more than about half a dozen numbers (or is poorly organized) will start to lose the readers' attention, depending some on what those numbers are and how the sentence presents them. Several consecutive sentences with numbers on the same related point will also start to become tedious for many readers, even if each individual sentence seems fine by itself. (Several consecutive sentences with numbers on different unrelated points is fine.) In these scenarios of text with a large amount of numbers, see what they would look like in a table (or a figure), and consider if they would be easier for the readers to digest in that form. You might then still decide to present those numbers in the text, but too often papers present a mess of numbers in the text simply because the authors were too lazy to make a table or never even considered it. The consequence is that the readers cannot easily digest that information from the text and start skipping over it. A table allows the readers to pause from the reading, to appraise the numbers in a visually easy and meaningful format for as long or briefly as they want, and then to return to reading.

If you are still unsure whether it would be better to present some set of your results in a figure or table or text, try making them all (or the two forms you are considering), show them to your co-authors, and ask them which they think is better. But *never* present the same set of results in your paper in more than one of these three forms – that is redundant, wastes the readers' time, and can lead to discrepancies too. Be decisive and make a choice for just one form.

This chapter opened by saying that there are two ways to think about the choice of presenting results in a figure, table, or text: a formal perspective and a functional perspective. The functional perspective considers the *function* that each set of results serves within your overall paper and takes into consideration all the other results you are also presenting. Most readers will give their highest attention to your figures, because people find pictures interesting to look at. Most readers will give medium attention to tables, because they can pause from reading and look at the table separately for as long as they want. (Of course, if a table looks long, disorganized, or boring, readers might simply skip over it altogether, but that is a separate issue.) And most readers will give their lowest attention to results in the text, because they will usually read them once without stopping and then keep rolling right along to reading the next sentence. That is just how people read. They move along to the next sentence, and they rarely stop or go back, unless something is really puzzling, confusing, or alarming. (And if the amount of numbers in the text seems heavy or cluttered, they might even skim or skip over them to get to the next sentence. But again that is a separate issue.) So given these differences in how much attention readers usually give to figures vs. tables vs. text, it is generally preferable to put your main results in figures, if that is possible. Numbers that are of the lowest importance should usually just be stated in the text, if possible, rather than being given the prominence of a table or figure. Such information usually includes statistical analyses that are not really results of your study but rather are formal assessments of the quality of your research, such as the rate of loss-to-follow-up or an assessment of how often two radiologists rated the x-rays identically in a clinical study. Between these two ends of the spectrum (main results in figures and least important information in text), there is open space to decide which results need more or less prominence in your paper, or what you want to emphasize more or less.

It is also important to think ahead about the expectations of your target journal(s). Most journals put a limit on the number of tables and figures, but the limits are quite variable between the journals, as is the actual enforcement of those limits. It is better to look up that information from the outset and plan your presentation accordingly. Although some journals will allow you to publish additional figures and tables as internet-only supplemental files, many people reading your article will not have immediate access to such supplemental files, and even those who do will often not bother retrieving them. So you should only make use of such internet-only supplemental tables and figures if you want to present additional information only for people with a strong interest in your topic (e.g. other researchers of the same topic) and you do not expect most other readers to ever look at them. Generally speaking, if you have more tables and figures than your target journal allows, you probably are trying to present too much information without sufficient selection. The journal limits on tables and figures are usually sufficient or even generous, so even if the journal does not enforce them, you should try to discipline yourself to adhere to them. On the other hand, you should use either figures or tables to present the bulk of your results. If you have a large amount of numbers in the text of your Results section and you have not reached the limits of your target journal(s) for figures and tables, then you probably need to spend more time trying to put those results into tables or figures instead.

This chapter has presented a formal and a functional perspective on how to chose between figures, tables, or text. You should keep both perspectives in mind, and try to find a balance between them. Moreover, these are in no sense "rules" to follow. You should use your own judgment. This chapter simply presents some guidance and a framework for thinking about how your readers will view your results in these various modes of presentation.

References

1. Wright DB. Making friends with your data: Improving how statistics are conducted and reported. Brit J Educ Psychol. 2003; 73: 123-136.
2. Durbin CG Jr. Effective Use of Tables and Figures in Abstracts, Presentations, and Papers. Respir Care. 2004; 49: 1233-1237.
3. Howie JW. How I read. BMJ. 1976; 2 (6044): 1113-1114.
4. Tufte ER. The Visual Display of Quantitative Information, 2nd ed. Cheshire, CT, USA: Graphics Press; 1983, 2001.
5. Tufte ER. Envisioning Information. Cheshire, CT, USA: Graphics Press; 1990.
6. Altman DG. Practical Statistics for Medical Research. Boca Raton, FL, USA: CRC Press; 1991, 1999.
7. Gillan DJ, Wickens CD, Hollands JG, Carswell CM. Guidelines for Presenting Quantitative Data in HFES Publications. Hum Factors. 1998; 40: 28-41.

Chapter 16
Tables

The purpose of a table is to advance the readers' understanding of the topic. To serve its purpose, a table must present a coherent set of results (or raw data) accurately, in a form that will engage the readers and increase their comprehension of the topic. Some tables do not advance the readers' understanding, despite the readers' efforts to look at the table, because the table contains unimportant information, lacks thematic coherence, is poorly organized, is typographically confusing, or various other reasons. Tables that do not advance the readers' understanding, despite the readers' efforts to review the table, do not serve the purpose that a table is meant to serve. They should be revised or fixed until they are able to fulfill their purpose. A table that most readers refuse to even look at – because it contains too much information, lacks relevance, is confusingly arranged, or any other reason – serves no purpose at all. If most readers are not going to even look at a particular table, then that table should be either replaced with a table that most readers will look at or just deleted altogether. (If some subgroup of readers would make good use of that table, it could be dumped to a supplemental internet-only file.) Some tables mislead the readers into a false or confused misunderstanding – because they contain miscalculated numbers, numbers that are inconsistent with the same results in the Abstract or Discussion, numbers that are based on inappropriate statistical tests, or other erroneous information. These kinds of confusing or misleading tables negate the goal of scientific research, which is to improve our understanding of the world. Every table should be double-checked to verify that its contents are accurate and consistent with the rest of the paper, so the readers will not become confused or misinformed. Tables that would mislead the readers into a false or confused misunderstanding should be corrected, replaced, or deleted. Tables accomplish their purpose by presenting accurate results (or raw data) in a form that enables the readers to review those results (or data) efficiently yet precisely. Tables accomplish their purpose even better by engaging the readers to discover more information in the table than is actually printed on the page, by making comparisons of the basic information within the table.

The first step in creating a table is deciding which contents it will present and why. Every table should have thematic coherence, and it should serve a specific role

© Springer Nature Switzerland AG 2019
M. Hanna, *How to Write Better Medical Papers*,
https://doi.org/10.1007/978-3-030-02955-5_16

within the overall paper. A table might present a variety of different variables and calculations, but there should be some reason why they all belong together in the same table and why the paper needs that table. The contents of a table should contribute toward answering the study's questions [1]. A table in a journal paper is not an appropriate place to dump a bunch of numbers simply because you have them available or have not figured out what to do with them otherwise.

A table in a journal paper should be neither too small, nor too large. If a table contains less than say a dozen cells of contents, it would probably be better to just present that information as text rather than as a table. At the other extreme, if a table takes up more than one page, consider whether all the information in the table is really necessary, and try to be more selective. Even a table that takes up more than one-third or half of a printed page is less likely to be read completely, partly because it contains too much information, and partly because it becomes difficult to see the entire table at once, especially on electronic screens. The most useful tables can be seen completely in one single visual field. So try to distill and/or compress your table down to under one-third or at most one-half of a page, if possible. If a table can be formed appropriately using portrait page-orientation, then do so, because many people will not bother reading tables in landscape page-orientation on electronic screens, because it requires rotating the page (or their head). (The fact that books and journals are printed on paper in portrait page-orientation is curious and unfortunate, considering that the human visual field is in landscape orientation.)

Whereas figures have a wide variety of different forms, tables all have essentially the same form or structure: a gridwork of columns and rows. So in contrast to making figures, the design of better tables involves only limited choices about the overall form. Instead, the design of better tables depends mostly upon careful editing of the visual details of the table, (as discussed later in this chapter). Nonetheless, the arrangement of the columns and rows has a major influence on the usefulness of the table. Regardless of whatever the contents of a table might be, people can read the table either by scanning across the rows or by scanning down the columns [2 (pp. 30–31), 3 (p. 179)]. If both directions of scanning are meaningful, many readers will indeed scan the table in both directions, even though this amounts to viewing the information in each cell twice. When people view tables, they are reading the information in each cell of the table, one by one. Yet their higher aim is to make comparisons between cells within each row or column, (or to look for patterns within rows or columns), if the table contents provides that kind of higher-order multicell information. So the main principle of good table design is to streamline the graphic presentation in ways that will make it faster and easier for readers to extract meaningful information from the table, especially as they scan across the rows or down the columns.

For any table, it is always possible to swap the rows and columns, but it is never the case that the presentation of the table's contents is equally good in either construction. So whenever you make a table, try switching the columns for the rows, to see which construction will be more natural and meaningful for the readers. The contents of the table, the portrait orientation of the journal page, and/or the general expectations and habits of readers will often impose a preference for constructing the table either vertically or horizontally. If no such preference is apparent, then it is usually better to put the numbers that you want the readers to compare into the same column, not the same row, because the eyes can scan and compare numbers faster and more efficiently in a column, because the digits are lined up vertically (**table 16.1**) [4 (p. 42), 5]. But if you are comparing two or more study groups, then

Table 16.1 Example of Constructing a Table in Two Different Directions. The two tables in this example present the mortality rate (per million inhabitants) due to a pandemic, for 7 geographic regions, divided by 7 age strata, plus "totals" (actually more like "weighted averages" here). The contents of tables A and B are the same; only the direction of organizing the contents has been swapped. (The regions are in order of decreasing total mortality rate; the age strata are in order of increasing age.) A legitimate case could be made for either orientation here, depending on the authors' intentions and the expectations about the readers, but ultimately version B is probably preferable in most contexts. In this example, it is possible in both tables to read either horizontally or vertically, in order to make comparisons either between age groups (within one region) or between regions (within one age group). Although both such comparisons are meaningful, most readers would probably choose the geographic region(s) of most interest to them, and then within that one region, look to see which age groups were affected worse. Most readers would probably not choose a particular age group to focus on, and then see which geographic region(s) were worse for that age group; (though some readers might do that, e.g. a pediatrics policy-maker might be curious which regions were safest for children under 10). For that reason, it is more sensible to make the geographic regions the column headers (as in version B), so readers can choose a region and then scan vertically to understand the age distribution of mortality due to this pandemic in that region of interest. However, version A does make it easier to compare the totals for the 7 regions and to see the ranking of which regions had the highest mortality rates for this pandemic. If the authors did not expect most readers to look at anything more than the totals, then version A might be more useful. In either case, the important point is that the authors consider how each orientation of table construction emphasizes different readings, and the authors make a conscious choice between them.

A)

		0–9	10–19	20–29	30–39	40–49	50–59	60+	Total
					Age				
	Oceania	0.62	0.29	1.13	1.41	1.62	2.10	1.61	**1.28**
	Africa	0.93	0.24	1.65	1.39	1.64	1.81	0.68	**1.13**
	UK	0.83	0.48	0.22	0.43	1.15	0.81	1.48	**0.83**
Region	USA	0.31	0.51	0.65	0.52	0.76	0.81	0.42	**0.56**
	East Asia	0.07	0.17	0.07	0.08	0.44	0.20	0.21	**0.16**
	South America	0.17	0.09	0.25	0.23	0.06	0.16	0.10	**0.16**
	Europe	0.44	0.25	0.00	0.13	0.12	0.00	0.08	**0.13**
	Total	**0.30**	**0.24**	**0.46**	**0.43**	**0.54**	**0.57**	**0.36**	0.40

B)

		Oceania	Africa	UK	USA	East Asia	South America	Europe	Total
					Region				
	0–9	0.62	0.93	0.83	0.31	0.07	0.17	0.44	**0.30**
	10–19	0.29	0.24	0.48	0.51	0.17	0.09	0.25	**0.24**
	20–29	1.13	1.65	0.22	0.65	0.07	0.25	0.00	**0.46**
Age	30–39	1.41	1.39	0.43	0.52	0.08	0.23	0.13	**0.43**
	40–49	1.62	1.64	1.15	0.76	0.44	0.06	0.12	**0.54**
	50–59	2.10	1.81	0.81	0.81	0.20	0.16	0.00	**0.57**
	60+	1.61	0.68	1.48	0.42	0.21	0.10	0.08	**0.36**
	Total	**1.28**	**1.13**	**0.83**	**0.56**	**0.16**	**0.16**	**0.13**	**0.40**

by convention they would usually be the column headings. After choosing the construction direction, scan the results in your table both horizontally and vertically, and ask yourself whether meaningful insights can be derived from the results in each of those reading directions without having to ignore or skip over numbers. If the answer is "no", consider revising.

Generally, tables in medical scientific papers should have only one level of headings for the columns and only one level of headings for the rows. Although it is possible to build tables with more than one level of headings for the columns and/or rows, any such second level of overarching or nested headings will disrupt the readers' ability to scan straight across the rows or straight down the columns. So those kinds of complex tables should usually be avoided in contemporary medical publications.

Whenever possible, the order of the rows and/or columns should not be arbitrary. Instead, the order of the rows and/or columns should be determined by the data, to make meaningful patterns appear. So arrange the information in a logical order, both from left to right and from top to bottom [4 (p. 42)]. From left to right, the most logical order is usually the order in which such information would be presented if it was written as a normal sentence. From top to bottom, the most logical order is often the order of decreasing magnitude, frequency, or importance of the results presented, (except for placing a "total" in the final row) [5, 6, 7 (pp. 244–247)]. For example, a table that lists the cost of treating a dozen different diseases should list the diseases in the first column, neither randomly nor in alphabetical order, but instead in the order of decreasing cost, (with the costs then shown in the second column). In this way, when the readers view the table, they see not only the actual financial data for each individual disease, but they also see a rank ordering of all the diseases by cost. For another example, a table listing harms in a clinical trial should not list them alphabetically, chronologically, or haphazardly. Instead, the table should list them in order of decreasing frequency and/or severity, so the readers see the most important harms first, as they read the rows from top to bottom (**table 16.2**).

Whenever you create a table, you must also spend time editing its layout. Your goal should be to make the table as simple and clear to read as possible, while also maximizing its meaningfulness. That requires reflecting on how to present the information as clearly and logically as possible, so the readers can focus on your results, rather than wasting time trying to decipher a messy table. Each table needs its own particular graphic editing, but the following tips provide a start for the most commonplace aspects.

First, tables should be carefully cleaned up, so the readers' eyes can scan smoothly across the rows and/or down the columns. Eliminate any irrelevant information or other unnecessary clutter in the table. Unit labels (such as "%" or "mg") should be placed in the headings of the column or row, not next to the results themselves [6, 8]. If such heading placements are not possible, then your table probably contains information that does not really belong together in the same table. Numerical results in a table should never be reported to more significant digits than is meaningful and scientifically warranted [5, 9]. All decimal points (including "invisible decimal points" for whole numbers) in each column of the table should be aligned vertically [9], so the table looks neat and the readers can immediately see, for example, that the "21.3" in row 4 is larger than the "4.58" directly beneath it in

Table 16.2 Example of Constructing a Table in a Meaningful Order. The two tables in this example present the rates of minor harms reported at the end of an open-label, phase IV trial of a medication, as assessed by clinical interview (N=523). (These harms were classified as "minor" because the patients had not needed immediate medical treatment for these experiences.) Table A presents the harms in alphabetical order; table B presents them in the order of decreasing frequency. Tables in alphabetical order are appropriate when it is expected that readers will only look up information for a limited number of rows but will never read the entire table, (such as tables spanning several pages in a reference manual). Here, version B is better, because the ordering makes it easier to see which harms occurred frequently and which ones were uncommon, and perhaps even to discern a pattern or reason underlying the reported frequencies. Tables should be constructed to make rank ordering or other patterns of the data apparent.

A)

	n	%
asthenia	74	14
constipation	110	21
dizziness	117	22
dry mouth	108	21
diarrhea	51	10
headaches	171	33
insomnia	134	26
muscle cramps	6	1
nausea	166	32
nervousness	46	9
respiratory difficulties	58	11
rhinitis	14	3
sinusitis	10	2
somnolence	210	40
sweating	42	8
tremor	64	12
none of the above	32	6

B)

	n	%
somnolence	210	40
headaches	171	33
nausea	166	32
insomnia	134	26
dizziness	117	22
constipation	110	21
dry mouth	108	21
asthenia	74	14
tremor	64	12
respiratory difficulties	58	11
diarrhea	51	10
nervousness	46	9
sweating	42	8
rhinitis	14	3
sinusitis	10	2
muscle cramps	6	1
none of the above	32	6

row 5, before even really reading those numbers. Yet the numbers should all contain the same number of digits after the decimal point, unless there is some reason why not (e.g. different kinds of numbers, measurements were not all made to the same degree of accuracy, p-values of different magnitudes, etc.) The use of footnotes in tables should be minimized, because the information they present is usually of little or no interest to most readers. But if a footnote must be used, try to put the footnote symbol in the nearest row or column header, not in the cell with the data or results.

Second, attention should be given to the graphic form of the table itself, as a container for the results or data. If you are going to emphasize anything visually with a bold font or other such graphic features, emphasize the results themselves, not the other elements of the table such as headings [2 (pp. 52–65), 3 (pp. 91–95), 7 (p. 25)]. Generally, such emphasis is not necessary unless the table contains more numbers than most people would read [10], though putting totals in bold is a sensible standard practice. If you can, downplay any inessential features that do not represent results (such as lines beneath headings or footnote symbols) by putting them in light gray or reducing their size/weight. Grid-lines should be avoided if possible or muted otherwise [3 (pp. 112–116)]. Spacing between the columns and proper vertical alignment is usually sufficient to make vertical grid-lines superfluous [5]. Similarly, horizontal grid-lines can usually be forgone if space is set between every 3–5 rows. If gridlines must be used, they should be razor thin and halftone gray, to minimize their visual prominence. Similarly, background tones should always be avoided (unless the table is very large and intended only for looking-up values, which is extremely rare in journal papers). An illustration of several of the graphic editing points above is provided in **table 16.3**.

Table 16.3 Example of Graphic Editing of a Table. The two tables in this example present the baseline demographic and health characteristics of two study groups (n=300 each) in a randomized comparative trial (of surgery vs. non-surgical treatment for chronic low back pain). Table A is before graphic editing; table B is after graphic editing. For the graphic editing, the following steps were taken in this order. 1) The column of p-values was deleted, because it is invalid to calculate p-values for baseline characteristics, as explained in the chapter, "The Results". 2) The information presented in each column was reduced to one single number, so the two groups can be compared more efficiently. Although it is commonplace to report more than one number in each column (e.g. both the n and the % or both the mean and the SD), visually this slows down or muddles the comparisons of the two groups, because the two numbers to compare always have another number between them. For example, the readers' eyes must skip over "56", to see that the rate of smokers in the two groups was 15% vs. 19%. Moreover, the information in each cell of the table is redundant. Most readers will not really make use of both the n and the %; either one is sufficient and acceptable. In this example, the % was retained, because it is more meaningful here than the exact number. Similarly, although the SD does add different information beyond the mean, most readers will not really make use of it. If an indication of data variability must be given, it would be preferable to add another row (and report the range). 3) Version A reports the mean ± SD for the age and pain duration, but it does not clearly label the results as the mean and SD. So the word "mean" was added in the first column. The abbreviation "yr" was replaced with "years", because saving the space or ink of three letters is pointless. 4) Version A reported the mean for pain duration, but the SD made it clear that the raw data was not Normally distributed for this variable. It was therefore inappropriate to report the mean. Version B replaces the mean with the median. 5) The results for BMI have been rounded off to one decimal place, because any more is excessive. Rounding to whole numbers would also be acceptable here. 6) Although it is not easy to notice this, spaces were added in front of the results for age, disability benefits, pain duration, and BMI, so all the numbers in each column aligned vertically. 7) All the footnotes were deleted. Although the information in the footnotes was neither meaningless nor irrelevant, it would not have made any real difference in the readers' understanding of how comparable the two study groups were to each other or to the population from which they were drawn. In other words, the footnotes went too far into detail in this context. 8) The word "Characteristic" was deleted as unnecessary and distracting. The characteristics are row headers and therefore do not need a column header. And it is self-evident that they are characteristics of the patient sample. 9) The use of bold typeface for the column headers was eliminated as unnecessary. 10) The word "gender" was replaced with "sex" as recommended by the ICMJE. 11) The word "female" was placed after the "%" because it is one of the answer options or data codes for this variable, not part of the name of the variable. For the same reason, "college" was placed after "%" and then it was replaced with the word "post-secondary", to be more comprehensible to international (non-USA) readers. 12) Borders around the table cells were eliminated. (Version A has heavy black lines around each cell of the table; whereas, version B has only the default light gray guidelines). Most publishers will eliminate table cell borders and take care of other such formatting issues, but it is better to bring the table as close to its intended final form as possible yourself. (Indeed, your version is exactly what readers will see, in cases of conference presentations, internet-only supplemental files, and author manuscripts in public repositories.) Although some of these changes may seem too nit-picky and others too drastic, altogether they add up to make a table (version B) that better achieves the goal of this kind of patient characteristics table for a randomized comparative trial. The original (version A) presents too many numbers and words that the readers either will not or should not really see. And that scatters their mental efforts in unproductive directions. By contrast, the edited table (version B) focuses their mental efforts on comparing the surgical and non-surgical treatment groups, so they can see that they were comparable groups of patients, which is important for a comparative trial.

A)

Characteristic	Surgery	Non-Surgical Treatment	p
Female Gender – n (%)	200 (67)	212 (71)	0.30
Age – yr	66.0 ± 10.0	66.1 ± 10.6	0.86
College Education – n (%)	201 (67)	199 (66)	0.98
Married – n (%)	198 (66)	198 (66)	0.98
Employed* – n (%)	116 (39)	102 (34)	0.42
Disability Benefits – n (%)	21 (7)	20 (7)	0.99
Pain Duration** – yr	9.6 ± 8.7	9.2 ± 8.9	0.87
BMI	29.134 ± 5.7	29.278 ± 6.7	0.91
Smoker† – n (%)	46 (15)	56 (19)	0.55
Depression – n (%)	56 (19)	42 (14)	0.16
Joint Problem – n (%)	175 (58)	169 (56)	0.72
Other Comorbidity – n (%)	121 (40)	113 (38)	0.58
Daily Narcotics – n (%)	64 (21)	69 (23)	0.68

*Employed full-time or part-time.

**Pain duration according to patient self-report at intake visit.

†Current smoker of tobacco or e-cigarettes.

B)

	Surgery	Non-Surgical Treatment
Sex – % female	67	71
Age – mean years	66.0	66.1
Education – % post-secondary	67	66
Married – %	66	66
Employed – %	39	34
Disability Benefits – %	7	7
Pain Duration – median years	7.3	6.9
BMI	29.1	29.3
Smoker – %	15	19
Depression – %	19	14
Joint Problem – %	58	56
Other Comorbidity – %	40	38
Daily Narcotics – %	21	23

Third, look at your entire table as a whole from a meter away (or however far is needed to make it too difficult to read the individual numbers), and ask yourself whether the table is pleasing to look at and well laid-out. If not, revise the layout and/or design.

Finally, when you are completely done designing your table, double-verify that all the numbers in the table are accurate, are not repeated in the text of the Results, and are consistent with any repetition of those numbers in the Discussion or Abstract. The worst table possible is one that contains erroneous numbers.

Guidance on what to write in the legends is provided in chapter 20 ("Legends").

The readers are not going to memorize all the numbers in your table. Indeed, they will probably have forgotten all the numbers in the table already by the time they find the spot in the main text to resume reading. So whenever you are done making a table, you should look at it again and ask yourself, "How does this table advance the readers' understanding?" Different readers will focus on different aspects of the table and with different levels of attention, but by the time they are done looking at it, there should be some simple idea that most readers will retain from the table. For example, a table about the study patients' baseline characteristics might lead a reader to conclude, "These patients are similar to the ones I treat except that they were older than my patients" or "The two study groups appear to have been sufficiently similar to each other." If a table does not lead to some such overall take-away message, above and beyond all the individual numbers or words in the table, then that table may not be serving its purpose well. If a table does lead to an overall take-away message but that message does not really contribute toward answering the study's questions, then that table is probably in the wrong paper. Every table in your paper should serve a table's purpose of advancing the understanding of the readers.

References

1. Van Damme H, for Editorial Board. Twelve Steps to Developing Effective Tables and Figures. Acta Chir Belg. 2007; 107: 237-238.
2. Tufte ER. Envisioning Information. Cheshire, CT, USA: Graphics Press; 1990.
3. Tufte ER. The Visual Display of Quantitative Information, 2nd ed. Cheshire, CT, USA: Graphics Press; 1983, 2001.
4. Altman DG. Practical Statistics for Medical Research. Boca Raton, FL, USA: CRC Press; 1991, 1999.
5. Ryder K. Guidelines for the presentation of numerical tables. Res Vet Sci. 1995; 58: 1-4.
6. Kotz D, Cals JWL. Effective writing and publishing scientific papers, part VII: tables and figures. J Clin Epidemiol. 2013; 66: 1197.
7. Cleveland WS. The Elements of Graphing Data. Murray Hill, NJ, USA: AT&T Bell Laboratories; 1994.
8. Hamilton CW. On the Table. Chest. 2009; 135: 1087-1089.
9. Cole TJ. Too many digits: the presentation of numerical data. Arch Dis Child. 2015; 100: 608-609.
10. Durbin CG Jr. Effective Use of Tables and Figures in Abstracts, Presentations, and Papers. Respir Care. 2004; 49: 1233-1237.

Chapter 17
Figures: General Guidance

Figures are a crucial component of most research papers. Unfortunately, judging by the published literature, most medical researchers do not give their figures much thought. Figures are used far less often than they could be, and they are often low quality. Figures present much of the evidence from most research studies, so they should be designed more thoughtfully. When made well, they can be very engaging and convincing to the readers. Indeed, some people will even look at the figures first, and use them as the basis for deciding whether or not to read the rest of the paper (regrettably). Thus good figures are a key part of your paper, and you should devote time and attention to them. To paraphrase Alice in Wonderland, "What is the use of a journal paper without pictures?" [1].

Although your statistical plan may have already started to do this, take a moment to plan out the figures that your paper will present. Each figure should make one clear point. In other words, you should be able to say in one short sentence what each figure shows or "proves". Each figure should be relevant and necessary for your paper. Do not throw in extra figures simply because one of your co-authors already made them for a conference presentation last fall. Choose your set of figures to illustrate the main points of your paper.

You can use one figure to illustrate your paper's topic or methods, if this seems appropriate. Some such examples are as follows: a study on a skin disease could show a photograph of an affected patient's skin; a study on a new medical device should have a photograph of that device; a laboratory study could present a schematic diagram of the experimental set-up; and so on. The Results section of a clinical trial should start with a flowchart of the patient recruitment and allocation [2–6]. Although study sample characteristics can be presented in a multipanel figure with small graphs, it is generally preferable to present that information in a table (or the text), because the study sample characteristics are not worth the prominence of figures and usually are too heterogeneous for a figure anyway.

Next, you should always have one major figure for your main results, whatever they are, if it is possible to present them in a figure [7 (p. 54)]. Then, you can create further figures for your secondary results, however seems most useful in your paper.

© Springer Nature Switzerland AG 2019
M. Hanna, *How to Write Better Medical Papers*,
https://doi.org/10.1007/978-3-030-02955-5_17

Think about several possible ways to graph your data, and choose the graph that best enables your readers to see what you found. Try to graph your raw data if possible, instead of graphing summary statistics. In other words, try to create graphs that show the outcomes for each individual patient, instead of calculations about the whole sample, such as the mean, especially if your sample size is small (ca. N<100). Graphing raw data can reveal important aspects of reality that vanish if summary statistics are graphed instead (e.g. that a small subset of patients actually got worse, not better). (The graphing of data is discussed in more detail in the next chapter.)

Whenever applicable, try to show picture results of your research, such as x-rays or histology slices. These kinds of images are highly engaging for readers, especially clinical professionals. Also these kinds of images usually convey a substantial amount of information, even though they are only illustrative examples from specific individual subjects. (Further guidance about such figures is presented in chapter 19, "Figures: Photographs and Images").

When you are done making all your figures, look at your figure files alone. If someone looked only at all your figures and legends, but never read the rest of the paper, would he or she still get the gist of what you found? If not, you probably need to work on your figures more. The figures should not be mere supplemental illustrations of certain parts of your paper. Instead, they should be a somewhat self-sufficient slide-show of your research report, if possible [7 (pp. 54–55)]. The figures will then serve as a visual backbone for the paper, providing support to the larger line of thinking you present.

Journals have tight word limits. A figure is surely not worth a thousand words, but it can present a substantial amount of information without using up the word limit of your text. Use good figures to say much more than you otherwise could.

References

1. Carroll L. Alice's Adventures in Wonderland. New York: Signet; 1865, 2000.
2. Schulz KF, Altman DG, Moher D; for CONSORT Group. CONSORT 2010 Statement: updated guidelines for reporting parallel group randomised trials. BMJ. 2010; 340: 698-702.
3. Moher D, Hopewell S, Schulz KF, Montori V, Gøtzsche PC, Devereaux PJ, Elbourne D, Egger M, Altman DG. CONSORT 2010 Explanation and Elaboration: updated guidelines for reporting parallel group randomised trials. BMJ. 2010; 340: c869.
4. Vandenbroucke JP, von Elm E, Altman DG, Gøtzsche PC, Mulrow CD, Pocock SJ, Poole C, Schlesselman JJ, Egger M, for STROBE Initiative. Strengthening the Reporting of Observational Studies in Epidemiology (STROBE): Explanation and Elaboration. PLoS Med. 2007; 10: e297.
5. Pocock SJ, Travison TG, Wruck LM. Figures in clinical trial reports: current practice & scope for improvement. Trials. 2007; 8: 36.
6. Durbin CG Jr. Effective Use of Tables and Figures in Abstracts, Presentations, and Papers. Respir Care. 2004; 49: 1233-1237.
7. Cleveland WS. The Elements of Graphing Data. Murray Hill, NJ, USA: AT&T Bell Laboratories; 1994.

Chapter 18
Figures: Data Graphs

Although figures are a crucial component of medical papers, most medical papers have rather low-quality graphs. They present substantially less information than they could. The information they do present is usually shown in a suboptimal or inappropriate form. And then visually the graphs are often cluttered with many other useless and distracting marks. Probably many researchers do not give much thought to the visual presentation of their data, since training in data visualization and graphic design is very rare in the medical scientific world. So this chapter starts by identifying some types of low-quality graphs that are often seen in medical papers and explains why and how to replace them. Next, this chapter will present some other types of higher quality graphs that could be used often but currently are rarely seen. Finally, this chapter discusses some graphic editing steps that can be used to improve any graph you make. By putting some thought and clarity into your graphs, you will greatly increase the interest and comprehension of journal Editors, peer-reviewers, and readers.

There are several types of graphs that are common in the literature but should never be used. First, any kind of 3D graph (**figure 18.1**) should not be used [1 (pp. 71, 77, 118)]. The third dimension here does not have any meaning and is visually confusing [1 (pp. 71, 118)]. These 3D graphs could always be flattened out to 2D, without any loss of scientific information [1 (pp. 71, 77)]. Researchers sometimes attempt to create 3D graphs where the third dimension does convey information about the data. This is scientifically acceptable, yet it is not advisable without the support of an experienced graphic designer. Because the graph is still presented on two-dimensional paper or screens, it can be difficult to create a 3D graph with exactly the right proportions to convey that much information accurately [2]. Although it is possible to convey three or more dimensions on two-dimensional paper or screens [3 (pp. 12–35), 4 (p. 193)], doing that successfully requires extensive professional training and experience in data visualization. Interestingly, successful visualization of a third variable on the 2D plane of the paper or screen almost never involves an illusion of 3D space.

© Springer Nature Switzerland AG 2019
M. Hanna, *How to Write Better Medical Papers*,
https://doi.org/10.1007/978-3-030-02955-5_18

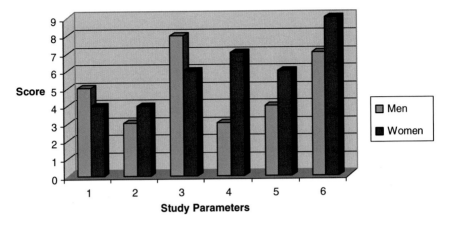

Figure 18.1 A 3D Graph. Three-dimensional graphs should never be used (unless the third dimension represents a third data variable). Here, the third dimension does not add any information and only creates optical distortions (the red columns occupy more 2D area on the page or screen than the blue columns because the sides of the red columns can be seen too, in another darker shade). The background shading and horizontal gridlines are also disruptive.

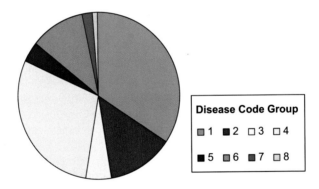

Figure 18.2 Pie Chart. Pie charts should not used. The relative sizes of the slices are difficult to compare. Instead, use a column graph or table, or just report the results in the text.

Second, do not use pie charts (**figure 18.2**). They present very little information for the space they take up. Furthermore, studies have shown that people cannot accurately perceive the relative proportions of the pie slices [1 (pp. 55–56, 69–73), 2, 4 (pp. 262–264), 5], probably due to the lack of a reference scale [4 (pp. 262–264), 5]. For these reasons, pie charts are not considered acceptable in scientific reports [1 (p. 178), 4 (pp. 262–264), 6]. Instead, if you are going to use a figure, you could use a column graph (**figure 18.3**). If there are only a few items (only a few pie slices), the information should probably just be reported in the text. If there are many items, it is probably best to present them as a table (in order of decreasing magnitude). As text or table, it becomes easy to add confidence intervals for each item (calculated through bootstrapping); whereas, such a feature on a pie chart would be quite confusing.

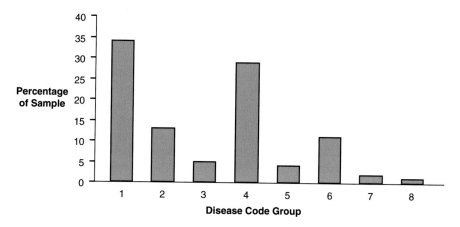

Figure 18.3   Column Graph. A standard column graph should be used instead of a pie chart. This one was made from the same dataset as figure 18.2. It could probably be improved further by ordering the 8 disease groups, from left to right, in descending order of their portion of the study sample. Notice also that the use of color in figure 18.2 has been eliminated here.

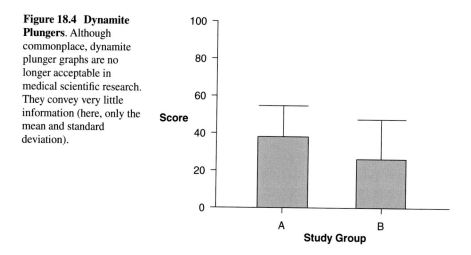

Figure 18.4   Dynamite Plungers. Although commonplace, dynamite plunger graphs are no longer acceptable in medical scientific research. They convey very little information (here, only the mean and standard deviation).

Third, **figure 18.4** presents a commonly seen type of vertical bar chart with whiskers, typically used to present the mean and SD or SEM. Because of their overall shape, these graphs are derisively referred to as "dynamite plungers". This kind of graph can be found quite frequently in the literature (especially in the laboratory sciences), but it is no longer considered acceptable [7–14]. Dynamite plunger graphs present very little information (only two numbers per column), and the ink at the base of the dynamite plunger does not correspond to any data. Instead of dynamite plungers, you should use box-and-whisker plots (**figure 18.5**). In a box-and-whisker plot, the middle bar is the median (the 50th percentile), the top of the box is the 75th percentile, the bottom of the box is the 25th percentile, the top whisker is the maximum, and the bottom whisker is the minimum. (Box-and-whisker plots sometimes

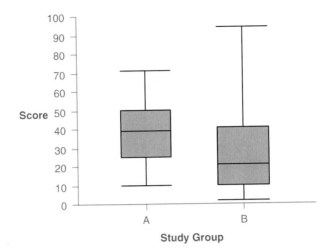

Figure 18.5 Box-and-Whisker Plot. A box-and-whisker plot should be used instead of a dyna-mite plunger. It shows the minimum, 25th quartile, median, 75th quartile, and maximum. (Many other variations are possible but rarely preferable.) This box-and-whisker plot was made from the same dataset as figure 18.4. The many differences between the two study groups are now revealed. (Additionally, the Y-axis has been graduated by 10s rather than 20s for greater accuracy. And the axes, ticks, and labels have been reduced from black to 50% gray, to give them less prominence than the results plotted in the graph.)

end the whiskers at various other cut-off points before the minimum and/or maxi-mum and then show any further subjects ("outliers") as individual dots beyond the whiskers [4 (pp. 139–143), 12, 15 (pp. 49–50)]. Although that approach is valid, it should usually be avoided, because it puts too much visual emphasis on those indi-vidual subjects for no good reason and distracts the readers away from the main results. It also makes the definition of the whisker ends more difficult to comprehend for most readers. So the whisker ends should just be the minimum and maximum values.) Box-and-whisker plots present more and better information than dynamite plungers, for the same amount of page space and ink. Figures 18.4 and 18.5 here have been generated from the same dataset. Notice how the two groups seem roughly similar in the uninformative dynamite-plunger graph (figure 18.4); whereas, the box-and-whisker plot (figure 18.5) reveals that the two groups have clearly different distributions of data. If the sample size is small enough (ca. n<50), it is usually even better to just plot all the raw data as individual dots, instead of the summary statistics of the box-and-whisker plot [7, 13, 14, 16 (pp. 40, 221–222, 488)].

More generally speaking: many researchers make graphs using their database spreadsheet software, but this usually contributes to low-quality [17]. Whenever possible, you should graph your data using the same software you use for statistical analysis or (even better) a program made primarily for graphing data. After making and revising the graph in that program, you can import the file to a vector graphic editing program to refine it further for visual elegance and clarity, (taking care to not alter the positioning of any marks representing results).

There are many ways you can create better quality graphs. The general goal is to transform your numerical data into a visual form that will quickly and clearly convey the pattern (or lack of pattern) in your data. The main barrier that prevents researchers from doing this is that they cannot imagine how that visual form would appear, because they have not previously seen such graphs often enough to have a model in their mind. So here are a few useful graphs that many researchers could use repeatedly.

First, you can use a scatter plot (**figure 18.6**) to present the distribution of data for any two continuous variables. Scatter plots can be used whenever there is some reason for looking at how much two variables relate to each other (or not); it does

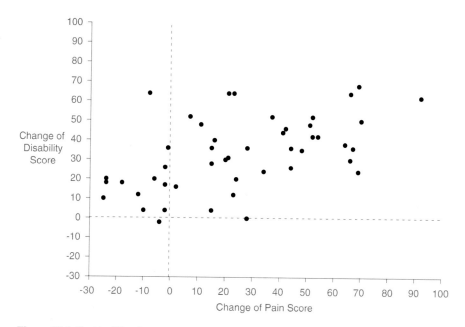

Figure 18.6 Scatter Plot. In a scatter plot, each dot represents one subject, and shows two variables for that subject. The overall pattern of dots shows the distribution of data for the two variables, as well as the correlation between them (or lack of correlation). There need not be an obvious pattern in the data to make use of a scatter plot, so long as the two variables have some reason to be shown together. In this example, from a small clinical trial, the X-axis shows the change in the pain score (on a visual analogue scale) from baseline to follow-up, and the Y-axis shows the change in the score from a disability questionnaire. Positive numbers represent improvement; negative numbers represent worsening. Each dot represents the outcomes from one patient. Dashed lines at "0" (no change) have been added to better distinguish between patients who improved versus worsened. This example scatter plot suggests a moderate relationship between the improvement in pain and the improvement in disability; (in fact, r=0.53, p<0.001). This example also reveals that the pain of some patients worsened, yet their disability improved nonetheless (upper left quadrant of the graph), thus showing that a patient's disability is not always directly dependent on their pain, as is often assumed in this field. Such insights would be lost in the typical approach of graphing summary statistics (e.g. mean and SD) at baseline and follow-up, separately for pain and for disability.

not matter whether or not the results actually show a correlation between the two variables. One advantage of this graph is that it gives the readers a quick and clear picture of the full distribution of the raw data (for two variables and their relationship), because each dot represents one single subject. Whenever you make a scatter plot (or other graphs using dots for each subject), consider replacing the dots with symbols that represent another relevant categorical variable [18], for example "M" and "F" for male and female [19].

Second, you can use a stacked column graph (**figure 18.7**) to present the distribution of categorical or ordinal variables such as disease severity or employment status. This kind of stacked column graph is often superior to the more commonly used cluster column graph (where a column for each category is placed side-by-side). In either graph, the viewers will mainly compare the vertical levels of the bars. Whereas a cluster column graph emphasizes comparisons within each group, a stacked column graph will emphasize comparisons between study groups, which is usually the main point.

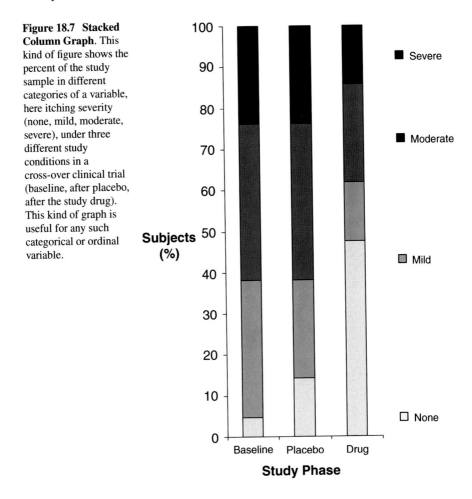

Figure 18.7 Stacked Column Graph. This kind of figure shows the percent of the study sample in different categories of a variable, here itching severity (none, mild, moderate, severe), under three different study conditions in a cross-over clinical trial (baseline, after placebo, after the study drug). This kind of graph is useful for any such categorical or ordinal variable.

Third, you can use a before-and-after paired-points graph (**figure 18.8**) to show the distribution of responses to an intervention. This graph has the advantage that it enables the readers to see an overall pattern of response while still being able to look at exceptions. When using a before-and-after paired-point graph, the length of the two axes must be chosen carefully, because they determine the slopes of the lines connecting the pairs of datapoints. The slopes of these lines in turn determine the implicit overall impression the graph gives the viewer about the change from the intervention. This graph is best suited for small sample sizes (say n<50), where readers can still look at all the individual pairs of datapoints. It can also work well in larger samples, if there is a clear overall pattern of response without notable outliers. Otherwise, histograms of the variable at pre-treatment and post-treatment and the magnitude of change would be clearer.

Fourth, the display of confidence intervals would improve many graphs in medicine. In most cases, when readers look at your figures, their primary interest is not really the data or results from your specific study sample. Instead, their real interest is the results they could expect to find in the larger population from which your study

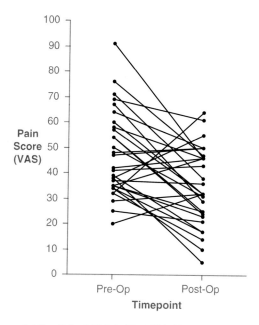

Figure 18.8 Before-and-After Paired-Points Plot. This kind of graph can be used for plotting the change of a variable from pre-treatment to post-treatment. Each subject in the study is represented by a line connecting two dots (here, one for their pre-op pain score, the other for their post-op pain score). This kind of graph is well-suited to showing the distribution of changes in the data, for a small to medium size sample. It is much more informative than graphs of summary statistics. Here we can see for example that although the patients improved overall or on average, some patients actually got worse. By contrast, any graph of summary statistics (such as a line graph of the mean and SD) would only show that the subjects got better (on average) while hiding the fact that some got worse.

sample was drawn. In other words, your readers generally do not really care what you found in your patients; instead, they want to know what your findings imply for their own patients. For this reason, whenever you make a figure, you should try to find a way to present the confidence interval for those results [20]. The confidence interval shows the readers what they might expect to find in their patient samples, (if their patient samples are drawn from the same larger population as yours). Confidence intervals often have a graphic appearance similar to the ubiquitous but less useful error bars that represent SD or SEM, so they should be easy for any researcher to make. Such error bars showing SD or SEM should be replaced with confidence intervals [4 (pp. 217–219)]. Graphically, it is easy to even show two different confidence intervals on the same graph (e.g. a 50% CI and a 95% CI, or a 90% CI and a 99% CI) [4 (pp. 217–219)], in situations where readers may want more than one CI.

There are many other good graphs you could use, depending on what you are trying to show with your data, but they cannot all be covered here. These examples are some of the most frequently useful graphs, and they should get you off to a good start. You can consult books of graphs to find more possibilities [1, 3, 4].

Finally, there are some general principles of how to make any graph convey information in a clear and scientifically acceptable way. Too many researchers simply use the graphs that their computer program spits out, without ever bothering to spend time cleaning up the appearance of their graphs. The consequence is predictable: messy graphs that readers cannot clearly understand or do not want to view for long. So spend some time looking carefully at each graph you make and visually adjusting and editing it. This should be done first in the program that generated the graph as far as possible and then refined further in a vector graphic editing program, taking care to not alter the positions of marks representing data.

The number one rule is to intensify the data presentation while simultaneously eliminating useless clutter [1 (pp. 91–105), 3 (pp. 36–65), 4 (pp. 25–54, 64–66, 110–111), 21 (p. 81)]. Graphs should always be visually clear. And depending on the data or results presented, they should be either simple or elegantly complex, but never complicated or cluttered [1 (p. 191)]. Eliminate any unnecessary marks and lines. In particular, many graphs add asterisks to indicate significance levels ($p<0.05$, $p<0.01$, etc.) But this is imprecise and clutters the graph unnecessarily [8]. The graph should put the main focus on the results themselves, (not on statistical tests about the results). If possible, the 95% CI should also be plotted on the graph itself; [22] otherwise, it can be reported in the figure legend. The exact p-values may also be reported in the legend, but they should not clutter the figure itself. Also, avoid using an insert box with a key to the symbols used in the graph for the various study groups; whenever possible, delete such insert boxes and label the results directly [4 (pp. 45–46), 21 (pp. 2, 81, 94–95)]. The ideal graph maximizes the data: ink ratio, by minimizing the amount of ink that does not represent actual data (also known as "chartjunk") [1 (pp. 90–121), 3 (pp. 33–35), 4 (pp. 25–30)]. Put another way, the best graphs minimize meaningless "noise" that does not refer to data and maximize meaningful "signal" that does refer to the data. Similarly, do not shade part or all of the background, because such shading does not represent data and decreases legibility by decreasing the contrast of the black ink of data against the white page.

Information that is of primary importance (data, results) should be shown in black, while information that is of secondary importance (axes, labels, error bars) should be shown in half-tone gray [2].

Many medical researchers use color in their data graphs (especially at conferences), but this is almost always a bad idea without any scientifically defensible justification. The use of color in data graphs almost never encodes meaningful information (at least not better than other graphic techniques), and it often has undesirable effects on viewer perceptions. Cleveland identifies only two uses of color that he believes do indeed improve graphs: encoding a third categorical variable (e.g. blood type) on an otherwise bivariate plot or encoding a quantitative variable in a surface plane (e.g. a topography map) [4 (pp. unnumbered frontispiece page with figures 1 and 2, 209–212, 230–231)]. The latter scenario occurs often enough in geology and other such earth sciences, but it is exceptionally rare in the medical sciences and can be accomplished better in grayscale than in colorscale anyway. So that leaves only one well-founded use of color in graphing data in the medical sciences: encoding a (third) categorical variable in a scatter plot or other such bivariate dot plot. In such a scenario, the color coding is genuinely beneficial, as Cleveland elegantly shows [4 (pp. unnumbered frontispiece page with figure 1, 210)]. Nonetheless, this function of color-coding can also be accomplished (though less well) by use of different symbols (e.g. "A", "B", "+", "O" for blood types) [4 (pp. 234–239)]. Ideally, such coding of a third variable should use both color-coding and symbols redundantly, in case the color cannot be perceived by some readers. Tufte's beautiful reflections on communicating information through color [3 (pp. 80–95)] do not obviously suggest any further applications for data graphing in the medical sciences beyond what is discussed by Cleveland (except perhaps for maps of epidemiological data). And while marveling over color in general, Tufte repeatedly warns against its many possible negative effects for scientific graphics, as though color were potentially quite toxic for data communication [3 (pp. 80–95)]. One other possible exception in the medical sciences might be to use one color (such as red or orange) in an otherwise black-and-white or grayscale graph, in order to draw the attention of the readers to some specific detail in a graph that is explicitly emphasized in the main text. For example, a paired-points graph such as figure 18.8 might use red for the three patients who had a major intraoperative complication, or it might use orange to identify the two patients that are presented in more depth as case examples. In such scenarios, color serves to highlight specific details, so the readers can find them faster and give them special attention. But aside from these few unusual exceptions, color serves no valid function in medical scientific graphs and should never be used. Beside the fact that some readers are color-blind, if anyone prints or copies your paper in black-and-white, the information you encoded with color will lose clarity [15 (p. 68), 22, 23]. Even when the color is clearly visible, it often looks garish and/or puts more emphasis on some parts than on others, usually for no good reason. So instead of using different colors, use clearly different gray tones, different geometric shapes, or different forms of patterning. Nonetheless, avoid stippling and stripes, because they cause distracting optical effects [1 (pp. 107–112, 120–121)] and look outdated.

The axes of a graph must be scaled correctly. They should not be truncated to the range of the data collected, and they should certainly never be truncated to "zoom in" on part of the data, such as the region of differences between two study groups. These kinds of truncations of the axes distort the overall visual impression the graph gives to the data, thereby leading to misinterpretation of the findings [24]. Instead, each axis should show the full range of possible values for that variable. For the same reason, you should avoid breaks in the axes. If it seems unmanageable to make a graph without a break in the axis, then that break should extend across the entire graph, effectively creating two panels [4 (pp. 104–109)]. Logarithmic scales distort the overall visual form given to the data, leading to misunderstandings. In Medicine, logarithmic scales should be avoided (except for odds ratios) because most readers do not see enough of them to interpret them well. If you feel there is some compelling reason to use a logarithmic scale, present the data first on the usual linear scale and then in another panel of the figure on a logarithmic scale [15 (pp. 68–69)]. In that way, readers can first see the results in the form they are accustomed to and then can see whatever it is you are trying to show through use of the logarithmic scale.

The ticks on the axes should not be any more frequent or specific than the precision of the raw data, because this may lead readers to infer greater precision from the graph than the data warrant [20]. For example, if estimated blood loss during surgery was only recorded to the nearest 100 mL, then the axis of a graph reporting that data should not included ticks every 10 or 50 mL; it should only include ticks every 100 mL. Nonetheless, tick-marks should be used in moderation [4 (pp. 39–41)]. If for example you are graphing patient height, there is no need to put 200 tick-marks on the Y-axis simply because you measured height to the nearest centimeter. Tick-marks should be placed outside the data-space formed by the axes, not inside [4 (pp. 31, 33–35, 37, 40)].

The formatting and style of the graphs should be consistent across all your figures in the paper, insofar as possible. For example, if squares represent cases and circles represent controls in one of your figures, do not reverse those symbols or use triangles for controls in another one of your figures [2].

Finally, remember that your graph will be shrunk to fit the space allotted on the journal page – typically about a quarter page. Although most journals handle this production aspect, you should make all your numbers and marks large enough that they will remain legible when reduced for the printed journal page [17]. The easiest way to do this is to think about how much space the journal will probably allot your figure [21 (pp. 104–111)], and then make your figure at that scale from the outset. Numbers or words inside the figure itself should often then be written a font size or two larger than you initially think is needed, to ensure their legibility.

High-quality graphs give power to your paper. Text, tables, and low-quality graphs *tell* your readers what you found, but high-quality graphs actually *show* your readers the evidence. They will get readers more engaged with your paper, because everyone likes to look at good figures. So high-quality graphs may also increase the chances that journals will want to publish your article. It is always well worth the extra time to reflect on your figures and improve their visual quality.

References

1. Tufte ER. The Visual Display of Quantitative Information, 2nd ed. Cheshire, CT, USA: Graphics Press; 1983, 2001.
2. Gillan DJ, Wickens CD, Hollands JG, Carswell CM. Guidelines for Presenting Quantitative Data in HFES Publications. Hum Factors. 1998; 40: 28-41.
3. Tufte ER. Envisioning Information. Cheshire, CT, USA: Graphics Press; 1990.
4. Cleveland WS. The Elements of Graphing Data. Murray Hill, NJ, USA: AT&T Bell Laboratories; 1994.
5. Hollands JG, Spence I. Judgments of Change and Proportion in Graphical Perception. Hum Factors. 1992; 34: 313-334.
6. Schriger DL, Cooper RJ. Achieving Graphical Excellence: Suggestions and Methods for Creating High-Quality Visual Displays of Experimental Data. Ann Emerg Med. 2001; 37: 75-87.
7. Tobias A. Dynamite plunger plots should not be used. Occup Environ Med. 1998; 55: 361-362.
8. Lane DM, Sándor A. Designing Better Graphs by Including Distributional Information and Integrating Words, Numbers, and Images. Psychol Methods. 2009; 14: 239-257.
9. Kick the bar chart habit. Nat Methods. 2014; 11: 113.
10. Streit M, Gehlenborg N. Bar charts and box plots. Nat Methods. 2014; 11: 117.
11. Krzywinski M, Altman N. Visualizing samples with box plots. Nat Methods. 2014; 11: 119-120.
12. Larson MG. Descriptive Statistics and Graphical Displays. Circulation. 2006; 114: 76-81.
13. Rockman HA. Great expectations. J Clin Invest. 2012; 122: 1133.
14. Weissgerber TL, Milic NM, Winham SJ, Garovic VD. Beyond Bar and Line Graphs: Time for a New Data Presentation Paradigm. PLoS Biol. 2015; 13: e1002128.
15. Bland M. An Introduction to Medical Statistics, 4th ed. Oxford: Oxford University Press; 2015.
16. Altman DG. Practical Statistics for Medical Research. Boca Raton, FL, USA: CRC Press; 1991, 1999.
17. Bullimore MA. Love the Data, Hate the Figures. Optom Vis Sci. 2004; 81: 642-643.
18. Schriger DL, Sinha R, Schroter S, Liu PY, Altman DG. From Submission to Publication: A Retrospective Review of the Tables and Figures in a Cohort of Randomized Controlled Trials Submitted to the *British Medical Journal*. Ann Emerg Med. 2006; 48: 750-756.
19. Hayes SN, Redberg RF. Dispelling the Myths: Calling for Sex-Specific Reporting of Trial Results. Mayo Clin Proc. 2008; 83: 523-525.
20. Wainer H. Depicting Error. Am Stat. 1996; 50: 101-111.
21. Briscoe MH. Preparing Scientific Illustrations, 2nd ed. New York: Springer; 1996.
22. Pocock SJ, Travison TG, Wruck LM. Figures in clinical trial reports: current practice & scope for improvement. Trials. 2007; 8: 36.
23. McDonald JC. Charts, Graphs and Tables – Reporting the Data. Radiat Prot Dosimetry. 2001; 95: 291-293.
24. Durbin CG Jr. Effective Use of Tables and Figures in Abstracts, Presentations, and Papers. Respir Care. 2004; 49: 1233-1237.

Chapter 19
Figures: Photographs and Images

Medical research sometimes makes use of a variety of photographs or images: photographs of a patient or part of a patient, x-rays and other forms of radiography, MRIs, CT scans, nuclear medical imaging, ultrasound images, histology slides, other micrographs, gels, blots, etc. These kinds of figures are generally quite engaging for readers and can be quite convincing too. For those reasons, you should present these kinds of figures whenever available and sensible. However, you must also be quite careful and vigilant to not present these kinds of figures in ways that could be viewed as misleading. Scientifically rigorous presentation of these kinds of figures has two aspects: unbiased selection of which images to present [1] and then not editing the images in ways that could be viewed as falsifying them [2–5].

With the exception of case reports or very small lab experiments, all research studies that collect photographs or other images will have far more images available than they can actually present. Consequently, figures that present photographs or other images almost always present mere examples. The readers are then supposed to assume that that example shown in the figure is representative of the other images that are not shown, unless the authors explicitly state otherwise. So photographs and images should be selected that are truly representative of the results generally obtained, (unless the purpose is precisely to illustrate an extreme or atypical case). It is biased and misleading to choose one of the best images (or images from the patients with the best outcomes) but then present it as "typical" or "representative". The most scientifically rigorous approach is to use an image that illustrates the median from the study sample. If space is available for further examples, the images with the best and worst results can also be shown. If a pair of images is shown to illustrate pre-treatment versus post-treatment, then images should be selected from a patient with the median amount of improvement from pre-treatment to post-treatment. The legend should in any case state clearly how the images presented were selected from all that were available, (e.g., "The MRI in the figure is from the patient with the median improvement on the main clinical outcome score.") Photographs and images from patients who are not part of the study sample should

© Springer Nature Switzerland AG 2019
M. Hanna, *How to Write Better Medical Papers*,
https://doi.org/10.1007/978-3-030-02955-5_19

never be used, unless there are no such photograph or images from the study sample, in which case, the legend should make that clear.

If you are using a photograph of a patient (or even just a part of the patient), you must obtain written permission from that patient to use his or her photograph. For practical reasons, it is better to seek that permission from the outset, before spending time working on that figure. The figure must also mask the identity of the patient, so that people who know that patient would still not recognize him or her. Merely masking the eye region is no longer considered sufficient in most cases [6].

Photographs and images are essentially raw data [3, 7, 8 (p. 21)], so they should not be edited in misleading or suspicious ways. Some graphic editing for clarity of presentation is acceptable and even preferable, but researchers are always at risk of wandering too far with such editing. Two important measures will protect you from accusations of falsifying your photographs or images. First, whatever editing you decide to do, document step by step what exactly you did. Anyone with access to your raw files, your editing documentation, and the software you used, should be able to reproduce the exact image you submitted for publication. The documentation should be made available as a supplemental file, so readers can check what visual editing you did on your figures. Second, you should also make the raw files of the unedited photographs or images available as a supplemental file for your paper, so readers can see what that visual data looked like before you edited it [9]. If you are unable or unwilling to make the original raw image available, then you should probably just not publish an edited version either. If the raw file is a photograph of a patient, then use a version that masks the patient identity, instead of the purely raw file.

With those two safeguards in place, it is entirely acceptable, even preferable, to perform some light visual editing on most photographs or images, to improve the clarity of presentation [2, 7]. All editing should take place in the TIFF file format, using software designed for image editing; other file formats or software programs will degrade the quality and accuracy of the images [3]. If two or more images are supposed to be compared to each other (e.g. experimental and control conditions, or pre-treatment vs. post-treatment), any editing they undergo should be equivalent for all images [3]. Files should be clearly labeled and well organized, so they do not get mixed up [5]. The first step of any editing is to make a copy of the original raw file; the original raw file should be retained untouched, while the editing is performed on a copy [3]. The next step is usually to crop the file, in order to remove irrelevant margins and focus the image on the area of interest. Such cropping should not remove any areas containing potentially relevant or meaningful content; it should only remove irrelevant space, background, borders, or entirely unrelated content. The cropping should also not remove context that changes the interpretation of what remains in the image [3]. Next, it may be necessary to adjust the brightness, contrast, or color balance, if the raw image was not clear. This should only be done to improve visibility; it should not alter the meaning of the image. If signal intensity/brightness or color conveys meaning, then such adjustments should not be made. Such adjustments of contrast or colors should never truncate the signal histograms of the original file [3]. Further editing may be acceptable, depending on the specific type of imaging being presented and the expectations of specialists in your field. Details within the image should never be cut out, erased, blurred, or otherwise modified, nor should anything ever be pasted in, duplicated, collaged together, or otherwise inserted. Any editing that is performed should be applied uniformly to the entire image that will be presented, not to only details or parts of the image [2–4]. Labels or arrows may be added if they do not obscure relevant details of the image [8 (pp. 22, 27–29), 10], but it may sometimes be better to just place arrows in the X and Y margins of the image, and let the readers find their point of intersection on the image. If applicable, a scale bar should be added directly into the figure (before any editing is performed), instead of stating the scale or magnification in the legend [3]. The final image submitted to the journal should be high resolution. If you zoom in to 1600%, the image should not become blurry or pixelated. If it does, the image resolution is too low and that file should not be used. In that case, go back to the raw file, which generally should have sufficient resolution for zooming in 1600%. If it does not, your original image acquisition was probably performed inadequately, but such issues of research methodology and data collection are outside the scope of this book.

Photographs and images are very engaging for readers, and they can be quite convincing. Researchers must be careful though to not select or present them in misleading ways. Legitimate visual editing can easily veer off into data falsification, especially if it is performed by people with no special training in such editing, as if a scientific image was no different than a holiday snapshot. The best protection against such suspicions is to make the raw image available to readers in supplemental files, along with meticulous step-by-step documentation of any editing that was performed.

References

1. Siontis GCM, Patsopoulos NA, Vlahos AP, Ioannidis JPA. Selection and Presentation of Imaging Figures in the Medical Literature. PLoS One. 2010; 5: e10888.
2. Suvarna SK, Ansary MA. Histopathology and the 'third great lie'. When is an image not a scientifically authentic image? Histopathology. 2001; 39: 441-446.
3. Cromey DW. Avoiding Twisted Pixels: Ethical Guidelines for the Appropriate Use and Manipulation of Scientific Digital Images. Sci Eng Ethics. 2010; 16: 639-667.
4. Rossner M, Yamada KM. What's in a picture? The temptation of image manipulation. J Cell Biol. 2004; 166: 11-15.
5. Neill US. Stop misbehaving! J Clin Invest. 2006; 116: 1740-1741.
6. International Committee of Medical Journal Editors. Recommendations for the Conduct, Reporting, Editing, and Publication of Scholarly Work in Medical Journals. Philadelphia: American College of Physicians; 1978, 2017. Accessed on 12 January 2018 at: www.icmje. org/icmje-recommendations.pdf
7. American Academy of Dermatology. Position Statement on Photographic Enhancement. 1997, 2007. Accessed on 11 May 2018 at: http://www.aad.org/Forms/Policies/Uploads/PS/ PS-Photographic%20Enhancement.pdf
8. Briscoe MH. Preparing Scientific Illustrations, 2nd ed. New York: Springer; 1996.
9. Pulverer B. When things go wrong: correcting the scientific record. EMBO J. 2015; 34: 2483-2485.
10. Aydıngöz Ü. Figures, tables, and references: integral but sometimes neglected components of scientific articles. Diagn Interv Radiol. 2005; 11: 67-68.

Chapter 20
Legends

Most researchers do not really know what to write in the legends for their tables or figures. Often they write nearly nothing. Sometimes they repeat the corresponding part of the Methods. Sometimes they comment on the meaning of the results. All these approaches are wrong and should be avoided. Instead, the legends should clearly explain how to decipher the information in the table or figure.

Legends for tables should start with a brief table title, which descriptively names the contents of the table (e.g. "Patient Characteristics"). The legend should then explain briefly what information is presented there, if it is not obvious from the table itself. The legend should end by defining any abbreviations or measurement units used. The legend should not repeat the study methods or start discussing the results in the table. Also try to avoid using footnotes with the table, because they look cluttered, are difficult to read, and rarely say anything of any real interest.

Similarly, legends for figures should start with a descriptive title that states clearly what the figure presents (e.g. "Heart rate and blood pressure of the study groups over time"), in order to identify it. Then, the legend should explain all the visual elements of the figure [1 (p. 59)]. Assume that your readers have never seen such a graph before, and explain simply to the readers what they are even looking at: what all the bars and dots actually represent. For example, do the whiskers on a box-plot represent the SD, the SEM, the 95% CI, the 5th and 95th centile, 2.5 SDs, the min/max, or something else? Do not belabor the explanation, but make sure no reader will sit there wondering, "What does that line there indicate?" The legend should enable the readers to translate all the visual elements of your graph into concepts and numbers that they can think about further. Indeed, that is the main purpose of the legend. It is not necessary though to repeat anything clearly marked in the figure itself.

Although many people will look at figures and tables without reading the rest of the paper, the legends should not be written under the assumption that people are not reading the rest of the paper. If someone does not understand the figures or tables correctly because he or she is not reading the full paper, then he or she has no one to blame but himself or herself. In particular, a figure legend should not repeat or

© Springer Nature Switzerland AG 2019
M. Hanna, *How to Write Better Medical Papers*,
https://doi.org/10.1007/978-3-030-02955-5_20

elaborate on the methods; [1 (p. 58)] that information belongs in the Methods section. Legends should be written for the people who are in the process of reading the full paper. Legends should not repeat information found elsewhere in the paper, because this makes them too long and tedious for all the good readers who are reading the full paper.

Good legends enable the readers to make sense of the information being shown in the table or figure. They do not consume the readers' time and mental energy repeating information in the main text, nor do they provide additional information that is inconsistent with the main text. Good legends just quickly explain, at the most basic level, what is being shown. And then they stop, so the readers can look at the actual table or figure instead.

Reference

1. Cleveland WS. The Elements of Graphing Data. Murray Hill, NJ, USA: AT&T Bell Laboratories; 1994.

Part III
Drafting

Chapter 21
Ethics of Scientific Writing

Introduction

Scientific writing is the process of putting information and thinking into a final permanent report, so it can be read and used by other people. For any given research study, there are innumerable various ways to legitimately write that report (depending on what exactly the authors want to say and how). But readers expect that each journal paper corresponds appropriately to the research reported. The amount of writing published about a research study should correspond appropriately to the amount and value of the actual research performed, and the writing about that research should be original, scientific, and truthful. Ethical problems arise whenever there is a gross disconnection between the writing activity of the authors and the actual research they have done. So ethical scientific writing involves several issues: 1) avoiding plagiarism – the copying of someone else's expressions or ideas, 2) writing a report that is accurate and unbiased, 3) maintaining patient confidentiality, 4) not writing too many papers from a research study – so-called "salami publication", and 5) not failing to actually write-up and publish a peer-reviewed journal paper about a completed study.

No Plagiarism

Plagiarism is the copying of someone else's expressions. Traditionally, it has been considered, along with fabrication and falsification (discussed in chapter 11), as one of the three major forms of research misconduct [1–3]. (Recent scholarship on research misconduct has displaced that traditional triplet with more useful taxonomies [3–6], but plagiarism is still viewed as serious misconduct.) Plagiarism usually refers to copying texts written by someone else or "borrowing" their underlying ideas, but it can also refer to copying their graphs, images, or other forms of expression. Plagiarism is a serious offense, and it can be sufficient grounds for retracting

© Springer Nature Switzerland AG 2019
M. Hanna, *How to Write Better Medical Papers*,
https://doi.org/10.1007/978-3-030-02955-5_21

a published article [1, 7, 8]. Indeed, it seems that a much greater portion of journals are explicitly concerned about plagiarism or duplicate publication than about data fabrication or falsification [9], perhaps because the publishers of the journals view plagiarism and duplicate publication as infringing directly on their business interests.

In chapter 2, it was asserted that all research misconduct has one of three vices as its root cause: ignorance, laziness, or greed. This explanation is clearly applicable to plagiarism. Some people (mostly students) plagiarize because they do not know it is serious misconduct or because they do not fully understand how to properly cite other works or otherwise avoid it [10 (pp. 191–192, 195)]. Other people (mostly early career researchers with poor motivations for being in research) are aware that they should not plagiarize but do it anyway, in order to reduce the amount of work they do to generate publications. And finally some people (mostly well-established researchers) plagiarize other people's work (especially unpublished cutting-edge ideas) to try to grab more resources (especially grants) for themselves. Whatever the cause of plagiarism, the consequence is that whenever someone is plagiarizing, he or she is failing to contribute anything new and instead is just taking credit for someone else's contributions. Plagiarism is essentially a form of theft of intellectual property – and the social recognition and material rewards that are received for that intellectual property [10 (pp. 196, 197, 275–276), 11, 12]. Interestingly, disdain for plagiarists appears to be deeply rooted in human beings' way of viewing the world; it is not something artificial first learned in the university. Clever studies have shown that children as young as 6 years old express less approval of "copy-cats" [13, 14].

It has sometimes been asserted that researchers who are not native speakers of English need to copy other people's papers in order to express themselves in good English [15, 16]. That argument is pathetic rubbish [17]. Although it does usually require more time and effort to write in a foreign language than one's native language, that is no excuse for stealing someone else's work. And there is no validity to anyone's claims that they are less capable of originally expressing their own ideas and/or less capable of upholding high ethical standards, simply because they grew up speaking some language other than English. *Au contraire*, people who speak English as a second (or third or fourth or fifth) language are oftentimes *more* capable of expressing their own thoughts in their own words than are native speakers of English, because people who learn a second language become consciously aware of the medium of language that we all use to communicate our thoughts. (And for that reason among many others, everyone should learn at least one other non-native language.) Several people who were not native speakers of English became famous for literary works they wrote in English – Joseph Conrad, Joseph Brodsky, Jack Kerouac, Chinua Achebe, V.S. Naipaul, Arthur Koestler, Salman Rushdie, Kahlil Gibran, Vladimir Nabakov, and many others.

Never copy phrases or sentences from another source without citing that source. It is equally illegitimate to copy a sentence while replacing words with other synonyms to try to hide the copying. In that scenario, the plagiarist is still copying something that someone else wrote, and stealing credit for that person's thoughts behind the specific word choices. When you are drafting your papers, look inside your own head, and figure out what it is *you* want to say. If you need to, talk aloud to yourself or to someone else, to help you figure out what you want to say. When you think you know what you want to say, type it – in your own words. If you find yourself getting stuck at the keyboard, make an audio recording of yourself talking (either to yourself or to someone else), and then type it later from the audio recording. Don't worry about how good it is. It is only a first draft. You can revise and edit it later.

If you can speak your own thoughts in English, you can also write your own thoughts in English, without plagiarizing someone else's text. But if you find it difficult to express yourself in English as a foreign language, just write the first draft of your paper in your own native language. Then you can also publish it in a journal of your own native language. Or if you really want to publish your paper in English, you can translate it into English (or have someone else translate it for you). Indeed, you can even do both: publish your paper first in your own native language, and then publish a translation in English. Just be sure to tell the journal Editors when you submit the manuscripts about the other version in the other language.

When you do finally have something written down, if you know someone else has already said something similar, put a citation to their work at the end of your sentence. However, there is probably no need to try to cite multiple "sources", if you are writing something generic (e.g. "The study was designed as a randomized controlled trial") or if you are writing something that has already been said so many times that it has become common knowledge (e.g. "The limbic system regulates emotions"). But even in these cases, do not copy anything from a specific source; write what you want to say in your own words without using someone else's text as a model.

If you need to use material from another work, charges of plagiarism can be avoided by citing the source that you are summarizing. If you are quoting the exact words that were written by someone else, you should put their copied words inside quotation marks and cite your sources in the references. Yet the use of such direct quotations is rare in medical science. Direct quotations are usually only used in medical science if: A) the source quoted is a higher authority (e.g. a government report or an official document from a professional society) and consequently it is important to use their exact wording, or B) the source text is being quoted in order to emphasize and discuss the way those original authors worded their ideas (e.g. disputing their way of talking about the topic). Otherwise, the preferred standard approach in medical science to cite someone else's text is to summarize (or at least paraphrase) their text, without quotation marks, and cite the reference. Typically this means writing just one sentence to summarize an entire paper.

Completeness and Balance

Research reports must be accurate, complete, and reasonably balanced [18]. In other words, errors, omissions, or bias are not merely low-quality work, they are viewed as unethical, just as carelessly providing sub-standard care to patients would also be viewed as unethical, not merely as low-quality medical services [19]. If you feel unable to write a research report that is accurate, complete, and reasonably balanced, seek out further education and/or training before continuing with research. Accuracy can usually be achieved almost completely by double-checking and triple-checking every detail of everything you do, and then checking it again a few more times, and then asking a few other people to do the same. Completeness is much easier to achieve – just do not intentionally exclude anything that could be considered important. Writing a paper that is reasonably balanced can be somewhat more difficult to judge. It does not require writing something that is neutral or agnostic about the topic. Researchers often have viewpoints about their topics, and these are a valuable component of scientific progress. But writing reasonably balanced reports requires thinking seriously about other competing interpretations of your results and other viewpoints and arguments about the topic.

Patient Confidentiality

Your research report must maintain the confidentiality of the patients' identities and/or obtain their permission to publish the information, depending on the details of the content. Any photographs of a patient that might enable someone to identify him or her must be masked to the extent possible and require the patient's written permission to publish. Published radiographic images should not contain the patient's name or date of birth on them, as they often do in routine clinical practice. Case reports or other narrative accounts of a patient's medical condition or treatment history usually also require the patient's written consent to publish.

Avoid Salami

Researchers are encouraged to avoid so-called "salami publication", which evokes the image of slicing a stick of salami into thin layers. "Salami publication" refers to the practice of unnecessarily dividing up the results of a study into two or more papers, for the main purpose of publishing more papers from a fixed amount of results [20, 21]. The consequence is that each paper contains less substantial content and readers have less information if they do not obtain and read the other papers. There may often be legitimate reasons to publish more than one paper from a study [21, 22], especially for major studies or if the target audiences are very different: for example, a multinational randomized controlled trial on a new treatment might yield one paper on the clinical outcomes for care-providers and another on the economic aspects for policy-makers. If instead the papers could be sensibly published all together but the investigators simply want to get more publications out of the study, then they are engaging in salami publication. Salami publication is not inherently unethical, but it is discouraged as a self-interested low-quality approach to reporting research [23, 24]. Journals usually also view it as wasteful of their resources [20, 24, 25]. And if readers and journal Editors are not clearly informed about the related papers, then salami publication is deceptive and unethical [25]. (If researchers report substantially overlapping data in two or more manuscripts or papers, then what they are doing is not "salami publication", but "redundant publication" – a more unethical issue discussed later in the chapter on the ethics of publication.) Although the term "salami publication" refers to publishing, the problem actually arises during the writing of a study (or even earlier during the planning of the writing). So whenever you are writing a first draft of your research, it is preferable to pack as much of the results as sensible into just one paper. Do not try to divide up your results from the outset, unless there are clear justifications inherent in the contents. Always inform the readers and journal Editors of any other related publications or manuscripts in preparation.

The Ethical Obligation to Write and Publish

Finally, if you conduct research, you have an ethical obligation to write it up and publish it. The ethical obligation to write up and publish the research is usually incurred because most researchers say they will conduct the research according to ethical guidelines and those guidelines usually state that the researchers are obliged to publish the research [18]. But in any case, the ethical obligation to write up and publish the research is essentially an implicit obligation or debt to the people (or the animals) that participated in the research and to the people who paid the costs of the research. Unless there is a scientifically legitimate explanation, failure to write up and publish a research study means that the efforts and risks of the participants (or the lives of animal subjects) and the funders' financial resources have gone to waste [26–28]. Failure to publish the research would be a betrayal of their trust and support.

It does not matter if the results were negative or inconclusive. All research should be published, regardless of the results or conclusions, to prevent publication bias from distorting the overall sum of evidence available in the literature [29–32]. The only exception is when the research had problems that were sufficiently substantial to render the results not publishable, from a scientific viewpoint.

"Publication" here means some kind of peer-reviewed report in an indexed journal, (or in some special cases in a book). The obligation to publish research is not fulfilled by publishing a conference abstract, self-posting a webpage or other internet document, or publishing in a periodical that is not peer-reviewed and indexed. (Nonetheless, some of those actions might preclude subsequent publication at many peer-reviewed journals – especially if the copyright has already been transferred to a third party.) It is generally accepted that research conducted for an academic degree need not be published beyond whatever the university requires, (though it remains questionable why not).

Unfortunately, many studies are never published, simply because the investigators run out of time, budget, and/or interest [33–36]. But those are not really ethically legitimate reasons to not write up and publish a study; they are more akin to poor excuses for leaving debts unpaid. Such researchers should not undertake any new research, until they have published all the valid data that they already have.

Conclusion

The ethical issues that arise during the writing phase – plagiarism, incomplete or biased reporting, failure to maintain patient confidentiality, "salami" publication, and non-publication are quite different from each other. Yet what they all have in common is disregard for the community of readers and failure to understand writing as a social service for that community. Think of it this way. Non-publication is a like a party guest who sits silently in a corner refusing to talk with anyone else. "Salami" publication is like someone who hogs the conversation by talking endlessly in detail about one small event. Incomplete or biased reporting is like someone who spins fisherman's tales that lead people astray about what actually happened. And plagiarism is like someone who, instead of adding something new to the dinner conversation, merely repeats what someone else just said ten minutes ago. So when writing your papers, try to keep an image in mind of the readers for whom you are writing. Then remember that writing is a social service you are performing for those readers, to share your new knowledge with them. They want you to be a good conversationalist. Writing is not merely the task of typing words on a computer to finish an assignment. Writing serves to communicate truthfully and socially with other human beings.

References

1. Office of Research Integrity – Office of Public Health and Science – U.S. Department of Health and Human Services. Managing Allegations of Scientific Misconduct: A Guidance Document for Editors. Rockville, MD, USA: U.S. Department of Health and Human Services; 2000. Accessed on 24 October 2017 at: https://ori.hhs.gov/images/ddblock/masm_2000.pdf
2. ALLEA – All European Academies. The European Code of Conduct for Research Integrity, Revised Edition. Berlin: ALLEA; 2017. Accessed on 5 November 2017 at: www.allea.org/wp-content/uploads/2017/04/ALLEA-European-Code-of-Conduct-for-Research-Integrity-2017.pdf
3. Organisation for Economic Co-Operation and Development, Global Science Forum. Best Practices for Ensuring Scientific Integrity and Preventing Misconduct. Accessed on 13 January 2018 at: www.oecd.org/science/inno/40188303.pdf
4. Fanelli D. How Many Scientists Fabricate and Falsify Research? A Systematic Review and Meta-Analysis of Survey Data. PLoS One. 2009; 4: e5738.
5. Council of Science Editors. CSE's White Paper on Promoting Integrity in Scientific Journal Publications, 2012 Update, 3rd Revised Edition. Wheat Ridge, CO: Council of Scientific Editors; 2012.

6. Smith R. Time to face up to research misconduct. BMJ. 1996; 312: 789-790.
7. International Committee of Medical Journal Editors. Recommendations for the Conduct, Reporting, Editing, and Publication of Scholarly Work in Medical Journals. Philadelphia: American College of Physicians; 1978, 2017. Accessed on 12 January 2018 at: www.icmje. org/icmje-recommendations.pdf
8. Amos KA. The ethics of scholarly publishing: exploring differences in plagiarism and duplicate publication across nations. J Med Lib Assoc. 2014; 102: 87-91.
9. Bosch X, Hernández C, Pericas JM, Doti P, Marušić A. Misconduct Policies in High-Impact Biomedical Journals. PLoS One. 2012; 7: e51928.
10. Booth WC, Colomb GC, Williams JM. The Craft of Research, 3rd ed. Chicago: University of Chicago Press; 1995, 2008.
11. Rosselot Jaramillo E, Bravo Lechat M, Kottow Lang M, Valenzuela Yuraidini C, O'Ryan Gallardo M, Thambo Becker S, Horwitz Campos N, Acevedo Pérez I, Rueda Castro L, Angélica Sotomayor M. En referencia al plagio intelectual: Documento de la Comisión de Ética de la Facultat de Medicina de le Universidad de Chile. Rev Méd Chil. 2008; 136: 653-658.
12. Maddox J. Plagiarism is worse than mere theft. Nature. 1995; 376: 721.
13. Olson KR, Shaw A. 'No fair, copycat!': what children's response to plagiarism tells us about their understanding of ideas. Dev Sci. 2011; 14: 431-439.
14. Yang F, Shaw A, Garduno E, Olson KR. No one likes a copycat: A cross-cultural investigation of children's response to plagiarism. J Exp Child Psychol. 2014; 121: 111-119.
15. Yilmaz I. Plagiarism? No, we're just borrowing better English. Nature. 2007; 449: 658.
16. Vessal K, Habibzadeh F. Rules of the game of scientific writing: fair play and plagiarism. Lancet. 2007; 369: 641.
17. Afifi M. Plagiarism is not fair play. Lancet. 2007; 369: 1428.
18. World Medical Association. Declaration of Helsinki – Ethical Principles for Medical Research Involving Human Subjects. Accessed on 10 January 2018 at: https://www.wma.net/policies-post/ wma-declaration-of-helsinki-ethical-principles-for-medical-research-involving-human-subjects/
19. Altman DG. The scandal of poor medical research. BMJ. 1994; 308: 283-284.
20. Abraham P. Duplicate and salami publications. J Postgrad Med. 2000; 46: 67-69.
21. Kassirer JP, Angell M. Redundant Publication: A Reminder. NEJM. 1995; 333: 449-450.
22. Bennie MJ, Lim CW. Salami publication. BMJ. 1992; 304: 1314.
23. Rogers LF. Salami Slicing, Shotgunning, and the Ethics of Authorship. Am J Roentgenol. 1999; 173: 265.
24. Huth EJ. Irresponsible Authorship and Wasteful Publication. Ann Intern Med. 1986; 104: 257-259.
25. The cost of salami slicing. Nat Mat. 2005; 4: 1.
26. Chalmers I, Glasziou P. Avoidable waste in the production and reporting of research evidence. Lancet. 2009; 374: 86-89.
27. MacCallum CJ. Reporting Animal Studies: Good Science and a Duty of Care. PLoS Biol. 2010; 8: e1000413.
28. Frank E. Publish or perish: the moral imperative of journals. CMAJ. 2016: 188: 675.
29. The PLoS Medicine Editors. An Unbiased Scientific Record Should Be Everyone's Agenda. PLoS Med. 2009; 6: 0119-0121.
30. Rosenthal R. The "File Drawer Problem" and Tolerance for Null Results. Psychol Bull. 1979; 86: 638-641.
31. Guyatt GH, Oxman AD, Montori V, Vist G, Kunz R, Brozek J, Alonso-Coello P, Djulbegovic B, Atkins D, Falck-Ytter Y, Williams JW Jr., Meerpohl J, Norris SL, Akl EA, Schünemann HJ. GRADE guidelines: 5. Rating the quality of evidence—publication bias. J Clin Epidemiol. 2011; 64: 1277-1282.
32. Chalmers TC, Frank CS, Reitman D. Minimizing the Three Stages of Publication Bias. JAMA. 1990; 263: 1392-1395.
33. von Elm E, Costanza MC, Walder B, Tramèr MR. More insight into the fate of biomedical meeting abstracts: a systematic review. BMC Med Res Methodol. 2003; 3: 12.

34. Weber EJ, Callaham ML, Wears RL, Barton C, Young G. Unpublished Research from a Medical Specialty Meeting: Why Investigators Fail to Publish. JAMA. 1998; 280: 257-259.
35. Sprague S, Bhandari M, Devereaux PJ, Swiontkowski MF, Tornetta P III, Cook DJ, Dirschl D, Schemitsch EH, Guyatt GH. Barriers to Full-Text Publication Following Presentation of Abstracts at Annual Orthopaedic Meetings. J Bone Joint Surg Am. 2003; 85-A: 158-163.
36. Smith MA, Barry HC, Williamson J, Keefe CW, Anderson WA. Factors Related to Publication Success Among Faculty Development Fellowship Graduates. Fam Med. 2009; 41: 120-125.

Chapter 22
The Introduction

The Introduction is a crucial part of every paper for four reasons. First, the Introduction serves to draw the readers into the paper, gradually orienting them to what this paper is really about. Second, the Introduction serves to frame the research that will be presented later in the paper. In other words, the Introduction provides a set of issues and meanings that the authors implicitly ask the readers to consider when assessing and interpreting the actual data. Third, the Introduction makes it clear why this research is important to read about. Fourth, the Introduction lets the readers know whether the paper will be engaging or boring to read. If the Introduction is confusing or dull, the readers will assume that the rest of the paper is also. They will then switch to skimming mode or jump to the conclusion and then put the paper down.

Unfortunately, many researchers sabotage their paper by leaving the Introduction underdeveloped or poorly utilized. Often they only write one short muddled paragraph, probably because they do not know what they should say in the Introduction. Most researchers seem unsure what to write in the Introduction, probably because there is comparatively little guidance about it in the literature and because general guidelines also provide rather thin information about the Introduction relative to other sections of the paper [1]. (Indeed, due to its empirical orientation, the scientific community in general seems to have a weak conception of what the Introduction is really for.) Some medical researchers, realizing that the Introduction ought to say something, write a long historical background or a summary of all the existing literature on the topic, neither of which is appropriate or useful. The Introduction should not be a history lesson (e.g. all the different treatments for a disease since 1883) and should not be a literature review of all past studies [2, 3].

Instead, the Introduction should lead the readers into the general topic, then lay out the set of specific problems that the scientific and/or healthcare community is trying to solve, and finally present the study that the authors conducted. Thus, the Introduction should normally have a beginning, a middle, and an end. For full-length papers, these three sections are normally one paragraph each [4], though the

© Springer Nature Switzerland AG 2019
M. Hanna, *How to Write Better Medical Papers*,
https://doi.org/10.1007/978-3-030-02955-5_22

middle might be longer, as discussed below. For shorter reports, these three sections still exist but are usually condensed into a single paragraph.

The beginning of the Introduction (i.e. the first paragraph for full-length papers) presents an overview of the *general topic*. It should be written as if the reader is someone far outside the authors' fields and knows little to nothing about the topic of the paper, (yet without being too tedious or pedantic for people who are in the field). Typically this paragraph or passage quickly defines and characterizes the disease or condition that is being studied, in very basic terms. It often presents background information on its epidemiology or economic dimension. The beginning of the Introduction should avoid saying anything complex or specialized. In a sense, it serves as a fast warm-up paragraph that situates the readers and lets them get comfortable with the paper, especially readers from other backgrounds. Yet the first paragraph is deceptively simple. Although it is written in a simple and clear way that anyone should be able to understand, the choices that the author makes about what exactly to say and how will have a profound influence on framing the rest of the paper and orienting the perspective of the readers. For example, an opening paragraph that matter-of-factly states the economic burden of treatment for a particular disease implicitly presents this economic dimension as a problem that needs to be addressed, and thereby creates a financial frame for all further information in the paper.

The middle of the Introduction (i.e. the second paragraph of full-length reports) serves to develop the *specific issue(s)* that this study will address. If the study is about a form of therapy, this paragraph or passage presents that therapy. If the paper is about some particular problem in medical care, this paragraph or passage explains what that problem is. If the paper is about some special group of patients, this paragraph or passage explains who they are and what their issue is. Normally, an integral part of this development is to summarize the relevant scientific literature on the subject. But the literature should not be summarized merely for its own sake, one paper after another, ("So-and-so et al. found that..... Other-person and colleagues found that.... Etc.") Instead, these passages should be explaining what the precise issue is, using citations and summaries of the literature to show that this specific issue really does exist and is not merely the authors' own opinions and imagination. In other words, the focus should be on the medical or scientific contents of those publications, not on the research studies or the papers themselves. It should provide the readers with a succinct awareness of what is already known about the topic. Equally important, it should also highlight what key points remain unknown. Yet when describing what remains unknown, you should always be careful to find recent publications stating that those points do in fact remain unknown; otherwise, whatever you are claiming remains unknown might often only be due to your own unfamiliarity with the recent literature [5]. Indeed, many papers have been entirely superfluous – addressing questions that had already been answered repeatedly and better in the previously published literature [1, 5–7]. While presenting the specific issue of the paper, the second paragraph or passage should also be explaining why it matters. It should make it clear what the real world stakes are and why a research study was needed on this topic.

As stated above, the Introduction always has a beginning, middle, and end, and three paragraphs is often sufficient for the Introduction of a full-length research paper. It is entirely permissible though to write more paragraphs if needed. More paragraphs in the middle might be necessary if the specific issue of the paper is complex or if the paper has several subtopics. For example, if the paper is about a clinical trial of a new drug in a subpopulation of patients that is refractory to conventional treatment, then it might be necessary to have three middle paragraphs instead of just one: one about the refractory subpopulation, another about the basic biological rationale underlying the novel therapy, and another about any previous clinical experience with this new drug. As can be seen in this example, these additional paragraphs would serve to lengthen the middle of the Introduction. If the Introduction is concise and coherent, the number of paragraphs does not matter; the three paragraph approach is simply a guide to ensure an adequate Introduction for full-length papers. Yet for research reports, it should never be necessary to use more than one paragraph for each the beginning and the end of the Introduction; it is only the middle that might need more.

The end of the Introduction (i.e. the last paragraph of a full-length report) serves to present the authors' research study. This paragraph or passage is usually brief and simple. It should summarize the type of study succinctly and generally, to make it clear to the readers what the study was. It should also state the aim of the study (or the aim of this specific paper, if multiple papers are being written from the same study). The study aim should not be a description of the study itself, (e.g. "The aim of our research was to report the rate of surgical complications in obese patients.") Instead, it should focus on the real world problem that you tried to illuminate, (e.g. "The aim of our research was to determine if obesity should be considered a relative contraindication to surgery for safety reasons.") If you conducted an experimental (i.e. laboratory) study, then you might state the hypothesis here, but hypotheses (which are more specific than study aims and also formulated in more statistical terms) are usually better placed in the Methods [1]. The final paragraph might also state what the researchers expected to find, prior to starting the research. But the Introduction should never present a summary of the study findings. Regrettably, many papers (especially in the life sciences) do summarize their findings toward the end of the Introduction, but that is unnecessary, unscientific, and uncollegial. It is unnecessary, because the findings were already summarized in the Abstract, which the readers just read 5 minutes ago. It is unscientific to summarize the findings in the Introduction, because this amounts to presenting the study outcomes before the readers have had the chance to examine the methods and assess the evidence. Thus it is also uncollegial, because it asks the readers to simply believe the authors, rather than using their own scientific education and experience to assess the veracity of the new knowledge presented. For all these same reasons, the Introduction should also not state any conclusion [8]. The final paragraph of the Introduction should limit itself to summarizing the nature of the study and the aims of the paper. Need be, it may elaborate on these points, but it should not jump ahead to presenting results or conclusions [9].

The study aims are in some sense the culmination of the Introduction. They truly do introduce the rest of the paper, by stating what the purpose or goal of the research was. The study aims should always be quite clear to the researchers, and furthermore special care should be given to formulating them. But strangely, many researchers write muddled study aims or too many of them, as if they were not really sure why they were doing their research. Every scientific paper should have one clear question that it aims to answer [2, 4, 9–11]. Although the study aim is normally formulated as a statement, not as a question, it should always be possible to say that the aim of the study was to provide an answer to the question "X". That is why we do research – to find answers to questions we have. If your study aim cannot be reformulated as a question (or if it is uninteresting as a question), then something is wrong – probably you are trying to report data without really knowing why. Some papers try to state more than one study aim, but usually this reflects a lack of mental focus by the authors more than a justified need to report on multiple study aims in one paper. If you find yourself drafting more than two or three study aims, you are going astray – probably you are trying to present too many different results in the same paper or you are formulating your study aims in the wrong way. If you have two or three study aims, but one of them seems clearly more important to you than the other(s), then the most important one is your study aim. Any other "secondary" study aims are probably not really study aims; they are probably only descriptions of other aspects of your results that you want to report. "Secondary study aims" should be either clearly labeled as such or not mentioned at all. If instead, you have two or three study aims that all seem equally important to you, then you might be formulating your study aims too specifically. Try to write one single study aim that encompasses everything you are trying to say with your two or three study aims. If you cannot formulate a single overarching study aim, then your paper probably lacks sufficient focus and unity. In that case, you would probably be better off writing two or three separate papers, each one focused on a specific question or aim. You should consider how the paper might be cut up into two or more papers, each with separate aims; (while still be careful to avoid "salami" publication). Of course, formulating a good study aim requires understanding why the research was actually conducted.

Many scientists are very good at the actual research that they do but not so good at understanding and explaining the relevance of the research they are doing. In other words, they know *what* they are doing, but they do not really know *why* they are doing it or why anyone outside their own specialty should care. Medicine exists to improve the health of real people, so medical research is always to some degree or other an applied science. Although medical researchers do experience scientific curiosity and pure wonder about the human body and health, ultimately all medical research is conducted to solve the problem of human illness. So when writing a paper, researchers should ask themselves, "What exactly is the specific (health) problem in the real world that this study tries to help solve?" Most researchers could probably find a good answer to this simple question, if they spent some time thinking about it. But because many researchers are engrossed in the technical or clinical details of their work and rarely stop to think about and discuss the larger context around their research, the relevance of their research often remains opaque to most everyone else. So always take a step back from your research study, look at the larger real world, and ask yourself, "What exactly is the one problem that this study tries to help solve?" Writing a good Introduction requires thinking for awhile about something bigger than your own clinic or laboratory, something bigger than your numerical data. If the specific problem addressed by your research sounds unimportant to you, then your research has probably become too technically specialized or too academic [12–14]. Reading papers of public health or health policy may help to reopen your field of vision and see better where your research fits into the big picture.

The Introduction as a whole should accomplish four goals. First, the Introduction should demonstrate command of the field of relevant scientific literature within which your paper is situated. Scientific medical research is mostly not an act of individual creative genius; it is a collective undertaking to build up knowledge piece by piece. Accordingly, each study must take into account what is already known about the subject and build logically upon that. Although the Discussion will also make use of the literature (in a slightly different way), the Introduction is the place where the authors provide an account of the state of scientific knowledge prior to their research and how that led logically to the research they conducted. Indeed, the Introduction should make it clear that the question addressed in the present study had not already been sufficiently answered by past research, because superfluous research on living subjects is considered unethical [1]. If the Introduction fails to demonstrate command of the literature, readers will assume that the authors are not sufficiently familiar with the scientific work that has already been done on the topic, nor with the current debates and interests of the scientific community. Reading a large number of papers relevant to your topic is the indispensable prerequisite to being able to write an Introduction that demonstrates command of the literature. But then the Introduction should be very selective, not comprehensive in the papers it cites. Citing many papers without clear reasons does not work well. And the goal of the Introduction is certainly not to just demonstrate that the authors have read the literature, like doctoral candidates trying to prove their erudition. The Introduction should make thoughtful choices about which previous papers are most relevant for presenting the current topic and the state of best evidence. Moreover, those papers should not be discussed in detail in the Introduction. They should be quickly cited as support for steps in your own thinking about what was known on the topic and what else still needed to be studied and why. Thus the Introduction as a whole should leave no doubt in the readers' minds that the authors have read the relevant literature, thought seriously about it, and know how their study relates to the still unsolved issues.

Second, the Introduction as a whole should provide the readers with at least an approximate sense of how *probable* it was, prior to your study, that the research would yield positive evidence [15, 16]. For example, if your study was a clinical trial on medicine D for disease Q, the Introduction should provide the readers with some approximate sense of how probable it was that medicine D would be effective treatment for disease Q. If your study hypothesized XYZ, then the Introduction should provide the readers with some approximate sense of how probable it was that your study would support hypothesis XYZ. If previous studies have already provided evidence on your specific treatment or hypothesis, it may be nearly sufficient to summarize and synthesize their findings. Additionally, you would then just add another sentence stating how probable you felt it was that your study would also yield evidence supporting your form of treatment, hypothesis, or whatever. If there are no previous studies on the same treatment, hypothesis, or whatever, then you may need to provide more reasoning and explanations. For example, you might need to discuss the underlying biological basis for the treatment or hypothesis you were testing and then state, numerically, how probable you felt it was that your research would support that new treatment or hypothesis. If your study is not testing a specific treatment or hypothesis but instead is more broadly exploring a study aim, it should still be possible to have a sense of how likely it was to find or confirm whatever you were exploring. Thus by the end of the Introduction, the readers should have some approximate sense – to about the nearest 10% – of how probable it was that your study would have positive findings, and why it was that probable (or improbable). Regrettably, only very rarely do medical scientific papers really fulfill this goal so far, but doing this is epistemologically important for understanding how your results relate to and alter the prior state of knowledge.

Third, the Introduction as a whole should also elucidate what the relevance of the study is. It should explain how the study will shed light on the real world problem identified by the authors. It should make it clear why the readers should care what the results were. If the authors do not make this chain of associations (real world problem – this study – future improvements), then it will remain difficult for most readers to fully understand why the study was done and what would be the relevance of the findings [17, 18 (pp. 45–48)]. Instead, the research will seem like an academic exercise that was done merely because the authors have a university job to conduct research on whatever obscure topics landed on their desks [2, 12, 19, 20] or simply are trying to not "perish" [21, 22]. Your research does not need to be earth-shaking news, but whatever you are researching, you should be able to explain why it matters. This step is really a crucial part of writing a paper, because it will have major influence on journal Editors' and peer reviewers' assessment of the value of the paper [13, 14, 23–26]. One of the key questions that Editors and reviewers always ask themselves is: "How *relevant* is this paper?" The "relevance" of your research is how it will improve patient health (or save resources or otherwise improve the world). Editors and peer reviewers want to know what difference each paper will make in the health of real people. They do not expect every paper to be a groundbreaking cure for cancer, but they do want to see how the paper will make some small improvement in a real world issue. If the authors do not elucidate the relevance of their research, it will remain opaque, and readers will feel that the paper is *irrelevant*. So you should always think clearly about the larger context surrounding your research and explain why your study is relevant to the real world.

Fourth, the Introduction should get the readers engaged with the paper and put them in a favorable open-minded mood for reading the rest of the paper [27 (pp. 32–33, 112)]. Providing a clear explanation of the paper's topic and relevance, as described above, serves as the foundation for accomplishing this goal. Writing in a quick and simple style, as described below, also makes it easier for the readers to get engaged with the paper. Yet the Introduction should also convince the readers to take the authors' viewpoint and listen openly to what will be said in the rest of the paper. Care must be taken to not put the readers in a defensive, oppositional, or close-minded mood already in the Introduction. One of the most common ways that happens is when the Introduction makes it seem that the authors either already had a conclusion in mind before doing the research or they now want to sell the readers on their conclusions. Introductions that reveal such bias by the authors make many people read the paper more critically and argue back in their minds every paragraph from the very start. Another common way of making readers oppositional already in the Introduction is to come across as pompous or arrogant. Again, that puts many readers in the mood of wanting to show that the authors are not as smart as they pretend, and thus it makes the readers more critical. The Introduction should avoid these kinds of effects, and instead it should convince the readers to read the paper cooperatively. An Introduction that is too brief and underdeveloped is a lost opportunity to get the readers more engaged and favorably disposed before revealing the methods and results.

The writing style of the Introduction should be comparatively simple and fast-flowing. It is less ponderous than the Discussion, (and of course it does not involve the technicalities, numbers, and details seen in the Methods and Results). Since the Introduction serves to present the background and rationale for the study, it is something that should be readily comprehensible to most anyone reading the paper. The Introduction achieves this comparative simple and fast-flowing style mainly be using shorter and less complex sentences. It minimizes the use of technical vocabulary and numbers when possible. It quickly summarizes and cites literature without belaboring what those past papers said. The use of figures, tables, insert boxes, and so on is very rare but is acceptable if truly needed and relatively simple. Above all, the Introduction does not dwell for long on any one point or idea; each sentence moves forward to the next link in the chain of thinking. There should not be any useless or superfluous sentences that go astray on tangents or dig too deep into details. The Introduction should pursue a clear sequence of thoughts, one sentence after another. It should already be clear to you what that sequence of thoughts will be, if you carefully wrote an outline, (like you should have), as described in chapter 9.

In sum, the Introduction should not be written as a barrier wall that makes people stop reading the paper. It should be written in a style that quickly guides them into the paper and prepares them for what will follow. By the end of the Introduction, the readers should be engrossed in the paper and eager to read the rest of it.

References

1. Altman DG, Schulz KF, Moher D, Egger M, Davidoff F, Elbourne D, Gøtzsche PC, Lang T, for CONSORT Group. The Revised CONSORT Statement for Reporting Randomized Trials: Explanation and Elaboration. Ann Intern Med. 2001; 134: 663-694.
2. Elefteriades JA. Twelve Tips on Writing a Good Scientific Paper. Inter J Angiol. 2002; 11: 53-55.
3. Howie JW. How I read. BMJ. 1976; 2 (6044): 1113-1114.
4. Branson RD. Anatomy of a Research Paper. Respir Care. 2004; 49: 1222-1228.
5. Jones R, Scouller J, Grainger F, Lachlan M, Evans S, Torrance N. The scandal of poor medical research: Sloppy use of literature often to blame. BMJ. 1994; 308: 591.
6. Chalmers I, Glasziou P. Avoidable waste in the production and reporting of research evidence. Lancet. 2009; 374: 86-89.
7. Moher D, Hopewell S, Schulz KF, Montori V, Gøtzsche PC, Devereaux PJ, Elbourne D, Egger M, Altman DG. CONSORT 2010 Explanation and Elaboration: updated guidelines for reporting parallel group randomised trials. BMJ. 2010; 340: c869.
8. Sharp D. Kipling's Guide to Writing a Scientific Paper. Croat Med J. 2002; 43: 262-267.
9. Saper CB. Academic Publishing, Part III: How to Write a Research Paper (So That It Will Be Accepted) in a High-Quality Journal. Ann Neurol. 2015; 77: 8-12.
10. Morris JA. Theory must drive experiment. BMJ. 1994; 308: 592.
11. Sand-Jensen K. How to write consistently boring scientific literature. Oikos. 2007; 116: 723-727.
12. Rothwell PM. Medical academia is failing patients and clinicians. BMJ. 2006; 332: 863-864.
13. Groves T. Why submit your research to the BMJ. BMJ. 2007; 334: 4-5.
14. Lundberg GD, Paul MC, Fritz H. A Comparison of the Opinions of Experts and Readers as to What Topics a General Medical Journal (JAMA) Should Address. JAMA. 1998; 280: 288-290.
15. Burke JF, Sussman JB, Kent DM, Hayward RA. Three simple rules to ensure reasonably credible subgroup analyses. BMJ. 2015; 351: h5651.
16. Pharoah P. How Not to Interpret a *P* Value? JNCI. 2007; 99: 332-333.
17. Drotar D. Thoughts on Improving the Quality of Manuscripts Submitted to the Journal of Pediatric Psychology: Writing a Convincing Introduction. J Pediatr Psychol. 2009; 34: 1-3.
18. Booth WC, Colomb GC, Williams JM. The Craft of Research, 3rd ed. Chicago: University of Chicago Press; 1995, 2008.
19. Tallis RC. Researchers forced to do boring research... BMJ. 1994; 308: 591.
20. Hanna M. Solo scientists are not all hippies. Intelligent Life. 2008 (Winter); 2 (2): 14.
21. Altman DG. The scandal of poor medical research. BMJ. 1994; 308: 283-284.
22. Angell M. Publish or Perish: A Proposal. Ann Intern Med. 1986; 104: 261-262.
23. Making the most of peer review. Nat Neurosci. 2000; 3: 629.
24. Kassirer JP, Campion EW. Peer Review: Crude and Understudied, but Indispensable. JAMA. 1994; 272: 96-97.
25. Pierson DJ. The Top 10 Reasons Why Manuscripts Are Not Accepted for Publication. Respir Care. 2004; 49: 1246-1252.
26. Marcus E. A New Year and a new Era for *Cell*. Cell. 2004; 116: 1-2.
27. Aristotle. On Rhetoric. [Translated from the Ancient Greek by Kennedy GA.] Oxford: Oxford University Press; (ca. 355 BCE), 2007.

Chapter 23
The Methods

Many researchers do not put much thought and effort into writing the Methods section, because they assume that most readers will skip over it anyway. While unfortunately this is often the case, the Methods section is still important, because the people who do read it will use it to judge the quality of the research. For experimental research, they may even use it to try to verify the results by replicating the study. Above all, peer reviewers often scrutinize the Methods section to find flaws in the research that will require revision or justify rejection [1, 2]. If the Methods section is weak or confusing, readers will view the results as unreliable. And a sloppy or senseless Methods section reflects sloppy or senseless research. So it is important to write the Methods section as rigorously as you conducted the actual research.

Ideally, you should draft the Methods section before you even start the research, as part of your study proposal or protocol. This will enable you to see clearly what your research will look like to the eyes of your readers. You should ask yourself what are the flaws, limitations, or shortcomings of this research. You should ask yourself how the methods could be improved. Is your study designed properly? Will your study have sufficient statistical power? Are you using the best outcome measures to address your study questions? Is your statistical plan appropriate? And so on. You and your co-authors should spend time scrutinizing your draft of the Methods section in the study protocol and should do everything possible to improve your methodology *before* you start the research. The Methods section is really the only part of a paper that cannot be substantially improved after the research has been done, so it is the one part of the manuscript that must be done right from the outset to avoid unsolvable major criticisms from reviewers.

Nonetheless, when it is time to write your final paper, it is best to first write the Methods section anew, without looking at your earlier study protocol or proposal. If you merely copy your earlier study protocol or proposal, you may introduce errors into the paper, because the methods may have been altered since that earlier document was written (even though they should not have been). After you have a new first draft of your Methods section, you can compare it to your earlier study

© Springer Nature Switzerland AG 2019
M. Hanna, *How to Write Better Medical Papers*,
https://doi.org/10.1007/978-3-030-02955-5_23

protocol or proposal, to make sure you did not make any mistakes or omit important information.

For full-length reports, most medical journals use a Methods section that is structured into subsections with subheadings. There are no absolute fixed rules about these subsections; you may choose whichever ones you need to present the relevant information on your study. Reporting guidelines are now available for most types of studies [3, 4], and those guidelines provide good indications about the most essential subsections of the Methods. It can also be helpful to look at several papers in your target journal with similar topics or designs, to see which subsections are in common use. Typically, a clinical paper might contain the following subsections: Ethics, Study Design, Subjects, Interventions (or "Treatment"), Outcome Measures, Statistical Analysis. Whichever subsections you use in the Methods, they should be presented in a logical order, which most often is their chronological sequence.

Thus the first subsection should be the one on Ethics, because of course none of the research should be done before the ethics have been squared away. Many papers omit the subsection on Ethics and simply throw this information in elsewhere or skip it altogether. But that is a sign of a low-quality Methods section. Most well-written papers in high-quality journals will have a separate subsection on Ethics, so your papers should too. The Ethics subsection is usually brief and to the point. At a minimum, it should have one sentence on who (which Research Ethics Committee) approved the study or determined that it was exempt from review, including any date or number assigned to that decision [5]. If the study was registered in a study registry, the paper should state which registry, the date of registration, and the registration number; (if the Methods contains a "Reporting" subsection as described below, information about study registration is better placed there). If informed consent was obtained from the study subjects, the Ethics subsection should state whether it was written or oral, and whether it was for participating in research or merely for the medical treatment. If any specific laws or ethical guidelines (such as the World Medical Organization's Declaration of Helsinki [6]) were explicitly reread and followed by all members of the research team, that should also be stated [5]. You should not cite any such guidelines or laws that you did not really read, reflect upon, and apply to your research.

Next, the Methods should have a subsection on the Study Design. Many papers omit this subsection too and simply throw this information in elsewhere. But again, that is a sign of a low-quality Methods section; most well-written papers will have a separate subsection for the Study Design, even if it is brief. This subsection should succinctly describe the design, using standard terminology (e.g. "prospective", "retrospective", "multicenter", "randomized", "single-blind", "cross-over", "cross-sectional", "cohort study", "survey", "mouse model", "pilot study", and so on) [7]. The timepoints for follow-up data collection can be stated here in the subsection on Study Design, if that information is simple and does not require specifying which types of data were collected at which timepoints. Otherwise, it is probably better to explain that later in a subsection on Data Collection.

For clinical and observational studies, the Methods should also describe the study setting, so readers can determine how applicable the study is to their own practice. The Study Setting subsection describes the kind of place where the research was conducted, in terms of the type of institution (e.g. "large university hospital", "small outpatient clinic"), level of care (i.e. general population, primary care, secondary care, etc.), financial accessibility (i.e. public vs. private), and the kind of geographic region from which that institution draws its patients (e.g. "rural European town", "large Asian city", and so on) [8, 9].

As discussed in chapter 14 ("Statistics: Common Mistakes"), researchers should always perform a sample size estimate or power analysis prior to starting the research, in order to estimate how much data is actually needed. Regrettably, only a minority of studies actually do this, and most of them fail to report it. Without this information, it is difficult to know whether statistically non-significant results are reliably negative or only reflect an inadequate sample size. So if you performed a sample size estimate or power analysis (as you should have), then your Methods should have a subsection (e.g. "Sample Size Planning") succinctly reporting those calculations [8, 9], especially if your main outcomes were not statistically significant. This subsection would typically report your expectations for the main outcomes, the resulting effect size sought, the α and β values used, and any adjustments to the target sample size to account for anticipated loss to follow-up or missing data. If no such power analysis was performed, then any information about the intended sample size may simply be reported in the subsection on Subjects. In any case, the Methods should not discuss the actual final sample size; (that belongs in the Results); the Methods should only discuss the intended minimum sample size. The Methods section should also not report any post hoc power calculations made from the actual data; those should be reported in the Results.

Next, there is normally a subsection on the Subjects. This subsection should explain clearly where, when, and how you recruited your subjects and the eligibility criteria for participation. Many researchers report here how many subjects were actually screened, excluded, and enrolled, and sometimes also their basic demographic characteristics such as sex and age, but all that is inappropriate for medical research. Any information that could not be known before the study was started should instead be presented in the Results (except for the selection of statistical tests, or other purely methodological decisions made after data collection) [5]. Instead, the Methods subsection for Subjects should focus on the methodological aspects: the eligibility criteria and the approach to recruiting [8–10]. If your paper reports an experimental study (on animals for example), then your study protocol probably did specify exactly how many subjects would be included and what their characteristics had to be. In that case, it is appropriate to report that information here in the Methods. But any further data that was determined only after selecting those subjects (animals or otherwise) should still be reported in the Results, not in the Methods.

The further types of subsections in the Methods become more variable here, depending on the topic and contents of the research. But most often the next subsection is about the "Treatment" or "Interventions". This subsection should explain clearly but succinctly what you actually did (for example, the medical treatment you provided). If your interventions (or aspects of them) are already well-known among practitioners, you should remain as brief as possible when summarize them. You do not need to explain at length anything that can be found in every introductory medical textbook; it is sufficient to provide a very brief summary and citations to those textbooks or past papers. Nonetheless, your summary of any medical treatment should provide exact details on the dosage, frequency, means of administration, and so on, with sufficient detail that someone else could provide the exact same treatment. If other imaginable accompanying treatments were prohibited or permitted, you should state that too.

The "Outcome Measures" subsection should explain which kinds of data you collected and how you measured them. Try to use and prioritize direct outcome measures that are comprehensibly relevant to the patients themselves. Whenever possible, avoid or subordinate any indirect outcomes, i.e. surrogate variables or physiological measurements that are not directly experienced by the patients and thus are only relevant to healthcare professionals and researchers [11]. This subsection should make it clear how all the variables in the database were coded (or the units in which they were measured) [12, 13]. In prospective clinical trials, this subsection should specify which variable(s) was considered the main outcome vs. which were secondary outcomes [8]. If the variables were measured at multiple timepoints, the Methods should specify which timepoint was considered the main outcome. If you used questionnaires, you should provide a brief description of them (number of items, types of contents, types of answer possibilities, number of scales, possible score ranges, etc.) for readers who are not familiar with those instruments. You should also cite any relevant literature about the validation, translation, or statistical properties of those questionnaires. If your outcome measures involved ratings by clinicians or other experts, you should specify what their qualifications were, whether they were blinded to study conditions or purposes, and how disagreements between them were resolved [8]. If applicable, you should also explain how harms were monitored and assessed [14, 15]; clinical trials may even need an entire separate subsection of the Methods for this.

Depending on the contents of your research, you might need further subsections on specific types of outcomes, such as "Radiological Imaging", "Hematological Labwork", "Genetic Analyses", and so on. If so, these subsections should just describe which kinds of data were collected, how it was analyzed, and so on. Generally speaking, if some other specialist was involved in analyzing a particular kind of data, then you probably need a separate subsection in your Methods to explain those procedures. Indeed, those subsections are often drafted by those specialists who did that particular kind of data analysis. But again, there is no need to explain the details of well-established standard techniques that can be found in any medical textbook; it usually suffices to present brief summaries and references for those textbooks or previous papers.

Next, your paper might need a subsection on Data Collection. This could specify the timepoints at which different kinds of data were collected (e.g. the follow-up timepoints) and how the data were actually collected (e.g. paper forms, electronic questionnaires, nurses taking blood samples, etc.) Alternately or additionally, your paper might need a subsection on Database Preparation and/or Quality Control.

This subsection might specify how the data was entered into a database and how the dataset was checked for errors or audited for accuracy.

Finally, nearly all papers have a subsection on statistical analysis. This subsection should start by stating how missing data was handled (e.g. ignored, last observation carried forward, maximum likelihood estimation, multiple imputation, etc.), unless there was none [9, 16, 17]. Most researchers forget to do this, because they simply ignore missing data, which is surely the weakest way of dealing with missing data. If there was absolutely no missing data, that fact can be stated early in the Results somewhere. The "Statistical Analysis" subsection should then state which statistical tests you used and why you choose those tests (e.g. due to the types of variables being analyzed, the distribution of the data, etc.) Although many papers state the threshold p-value deemed statistically significant, that is a practice that should be abandoned, as explained in chapter 14 ("Statistics: Common Mistakes"). If space permits, it is not irrelevant to state which software you used for the statistical analysis, because different programs do sometimes come to slightly different outputs depending on their models and ways of handling data. Readers may also want to feel reassured that you used reliable statistical software.

Although almost no one does this yet, the Methods section should often end with a subsection "Reporting", placed after the subsection "Statistical Analysis". This subsection should name and cite any reporting guidelines that were read and followed (e.g. CONSORT). It should identify and cite any other publications or gray literature about the same study, such as trial registry entries, study protocols, conference abstracts, prior related publications, or translations; forthcoming publications should also be mentioned. Any other such information that is relevant to how the study has been written up and reported could also be placed in this subsection.

Researchers often wonder how much detail their Methods section needs, or what must be reported and what should be left out. One rough and dirty way to get an initial answer to this question is to just look at the word count of your Methods section compared to the total word limit set by your target journal in their Instructions to Authors. If you Methods section is more than about one-third of the total word count limit, you are probably reporting too many details (or writing them too wordily). On the other end, if your Methods is less than about one-fifth of the total word count limit, you are probably either not providing enough detail or are omitting important kinds of information altogether. However, looking at the word count is merely a rough initial guide; what really matters is the contents of what you wrote compared to the expectations of the scientific community. In that regards, the expectations are quite different, depending on whether your research was an experimental study versus a clinical or observational study.

Experimental studies aim to demonstrate causal relationships by showing that when someone does ABC under conditions LMN, the result is always XYZ. Experimental studies are not intended as descriptions of one-time real-world events that happened at a specific time and place. They are intended as timeless, placeless demonstrations of natural relationships between things, which can be repeated again and again, as often as anyone wants. Accordingly, an essential feature of experimental science is that other research teams must be able to repeat the same experiment at another time and place and obtain the same results, in order to verify the causal relationships. If they repeat the experiment but obtain different results, this is usually sufficient to invalidate the earlier study, or at least throw it into question. So if you are reporting an experimental study, you must report enough details of your Methods that another research group will obtain the same (or at least consistent) results if they replicate your research. If another research group cannot repeat your research because they are not sure what exactly you did, or if they obtain contradictory results because they had to guess about some details of your research, then your paper did not report enough details about its methods. The irreproducibility of vast amounts of experimental research has recently been recognized as a major problem in the life sciences [18–21]. So if you are reporting an experimental study, ask a few colleagues (who were not involved in your research) to read your Methods section and tell you if they believe they could repeat your experiment exactly enough to obtain the same results. If they do not believe they could, add the details that they say are lacking.

Clinical and observational studies, by contrast, follow different epistemological principles. They are studies conducted at a single specific time in history and a single specific place in the real world. No one will ever attempt to replicate them exactly. It would be impossible to control all the confounding variables in the real world anyway, so it would be futile to aim for such reproducibility in the clinical, health, and social sciences, as we do in the experimental sciences. Even if someone attempts to repeat a study but obtains contradictory results, this does not disprove the earlier study, the way it would for an experimental study. In clinical and observational research, evidence merely piles up, even if it is inconsistent or contradictory. Whereas the experimental sciences use replication in an attempt to obtain consistent results that demonstrate some inherent law of nature, the clinical, health, and social sciences instead use metanalysis and other forms of evidence synthesis to try to obtain a relatively reliable understanding of the way the *human* world usually works. Accordingly, there is no need in the clinical and health sciences to report all the nitty-gritty details of what exactly you did and how, because no one is ever going to try to repeat your research exactly and no one is interested in reading every last banal detail of how you did everything. But at a minimum, readers do need to know all the essential methodological features that might have had a noteworthy influence on your results or their meaning. So you should present your methods in enough detail that readers can understand what you did and can assess the validity of your results. If certain details about the methods would not really change your results or their meaning, then those details are probably irrelevant and should be skipped. Furthermore, your Methods section should report all the details that anyone would need to know if they wanted to include your research into a systematic review, meta-analysis, or other form of evidence synthesis *and grade the methodological quality of your evidence* [22]. So look at recent systematic reviews and metaanalyses in your area, and try to see which kinds of methodological information they examined, and what complaints they made about inadequate reporting. In sum, experimental studies need to report enough methodological detail to be *reproducible*, while clinical studies need to report enough methodological detail to be *synthesizable*. And both modes of research need to provide enough information about the methods that the readers can assess the validity and meaning of the results reported. But anything beyond that is unnecessary clutter that does not belong in a journal paper.

Regardless of whether you are reporting experimental or clinical research, if part of the methodology you used has been presented in an earlier publication, you can and should refer readers back to that earlier publication for the full explanation. Then you should present just a brief summary of those methods, so readers will not be lost if they do not read that earlier publication. If a study protocol is available somewhere, the paper should explicitly tell readers where they can access that protocol [8]. If the methods reported in the paper differ from the study protocol, the differences should be explained in the paper [8].

In the Methods section you can also present brief justifications and explanations. If you choose to do things one way rather than another, you should probably explain why you made that choice, especially if many researchers would have done it another way. If you used questionnaires, you should always briefly describe and explain them, because readers cannot be expected to be sufficiently familiar with all the hundreds of questionnaires that exist. If you used uncommon statistical methods, it is helpful to briefly explain and/or justify them, rather than expecting the readers to go consult a textbook of statistics or remain in the dark. Nonetheless, the Methods section is not the place to provide long defenses of your methodology, especially if you used suboptimal methods that reduce the validity of your results. That kind of longer defense of your Methods belongs in the Discussion section. Ideally, it is avoided altogether by improving your methods before you even start the research.

The Methods section is normally written in a matter-of-fact technical style. Its most characteristic feature is that it is usually written in the passive voice with the object of the action being the subject of the sentence (e.g. "The patients were randomly assigned to three study conditions" or "The test-tubes were centrifuged for two minutes"), not in the active voice with the subject of the action being the subject of the sentence (e.g. "We randomly assigned the patients to three study conditions" or "We centrifuged the test-tubes for two minutes"). Elsewhere, the passive voice is not preferable, but the rationale for using it in the Methods section is to put the readers' attention on what was actually done (e.g. "randomly assigned" or "centrifuged") and the objects to which it was done (e.g. "patients" or "test-tubes"), rather than on the doer (e.g. "We"). If you have a reason why you want to use the active voice in a specific sentence, you may, (e.g. to put the emphasis on why *you* chose to do something one way rather than another). Otherwise, just stick to the convention of using the passive voice in the Methods. Aside from that, the Methods section is written in a plain and simple way. Its goal is to transmit essential technical information, including all necessary details. The best way to do that is to state the information as directly and precisely as possible, without any unnecessary embellishment or complexity.

Overall, your Methods section should convince the readers that you have done rigorous research and that your results are reliable. That depends mainly on actually doing high-quality research in the first place, (which in turn depends on thoroughly thinking through everything that you will have to report later in your Methods section). But once the research is done, convincing readers that your results are reliable depends on writing up a rigorous Methods section. That requires presenting all the relevant technical details, concisely, in a logical order, without any additional fluff or useless information. If you do that, then readers will read your Results section with confidence that your findings are reliable.

References

1. Byrne DW. Common Reasons for Rejecting Manuscripts at Medical Journals: A Survey of Editors and Peer Reviewers. Sci Ed. 2000; 23 (2): 39-44.
2. Kassirer JP, Campion EW. Peer Review: Crude and Understudied, but Indispensable. JAMA. 1994; 272: 96-97.
3. Simera I, Altman DG. Writing a research article that is "fit for purpose": EQUATOR Network and reporting guidelines. Ann Intern Med. 2009; 151: JC2-2 to JC2-3.
4. Simera I, Moher D, Hoey J, Schulz KF, Altman DG. A catalog of reporting guidelines for health research. Eur J Clin Invest. 2010; 40: 35-53.
5. International Committee of Medical Journal Editors. Recommendations for the Conduct, Reporting, Editing, and Publication of Scholarly Work in Medical Journals. Philadelphia: American College of Physicians; 1978, 2017. Accessed on 12 January 2018 at: www.icmje.org/icmje-recommendations.pdf
6. World Medical Association. Declaration of Helsinki – Ethical Principles for Medical Research Involving Human Subjects. Accessed on 10 January 2018 at: https://www.wma.net/policies-post/wma-declaration-of-helsinki-ethical-principles-for-medical-research-involving-human-subjects/
7. Haynes RB, Mulrow CD, Huth EJ, Altman DG, Gardner MJ. More Informative Abstracts Revisited. Ann Intern Med. 1990; 113: 69-76.
8. Moher D, Hopewell S, Schulz KF, Montori V, Gøtzsche PC, Devereaux PJ, Elbourne D, Egger M, Altman DG. CONSORT 2010 Explanation and Elaboration: updated guidelines for reporting parallel group randomised trials. BMJ. 2010; 340: c869.
9. Vandenbroucke JP, von Elm E, Altman DG, Gøtzsche PC, Mulrow CD, Pocock SJ, Poole C, Schlesselman JJ, Egger M, for STROBE Initiative. Strengthening the Reporting of Observational Studies in Epidemiology (STROBE): Explanation and Elaboration. PLoS Med. 2007; 10: e297.
10. von Elm E, Altman DG, Egger M, Pocock SJ, Gøtzsche PC, Vandenbroucke JP, for the STROBE Initiative. The Strengthening the Reporting of Observational Studies in Epidemiology (STROBE) Statement: Guidelines for Reporting Observational Studies. Ann Intern Med. 2007; 147: 573-577.
11. Guyatt GH, Oxman AD, Kunz R, Woodcock J, Brozek J, Helfand M, Alonso-Coello P, Falck-Ytter Y, Jaeschke R, Vist G, Akl EA, Post PN, Norris S, Meerpohl J, Shukla VK, Nasser M, Schünemann HJ; GRADE Working Group. GRADE guidelines: 8. Rating the quality of evidence—indirectness. J Clin Epidemiol. 2011; 64: 1303-1310.
12. Bagley SC, White, H, Golomb BA. Logistic regression in the medical literature: Standards for use and reporting, with particular attention on one medical domain. J Clin Epidemiol. 2001; 54: 979-985.
13. Lunt M. Introduction to statistical modelling: linear regression. Rheumatology. 2015; 54: 1137-1140.
14. Ioannidis JPA, Mulrow CD, Goodman SN. Adverse Events: The More You Search, the More You Find. Ann Intern Med. 2006; 144: 298-300.

15. Ioannidis JPA, Evans SJW, Gøtzsche PC, O'Neill RT, Altman DG, Schulz K, Moher D; for CONSORT Group. Better Reporting of Harms in Randomized Trials: An Extension of the CONSORT Statement. Ann Intern Med. 2004; 141: 781-788.

16. Li T, Hutfless S, Scharfstein DO, Daniels MJ, Hogan JW, Little RJA, Roy JA, Law AH, Dickersin K. Standards should be applied in the prevention and handling of missing data for patient-centered outcomes research: a systematic review and expert consensus. J Clin Epidemiol. 2014; 67: 15-32.

17. Little RJ, D'Agostino R, Cohen ML, Dickersin K, Emerson SS, Farrar JT, Frangakis C, Hogan JW, Molenberghs G, Murphy SA, Neaton JD, Rotnitzky A, Scharfstein D, Shih WJ, Siegel JP, Stern H. The Prevention and Treatment of Missing Data in Clinical Trials. NEJM. 2012; 367: 1355-1360.

18. Landis SC, Amara SG, Asadullah K, Austin CP, Blumenstein R, Bradley EW, Crystal RG, Darnell RB, Ferrante RJ, Fillit H, Finkelstein R, Fisher M, Gendelman HE, Golub RM, Goudreau JL, Gross RA, Gubitz AK, Hesterlee SE, Howells DW, Huguenard J, Kelner K, Koroshetz W, Krainc D, Lazic SE, Levine MS, Macleod MR, McGall JM, Moxlex RT III, Narasimhan K, Noble LJ, Perrin S, Porter JD, Steward O, Unger E, Utz U, Silberberg SD. A call for transparent reporting to optimize the predictive value of preclinical research. Nature. 2012; 490: 187-191.

19. Marcus E. Credibility and Reproducibility. Cell. 2014; 159: 965-966.

20. Collins FS, Tabak LA. NIH plans to enhance reproducibility. Nature. 2014; 505: 612-613.

21. The long road to reproducibility. Nat Cell Biol. 2015; 17: 1513-1514.

22. GRADE Working Group. Grading quality of evidence and strength of recommendations. BMJ. 2004; 328: 1490.

Chapter 24
The Results

It seems that most researchers are already convinced that the Results section is an especially important part of their paper. After all, it is the part where they talk the most about their own work and the least about anything else, so it must be the most important part. Accordingly, many researchers simply present whatever they feel is interesting, in the way they feel is best. But the reality is a little bit different, requiring a bit more humility and social awareness. The Results section is indeed the only part of the paper where you are providing truly new information that no one else already knows, and therefore your Result section is increasing the amount of knowledge available to the scientific and healthcare communities. But if the Results section is somewhat more important than the other sections, the real reason is because the Results section is where most readers will form their judgment about what this particular paper adds to the existing body of knowledge already available in the scientific literature. Thus although you are the expert in your Results section, your role is more akin to that of an expert witness in a court trial, while the readers are the jury who may or may not give weight to your evidence. So it is crucial to write your Results section in a way that is clear, focused, comprehensible, and compelling for the readers.

To help you in that regards, most medical journals use a Results section that is structured into subsections with subheadings. There are no absolute fixed rules about these subsections; you may choose whichever ones you need to present the relevant information on your study. Reporting guidelines are now available for most types of studies [1, 2], and those guidelines provide some indications about important subsections of the Results. It can also be helpful to look at several papers in your target journal with similar topics or designs, to see which subsections are in common use. Typically, a clinical study might contain the following subsections: Data Collection, Study Sample, Main Outcomes, Secondary Outcomes, Harms. Whichever subsections you use, they should be presented in a logical order.

The very first subsection should be a brief presentation of the data completeness and accuracy. For a clinical trial, this would start with information about the number of patients screened, enrolled, assigned, treated, and then seen at follow-up [3].

© Springer Nature Switzerland AG 2019
M. Hanna, *How to Write Better Medical Papers*,
https://doi.org/10.1007/978-3-030-02955-5_24

A flowchart can be helpful if this information involves more than a half-dozen or so numbers [3–7]. If possible, present a brief analysis of whether excluded and/or non-participating subjects differed demographically or clinically from subjects enrolled in the study. Studies that were not clinical trials usually have some kind of analogous information to present on the number of subjects or the amount of data collected. Above all, this subsection should make it clear how much missing data there was, due to loss to follow-up, subjects not answering items on questionnaires, radiographic imaging not always being done, or whatever else. If the rate of missing data is high (say >10%), there should be an analysis of whether the data was missing at random or whether subjects with incomplete data (e.g. "drop-outs" in a longitudinal study) differed from subjects with complete data (in terms of demographic or clinical characteristics) [8–12]. All this information can normally just be presented in the text itself. This subsection of the Results might also provide a brief analysis of data accuracy, if needed. This might be an assessment of the accuracy of a new measuring device you used or an analysis of how often two radiologists rated the study x-rays in agreement. Alternately, such statistics of data accuracy might be presented at the start of the subsection of the Results where that data is actually presented (e.g. a statistical analysis of how often two radiologists' ratings of x-rays agreed could be presented at the start of the subsection on radiographic outcomes). This "Data Collection" subsection of the Results is essential, because it enables readers to understand the completeness and accuracy of the database underlying the rest of the results they will see. Unfortunately, many researchers completely skip this subsection, due to lack of awareness. This lowers the quality of their papers.

Next, in the subsection "Study Sample" (or "Subjects" or "Patients") characterize your study sample as best you can. Your study's results may not apply equally to everyone in the world. Readers need to form a sense of who your study sample was, so they can assess how applicable your results would be to their patients [3]. Start by presenting the demographic characteristics of the study subjects: sex (not "gender" [13]), age, ethnicity, education level, employment, socioeconomic status, etc. You should present not only means or medians but also an indication of the data spread (standard deviation, range, interquartile range, etc.), because many people are not exactly an "average" person. Then continue with the relevant baseline clinical or health characteristics. Again, the goal is to give the readers a clear picture of who your study sample was, medically, at the start of your study. The characterization of the study sample is normally presented in a table because it is far from the most important information and because readers usually want to know the exact numbers for this information. If you are comparing the baseline variables of two or more study groups, you should never make the commonplace mistake of reporting p-values for those differences [3, 5, 14–16, 17 (pp. 461–462)], because dissimilar groups will have statistically non-significant p-values in small studies while adequately similar groups may have statistically significant p-values in studies with large sample sizes [14]. Moreover, the p-value, even if it was reliable, would be irrelevant, because the difference between your two study groups really did exist in your study, regardless of whether or not that difference would be found in the larger population from which your sample was drawn. In other words, there is no meaningful null hypothesis here for which to calculate a p-value. Instead, you should simply compare the results of the baseline characteristics themselves and decide whether the magnitude of the difference between the two groups is meaningful or not [14]. If it is meaningful, you may need to control for that variable in your further statistical analysis of the study outcomes. Although rarely done, what is surely more important than comparing the study groups to each other is comparing the entire study sample, at least qualitatively, to the general patient population they supposedly represent. Thus if you notice that your study sample differs demographically from the usual patient population (e.g. the median age is a generation higher in your study sample than in the general patient population for that condition), then you should point this out during the characterization of your study sample (or address it in the Discussion).

Then you come to the major subsection of your Results: the "Main Outcomes" of your study. As mentioned earlier, you should choose the results that will address the study aims and questions you stated in the Introduction. The worst mistake anyone can make in the Results section is to do a "data dump". This occurs when researchers present lots of data, figures, tables, and statistical calculations without adequate reasoning and selectivity about what to present and what not to present. Chose the findings you need to address your paper's aims, and save the rest of your numbers and statistical analyses for some other paper or lecture [18]. Similarly, the Results section should put the main focus on the results that respond to the question(s) that the study was designed to answer, regardless of whether those results were positive or negative, and regardless of whether they were statistically significant or not. The Results section should not switch its main focus to some other set of findings simply because they had lower p-values [3]. If at all possible, it is best to present your main results as figures, because most readers will give more time and attention to figures and are more likely to remember information in figures.

All but the most experienced research teams usually have a particular shortcoming in the presentation of their main outcomes: they rush on to something else too soon. It is usually possible to dwell on your main outcomes longer, in the sense of providing further supplementary statistical analysis of the same data. For example, in a clinical study comparing two treatments, researchers would typically present a figure showing their main clinical outcome results for the two study groups at baseline and follow-up. And that is fine. Regrettably, most researchers would then just move on to showing figures or tables for the other secondary outcomes from their study, but rushing onwards is usually suboptimal. If the study is mainly about that main clinical outcome and that main clinical outcome data is what will answer the study aims, then it is often sensible to spend more time analyzing that data, and reporting more statistics about it, rather than rushing to report the basic results of some other less important study variable. Returning to the example of a clinical study, the figure just mentioned would provide only a rough sense of the magnitude of the treatment effect size, and it certainly does not provide a 95% CI for that treatment effect. So those numbers can and should be calculated and reported in the text [3, 19]. Similarly, calculating the number needed to treat (NNT) might help readers interpret the practical implications of the main outcomes shown in the figure [19–22, 23 (pp. 108–109)]. It might also be useful to present alternative analyses, for example, how much would that main outcome change if we assumed that none of the 8% of patients lost to follow-up had any benefit from treatment? Running a regression analysis on the main outcome is almost always highly informative, assuming the sample size is large enough to support such an analysis. If your main results were not statistically significant, you should calculate and report a post hoc power analysis [24–26], to assess how conclusive or inconclusive your findings are, though this should usually be presented in its own separate subsection. (Although confidence intervals also give a sense of this [27], a post hoc power analysis is more explicit and informative for most readers.) These are just a few hypothetical examples; the specifics will depend on the topic of your study and the kind of main outcomes data available. But the general point is that it is often possible to run additional meaningful statistical tests on your same main outcome data, in addition to your basic presentation of that result. Chosen thoughtfully, those additional analyses will help you and your readers dig deeper into your main outcome and understand it better. Lingering on your main outcome will also help ensure that it remains central in your readers' minds.

After your main outcomes, you should present your relevant secondary outcomes. Certainly this would include any secondary measures directly related to your main topic. In clinical trials, there might also be subsections on radiographic findings, results of laboratory tests (bloodwork, genetics, histology, etc.), quality-of-life measures, patient satisfaction, etc., if these were not the main focus of the study. It might also include deeper analysis or modeling of the data to understand what is happening, for example through regression analysis. You can also present other results that are important to know even though not directly related to your main themes. If you found anything unusual or unexpected, you can include it here toward the end of your Results, though it may be better to save it for another paper or try to confirm it in further research. There might also be subgroup analyses, but caution is needed in presenting these. Generally, subgroup analyses should only be performed and presented if they were planned in the study protocol and are reported according to guidelines [28]. Unplanned subgroup analyses are unreliable and should be avoided [3, 16, 17 (pp. 466–467), 23 (pp. 123–124), 28–31]. If you found something interesting from an unplanned subgroup analysis, it is probably best to save it to use as the basis for your next study. All these different kinds of secondary results should each be presented in their own separate subsections, not all lumped together. They should be presented in a logical order. And take care that you do not bury your main results underneath too many secondary or tangential findings. On the contrary, secondary results should work to support and further develop the main themes of the paper as expressed by the study aims and main outcomes. Secondary outcomes that have no clear relation to the study aims should perhaps be dropped (or dumped into a supplemental file). Secondary outcomes might be presented in figures, tables, and/or text, depending on which is most suitable to each result and how important that result is in the overall paper.

Last but not least, you certainly must report on any harms that were observed. These should be descriptively named (e.g. "tension headaches", "nausea", "cardiac arrhythmia"), and their duration should be specified. They can also be graded as "mild", "moderate", or "severe", and also specified as "treatment-related" or probably not [32, 33]. But if these judgments are made, then explanations should be provided (in the Methods) about how they were made and by whom. What you then did to treat these harms is usually not really relevant, especially if that treatment was standard procedure for such a harm; what matters is the description of the harm itself, so patients and other healthcare providers are aware of the risks. If there were more than say about a half-dozen harms, then it is probably best to present them in a table. If such a table would take up more than a page, you might simply summarize the frequency of various types of harms (by organ system or severity or treatment-relation) and offer the readers more details upon request or in an internet-only supplemental file. But failure to report at all on known harms (or reporting them in an overly vague way) is a form of falsification of the results, which can endanger future patients, and thus is serious research misconduct. So reports of clinical studies should always have a subsection on harms.

There are two things that should not be done anywhere in the Results section: repeating the methods or discussing the results. Unfortunately some researchers sometimes do one or both of those. Reread your Results section. If you have summarized what you did anywhere, delete it or move it up to the Methods section. If you have commented on your Results or started discussing them, cut those passages out or move them down to the Discussion.

Many medical papers present results of advanced level statistical analysis without any explanation of how to understand them. Many authors do this without awareness; others do it to show off how smart they are (or believe they are). In any case, this is always a serious mistake and unscientific. The goal of a scientific paper is to increase the readers' understanding of the topic. Statistical results that are too advanced or unfamiliar for the readers will probably not be understood by them, unless clear and simple explanations are provided. In most cases, those readers will simply skip over those parts of the paper and feel confused. So any paper that presents statistical results that are too advanced or unfamiliar for the typical readers of that journal, without providing further explanations, does not fulfill the goal of a scientific paper. Therefore, if you are presenting results from any kind of advanced or unusual statistical technique, you should present the results twice: first, present them in the usual form that other advanced researchers would expect for presentation of those results, and then present and explain them again in basic layperson terms that any second-year university student could comprehend [18]. When doing this, care must be taken to only restate and explain the results in simple terms, and not to veer off into interpreting the results or commenting on them. If you cannot explain your results in a way that any student can understand, then you probably do not sufficiently understand them yourself. Scientific truth is always clear and simple, never complex and muddled.

So for example, if you performed a multivariable logistic regression to assess if the likelihood of having a reoperation depended on patient age, sex, and body mass index (BMI), then you might normally present the main results as follows. "In the multivariable logistic regression analysis, the likelihood of having a reoperation depended on patient age (OR=1.04, 95% CI: 1.02 to 1.07, p=0.002) and sex

(OR=0.5, 95% CI: 0.2 to 0.9, p=0.04) but not on BMI (OR=0.8, 95% CI: 0.4 to 1.8, p=0.6)." Yet even in this somewhat simplified or minimal form, it would be reasonable to suspect that many readers of medical journals would not understand that sentence well enough to explain what exactly it all meant. So it would be sensible to provide further explanation, such as with the following sentences. "In other words, for each additional year of age, a patient's odds of having a reoperation rose cumulatively by 4% (i.e. OR=1.04), thus a likelihood of reoperation about 48% higher for patients a decade older (1.04^{10}). Compared to men, women had half the odds of having a reoperation (OR=0.5), though in the larger patient population from which our study sample was drawn, women's odds of reoperation may have been, with 95% confidence, anywhere from 20% to 90% the odds of reoperation for men (95% CI: 0.2 to 0.9)." Notice that the explanations are selected in such a way to focus the readers' attention on the key findings and make those comprehensible, while simultaneous serving as a model to decipher other parts. If results need more explanations than would be sensible in the text, then it is preferable to present the results in a table and use the table legend to explain in detail how to understand those results.

So how do you decide if some result you are reporting is "advanced" or "unusual" and needs this kind of accompanying explanation? Well, it is worth keeping in mind that most readers of medical journals are not researchers; they are practicing healthcare professionals, with little or no formal training in statistical analysis [34]. Accordingly, almost everything beyond basic descriptive statistics might potentially need further explanation in plain English. Even if readers do already have some understanding of the results when reported in the standard style of researchers and statisticians, most readers will appreciate the support of hearing the results explained again in everyday language. Yet readers' lack of familiarity with a particular method or technique is never a reason to avoid using that method or technique. The choice of techniques should depend only on what is methodologically most appropriate and valid.

Aside from the foregoing, all the information in the Results should be written succinctly. Many researchers make the mistake of talking too much in the Results section. Just show your results and get on with it. There is no need to belabor the Results section, (except for providing clear explanations, as described above). In fact, if you present your data well (in figures and tables), there is usually little need to say much more. Your Results section can become very short and easy to read. In other words, let your results speak for themselves, and cut out any unnecessary fluff and chatter.

There is a tiny but frequent error in reporting numbers that must be diligently avoided: many researchers report their findings with too many decimal places. Most readers will not take in more decimal places than are relevant for understanding the meaning of the results. But it is mentally taxing for readers to round off numbers themselves. For example, if someone writes that the patients' mean body weight was 74.875 kg, most readers will simply register that the mean body weight was 75 kg. Therefore, round off all your numbers to the maximum number of digits that remains meaningful (here: 75 kg), so readers can actually read your paper [17 (pp. 18, 487–488), 23 (pp. 58–60), 35–37]. Nonetheless, your data should always be measured and recorded as precisely as possible [23 (p. 314)], and statistical analysis should then be performed to as many decimal places as possible. Only at the last minute – when writing up results in the paper – should the numbers be rounded off to the appropriate number of significant digits. Rounding off should never be performed earlier, neither during the research, nor during the statistical analysis [17 (pp. 17–18)]. But at this final stage of the write-up, the results should always be rounded off appropriately; results should never be reported to more significant digits than needed.

The contents and form of the Results section depends substantially on how the statistical analysis was performed, so the earlier chapters about statistical analysis contain a large amount of information that is relevant to the write-up of the Results section. Nonetheless, the following basic point is worth repeating here, because it applies to almost all medical research. Whenever you report a p-value, be sure to report the actual result to which that p-value refers and also a confidence interval (usually the 95% CI) for that result [14, 38–42]. Furthermore, avoid interpreting the results as "significant" vs. "non-significant" in the Results section; instead, just report the numbers themselves, and save your interpretations about statistical significance for the Discussion.

Ideally, you want your Results section to be *compelling*. (Even if your results are negative, you still want them to be compelling. For example, if your research found that NewDrug does not work, then you want your results to convincingly show that NewDrug does not work.) So what makes results compelling? The main characteristic of compelling results is beyond your influence: strong results (e.g. large, clinically meaningful effect sizes) with undeniable statistical significance [43]. But four other features of compelling results depend largely on your efforts. First, your analysis must be rigorous. You must select the right statistical methods, apply them purposefully, and report the right details that demonstrate that you know what you are doing. If you feel unsure about the statistical analysis you are doing, seek support from a statistician, because even readers who themselves do not have a strong understanding of statistics will notice if your analysis was amateurish. In particular, although most readers do not appreciate it, 95% CIs that are narrow enough that the conclusions would not change if the results were anywhere else inside that CI should make the results much more compelling. Second, strive for a sparse presentation of your results without any fluff or chatter. Although some surrounding text is useful to describe what you are presenting or explain it to non-statisticians, try to keep the text minimal, so the readers can focus on the results themselves. Third but very importantly, clear figures are often what makes results compelling, especially when they make distinct patterns in the raw data undeniably visible. If you can show clear and meaningful patterns in your raw data, it is difficult for readers to ignore or refute that, and often they will not want to anyway. So it is always worth the extra effort to think about how you could present your main results in the figures. Fourth and most importantly, if you want your results to be compelling, there must be a logical selection and presentation of your results. Behind each result you present, there must be a clear reason why you are presenting that result, in that form, at that point in the paper. The Results section should never be a thoughtless and disorganized dump of findings [18]. There should be an underlying silent rational for what is presented in the Results, when, and how. So altogether, if you reflect carefully on these four features, your results should become as clear and convincing as they can be. And if your results are compelling, you will be in a strong position to influence your readers' thinking on the topic during the Discussion.

References

1. Simera I, Altman DG. Writing a research article that is "fit for purpose": EQUATOR Network and reporting guidelines. Ann Intern Med. 2009; 151: JC2-2 to JC2-3.
2. Simera I, Moher D, Hoey J, Schulz KF, Altman DG. A catalog of reporting guidelines for health research. Eur J Clin Invest. 2010; 40: 35-53.
3. Moher D, Hopewell S, Schulz KF, Montori V, Gøtzsche PC, Devereaux PJ, Elbourne D, Egger M, Altman DG. CONSORT 2010 Explanation and Elaboration: updated guidelines for reporting parallel group randomised trials. BMJ. 2010; 340: c869.
4. Schulz KF, Altman DG, Moher D; for CONSORT Group. CONSORT 2010 Statement: updated guidelines for reporting parallel group randomised trials. BMJ. 2010; 340: 698-702.
5. Vandenbroucke JP, von Elm E, Altman DG, Gøtzsche PC, Mulrow CD, Pocock SJ, Poole C, Schlesselman JJ, Egger M, for STROBE Initiative. Strengthening the Reporting of Observational Studies in Epidemiology (STROBE): Explanation and Elaboration. PLoS Med. 2007; 10: e297.
6. Pocock SJ, Travison TG, Wruck LM. Figures in clinical trial reports: current practice & scope for improvement. Trials. 2007; 8: 36.
7. Durbin CG Jr. Effective Use of Tables and Figures in Abstracts, Presentations, and Papers. Respir Care. 2004; 49: 1233-1237.
8. Altman DG, Bland JM. Missing data. BMJ. 2007; 334: 424.
9. Shih WJ. Problems in dealing with missing data and informative censoring in clinical trials. Curr Control Trials Cardiovasc Med. 2002; 3: 4.
10. Little RJ, D'Agostino R, Cohen ML, Dickersin K, Emerson SS, Farrar JT, Frangakis C, Hogan JW, Molenberghs G, Murphy SA, Neaton JD, Rotnitzky A, Scharfstein D, Shih WJ, Siegel JP, Stern H. The Prevention and Treatment of Missing Data in Clinical Trials. NEJM. 2012; 367: 1355-1360.
11. Ibrahim JG, Chu H, Chen M-H. Missing Data in Clinical Studies: Issues and Methods. J Clin Oncol. 2012; 30: 3297-3303.
12. Li T, Hutfless S, Scharfstein DO, Daniels MJ, Hogan JW, Little RJA, Roy JA, Law AH, Dickersin K. Standards should be applied in the prevention and handling of missing data for patient-centered outcomes research: a systematic review and expert consensus. J Clin Epidemiol. 2014; 67: 15-32.
13. International Committee of Medical Journal Editors. Recommendations for the Conduct, Reporting, Editing, and Publication of Scholarly Work in Medical Journals. Philadelphia: American College of Physicians; 1978, 2017. Accessed on 12 January 2018 at: www.icmje.org/icmje-recommendations.pdf
14. Cummings P, Rivara FP. Reporting Statistical Information in Medical Journal Articles. Arch Pediatr Adolec Med. 2003; 157: 321-324.
15. Knol MJ, Groenwold RHH, Grobbee DE. *P*-values in baseline tables of randomised controlled trials are inappropriate but still common in high impact journals. Eur J Prev Cardiol. 2011; 19: 231-232.
16. Assmann SF, Pocock SJ, Enos LE, Kasten LE. Subgroup analysis and other (mis)uses of baseline data in clinical trials. Lancet. 2000; 355: 1064-1069.
17. Altman DG. Practical Statistics for Medical Research. Boca Raton, FL, USA: CRC Press; 1991, 1999.

18. Wright DB. Making friends with your data: Improving how statistics are conducted and reported. Brit J Educ Psychol. 2003; 73: 123-136.
19. McGough JJ, Faraone SV. Estimating the Size of Treatment Effects: Moving Beyond P Values. Psychiatry. 2009; 6(10): 21-29.
20. Sackett DL, Cook RJ. Understanding clinical trials. BMJ. 1994; 309: 755-756.
21. Citrome L. Compelling or irrelevant? Using number needed to treat can help decide. Acta Psychiatr Scand. 2008; 117: 412-419.
22. Barratt A, Wyer PC, Hatala R, McGinn T, Dans AL, Keitz S, Moyer V, Guyatt G; for Evidence-Based Medicine Teaching Tips Working Group. Tips for learners of evidence-based medicine: 1. Relative risk reduction, absolute risk reduction, and number needed to treat. CMAJ. 2004; 171: 353-358.
23. Bland M. An Introduction to Medical Statistics, 4th ed. Oxford: Oxford University Press; 2015.
24. Running the numbers. Nat Neurosci. 2005; 8: 123.
25. Detsky AS, Sackett DL. When Was a 'Negative Clinical Trial Big Enough? How Many Patients You Needed Depends on What You Found. Arch Intern Med. 1985; 145: 709-712.
26. Bailar JC III. Science, Statistics, and Deception. Ann Intern Med. 1986; 104: 259-260.
27. Guyatt G, Jaeschke R, Heddle N, Cook D, Shannon H, Walter S. Basic statistics for clinicians: 2. Interpreting study results: confidence intervals. CMAJ. 1995; 152: 169-173.
28. Wang R, Lagakos SW, Ware JH, Huner DJ, Drazen JM. Statistics in Medicine—Reporting of Subgroup Analyses in Clinical Trials. NEJM. 2007; 357: 2189-2194.
29. Burke JF, Sussman JB, Kent DM, Hayward RA. Three simple rules to ensure reasonably credible subgroup analyses. BMJ. 2015; 351: h5651.
30. Sterne JAC, Smith GD. Sifting the evidence–what's wrong with significance tests? BMJ. 2001; 322: 226-231.
31. Guyatt GH, Oxman AD, Kunz R, Woodcock J, Brozek J, Helfand M, Alonso-Coello P, Glasziou P, Jaeschke R, Akl EA, Norris S, Vist G, Dahm P, Shukla VK, Higgins J, Falck-Ytter Y, Schünemann HJ; GRADE Working Group. GRADE guidelines: 7. Rating the quality of evidence—inconsistency. J Clin Epidemiol. 2011; 64: 1294-1302.
32. Ioannidis JPA, Evans SJW, Gøtzsche PC, O'Neill RT, Altman DG, Schulz K, Moher D; for CONSORT Group. Better Reporting of Harms in Randomized Trials: An Extension of the CONSORT Statement. Ann Intern Med. 2004; 141: 781-788.
33. Dindo D, Demartines N, Clavien P-A. Classification of Surgical Complications: A New Proposal With Evaluation in a Cohort of 6336 Patients and Results of a Survey. Ann Surg. 2004; 240: 205-213.
34. Doctors and medical statistics. Lancet. 2007; 370: 910.
35. Cole TJ. Too many digits: the presentation of numerical data. Arch Dis Child. 2015; 100: 608-609.
36. Altman DG, Bland JM. Presentation of numerical data. BMJ. 1996; 312: 572.
37. Larson MG. Descriptive Statistics and Graphical Displays. Circulation. 2006; 114: 76-81.
38. Cohen J. The Earth Is Round ($p < .05$). Am Psychol. 1994; 49: 997-1003.
39. Gardner MJ, Altman DG. Confidence intervals rather than P values: estimation rather than hypothesis testing. BMJ. 1986; 292: 746-750.
40. Braitman LE. Confidence Intervals Assess Both Clinical Significance and Statistical Significance. Ann Intern Med. 1991; 114: 515-517.
41. Bahrami H. The Value of p-Value. Am J Gastroenterol. 2005; 100: 1427-1428.
42. Cals JWL, Kotz D. Effective writing and publishing scientific papers, part II: title and abstract. J Clin Epidemiol. 2013; 66: 585.
43. Guyatt GH, Oxman AD, Sultan S, Glasziou P, Akl EA, Alonso-Coello P, Atkins D, Kunz R, Brozek J, Montori V, Jaeschke R, Rind D, Dahm P, Meerpohl J, Vist G, Berliner E, Norris S, Falck-Ytter Y, Murad MH, Schünemann HJ; GRADE Working Group. GRADE guidelines: 9. Rating up the quality of evidence. J Clin Epidemiol. 2011; 64: 1311-1316.

Chapter 25
The Discussion

The Discussion is probably the most important part of the main text of research papers, because it serves three crucial functions. First, the Discussion provides another opportunity (along with the Introduction) to define some important issue in medicine that people really need to learn something new about. Second, this is the place where researchers can provide an interpretation of the *meaning* of their data, as it relates to the study questions or aims. Third and most importantly, the Discussion is your main opportunity to actually influence the way readers think about something or the way they do something. Unfortunately, the Discussion is also the section that most researchers have the most difficulty knowing what they should write, or not.

When researchers do not know what they really should say in the Discussion, they commonly take one of the three following approaches, all of which are major blunders. One of these three blunders is that they merely repeat the Results section in some other words. There is never any need for this – if you reported your results in the Results section, you do not need to repeat them in the Discussion section. In the Discussion section, you should *comment* on the *meaning* of your results. The results rarely speak for themselves. They require interpretive commentary to acquire meaning for the readers. And explaining the meaning of the results definitely requires much more than repeating numbers and figures in words. It requires saying something *additional* that is not already apparent in the Results section itself. Another major blunder researchers commonly make is to launch into a review of all the literature ("So-and-so et al. reported that… Other-person and colleagues found that… Etc."). The Discussion section should never be a literature review, and the readers do not need a summary of all past studies, one after another, with no rationale for their presentation. The Discussion can and should use past studies to support its exposition on the topic under discussion. It may compare the results to those of closely similar studies. But the Discussion does not need to cover all past studies [1], and the focus of the Discussion should not become the past studies themselves. The focus of the Discussion should remain the topic that your paper (and previous papers) studied. A third common blunder is that some authors simply ramble on

© Springer Nature Switzerland AG 2019
M. Hanna, *How to Write Better Medical Papers*,
https://doi.org/10.1007/978-3-030-02955-5_25

more generally about the medical topic at hand from their own clinical experience. But a scientific research report is not the place to discuss one's clinical experiences and opinions, nor to write a general review of the medical topic. It is sometimes okay to briefly mention one's clinical experience to suggest an explanation for some particular finding in the report. But otherwise, discussing one's personal clinical experience quickly becomes quite vague and unscientific. So personal clinical experience should be saved for "viewpoint" type articles, letters to the Editor, conference presentations, or brainstorming your next research proposal, while general reviews of a medical topic should be saved for book chapters or teaching students. Researchers fall into these three common blunders – rehashing results, academic literature reviews, and personal clinical rambling – when then they have not given enough thought to what they really want to say in their Discussion. If you are not sure what to write about in your Discussion section, have a brainstorming session with your co-authors, to determine what are the key issues and what are the main points you want to make.

The advice literature consistently provides a certain model for how to write the Discussion section [2–5], which will be referred to here as the "template" Discussion. The template Discussion is certainly better than any of the three common naive blunder approaches just mentioned, but otherwise it is of limited value. The template approach prescribes a fixed topic for each paragraph of the Discussion, and authors are expected to simply fill in the contents from their research for each of those pregiven topics, (thus the label "template"). In the template approach, the first paragraph of the Discussion should summarize the key findings of the study. The second paragraph of the template Discussion should try to provide an interpretation or explanation for those results, for example, in terms of the underlying biological mechanisms. The third paragraph of the template Discussion should then compare the results of the study to the findings from similar previous studies. In the fourth paragraph of the template Discussion, the authors are expected to discuss the limitations of their study, which are usually supposed to be about three in number. Since most people are averse to actually doing this, many authors also quickly rebut or downplay those limitations and also list the main strengths of their study. The fifth paragraph of the template Discussion should suggest some of the possible implications of the study for further research or clinical practice. There are some variations on the contents of this template, but those are the basic elements that are usually found in advice papers recommending a template approach for the Discussion section.

The template approach to the Discussion is certainly not "wrong", and it is indeed better than the three kinds of common naive blunder approaches to the Discussion mentioned above. If you are a basic scientist (where this template originated and still predominates), or if you are a novice researcher (i.e. have not yet published at least five papers) who has also not had any much formal training in writing essays, then it is probably a good idea to just start with that safe and easy template approach to the Discussion until you gain more experience writing. That kind of template Discussion usually makes it easier to draft the Discussion, especially if you are having difficulty thinking of what to say, and it usually yields a Discussion section that is safe from major criticisms of the composition.

But the template approach inevitably produces Discussions that are relatively dull and predictable, much like a paint-by-number picture or anything else that is mass-produced from a pre-given template. Furthermore, the individual paragraphs of the template Discussion often seem like an unrelated series of dead-end statements that do not add up to anything. So most medical researchers who have already published some papers will be better off ignoring that template and instead writing a more expository Discussion, modeled upon the kind of essay writing used in the Social Sciences. Researchers should start from a blank page, with no pregiven pattern, put on their thinking cap, and try to write an original, custom-tailored Discussion from their own scientific mind. That may often yield a Discussion with some of the same elements as the template approach, but the overall effect is more robust and more thought-provoking.

Instead of the disjointed template approach, the Discussion should be a unified, rigorously scientific argument about what your research means for the real world. The goal is to advance the knowledge and practices of the medical and/or scientific communities. So before you start writing, think seriously about what it is that you really want to say to the medical and/or scientific community. Need be, brainstorm with your co-authors about what are really the essential themes and messages of the paper. That essential theme or message should then be developed across the entire span of the Discussion. Of course, you should have already written a detailed *outline* of your Discussion long before you start to draft the actual discussion (see chapter 9, "The Outline"). One of the worst ways to write a Discussion is to simply type up a jumble of various thoughts about the topic and the data, as often happens when people do not write an outline and have no clear plan about what they want the Discussion to say. The outline should make it possible to see and plan how you will develop a unified commentary, argument, line of thinking, or message across the span of the Discussion. Thus the Discussion should have a beginning, middle, and end that work together; it should not simply switch from one unrelated topic to the next, as the template approach often seems to do.

The beginning of the custom-tailored Discussion should start by presenting the big picture that contextualizes your results and gives them relevance. The first paragraph of the Discussion should never be about your own study, much less about merely your data; your Discussion should not even mention them at all in the first paragraph. Save that for later. Instead, the beginning of the Discussion should present some larger context that bestows meaning and relevance upon the study. In other words, the start of the Discussion should be about the topic you are going to discuss. And the topic you are going to discuss is not really your study or your data. The topic is something larger, which your study findings shed light on. So the Discussion should just use your study's findings to discuss the larger topic that makes them relevant. For a simple example, if you conducted a clinical trial of a new low-cost treatment, your Discussion might start by reviewing the fact that many patients do not use the available treatments, because the cost is high. The beginning of the Discussion should be consistent with and aligned with the Introduction of your paper, but it should not simply repeat the Introduction in other words. Oftentimes, one engaging way for the beginning of the Discussion to "set the stage" without merely repeating the Introduction is to find some recent major publication on the topic, such as a government report, and review how they presented the issues and problems that your study now tries to address. But however your approach it, the beginning of the Discussion should reawaken the readers' minds to why your empirical findings make any difference to the real world.

The middle of the custom-tailored Discussion should then develop your line of thinking about what your study means for the issue it addresses [6]. This line of thinking will probably include many of the elements traditionally seen in template-style Discussions, but it might not. Almost certainly, it will include a synopsis of your key results, your interpretation of those results, and commentary upon their meaning for the real world issue. This should include clear answers to your study questions or aims. Your discussion might also comment on methodological aspects of your research if these are needed to understand your findings. Your Discussion will probably also draw upon past literature (either on the same topic or other related topics) to elaborate your thinking on the issues. If there are other well-known studies of comparable quality on the same issue, your Discussion will probably cite them briefly as further support or provide possible explanations for divergences between them. But as stated above and contrary to an older opinion still heard sometimes [7], you are not obliged to review all previous studies on the topic. If the medical community wants a comprehensive review of all the literature on a topic, they will fund a team of people to write a review paper. Your Discussion should focus on discussing your research findings, which may or may not require comparisons to previous studies. Your Discussion section might also contain recommendations for clinical practice, healthcare policy, or subsequent research. If so, you should carefully consider whether or not your study really provides enough evidence to support such recommendations. (In most situations, a single study by itself does not.) In contrast to the template Discussion, all these elements are not included into the Discussion for their own sake and merely because someone said they should be. Instead, they are included (if they are included) for the purpose of developing a line of thinking about what your results mean for the issue. Accordingly, they should be ordered in the way that best develops your line of thinking.

Present your case like a lawyer. Explicitly or implicitly, every Discussion that says anything meaningful is presenting an argument for or against something, however moderately. Your Discussion should present your line of reasoning, based on the past literature and your current findings. This argument that you present should be logically ordered (like a lawyer presenting a case for something) and be well-reasoned, so readers will be persuaded [8]. Researchers must be objective, but this does not mean they must be "neutral". Researchers always have viewpoints about the way things are or should be, and there is no point in trying to suppress or hide this in a report. Yet (unlike lawyers) scientists cannot present spurious arguments to support their viewpoints. So your Discussion must present a fair and rigorous interpretation of your results; you should not spin the presentation of your results to support the conclusion you want while ignoring equally plausible interpretations. Be careful to not generalize your study findings to other types of patients or settings to which they might not apply [2, 4]. And do not make unsupported claims [2].

In any case, your readers are not stupid, so the best way to convince them of anything is to present a tight, rational, and fair discussion of your study.

Traditionally, many researchers have felt obliged to discuss the limitations of their study, but generally this winds up being a useless waste of the Discussion, especially considering the word limits imposed on most journal papers. Because most authors do not really want to do this, they reluctantly admit three (or fewer) limitations of their study and then immediately refute each limitation and downplay its relevance anyway. The real limitations of most studies are usually points that the authors are unable to recognize, so the limitations they do mention are often points that are either already apparent to readers or too trivial to make any difference, thus pseudo-limitations. This kind of dutiful listing of some minor limitations and immediately rebutting them generally does nothing much to enrich the Discussion. It is merely a boring formality from an older academic era, which should be avoided. Certainly, you should spend some time thinking about the methodological limitations of your study – ideally before you even start the study so you can correct those limitations before it is too late. At the write-up phase, if you genuinely want to restrain how your readers interpret your data, or if you feel there really is an important problem in your study methodology that should be explicitly emphasized, then certainly bring up this limitation in your Discussion. But otherwise, just stick to the case you are making about the topic you are discussing. No one needs to hear you state, for example, that your study was only conducted at one location and therefore may not be applicable to other locations. That is true of all single-site studies (which are the vast majority of studies), and everyone should already know that there might be geographic differences. If the journal Editor or peer-reviewers insist that you mention some particular study limitation, you can always add it in later, after they request it. Until then, remember that medical papers have tight word limits. So initially, save your precious few allotted words for saying something meaningful that you want to say about your topic, rather than commenting on minor methodological issues that obviously did not bother you enough to make you do the study differently. You do not need to write about your study limitations simply because someone else said that every paper should do so – use your own judgment to decide what is most relevant to your Discussion. That all said, one final point should be added. If you have a strong command of methodology, it can be quite effective to openly identify all the substantial limitations of your study, without apology or minimization. If you know exactly how much validity your results still retain after acknowledging their limitations, then it is easy to draw corresponding conclusions from those results without any much further objection. But it is very rare that anyone can actually strengthen their argument by hitting the limitations head on in this way. If you are going to do this, you should do it early in the Discussion to get it out of the way [6]. And again, really the best way to handle limitations is to prevent or correct them before you ever start writing your paper, so there is nothing much left to discuss about them.

The end of the custom-tailored Discussion should be its conclusions. Some journals have a separate "Conclusions" section at the end of each paper; most journals do not. For the authors writing a paper, this makes no difference. The last paragraph of your Discussion should be your "conclusions" paragraph. If the journal uses a separate "Conclusions" section, then you or the journal editorial team will simply insert the heading "Conclusions" between the last paragraph of your Discussion and the preceding paragraph. In either case, the content you write, should be the same, (especially since you may need to resubmit to another journal with the other format). The conclusion paragraph should be clear, direct, simple, and brief: three to five short sentences usually suffice, especially since the rest of your Discussion should have been driving home toward this conclusion.

There are a few things the conclusion should not do. First and foremost, the conclusion paragraph should not be a summary of the entire study; the Abstract serves that purpose [6]. Second, do not bring up some new point or topic that you have not already discussed. The conclusion paragraph should be the logical culmination of the rest of the Discussion (and the entire paper). Third, do not state "conclusions" that go far beyond the evidence you have presented or otherwise are not supported well by your findings and the overall body of literature [2]. Unsupported conclusions are quickly dismissed and forgotten by readers, (if they even make it through peer-review at all). In particular, do not conclude that your study shows that the medical treatment used there is "safe", "well-tolerated", "low-risk", etc. Most medical studies do not have a sample size even remotely close enough to draw any such inferences, and making such claims can endanger patients. You can conclude that a medical treatment is "unsafe", "harmful", etc. if that is what your data showed, but a lack of evidence of harm can almost always be attributed to insufficient sample size (and possibly inadequate safety monitoring and loss-to-follow-up too). Finally, unless your study was indeed inconclusive, do not conclude in one way or another that "further research is needed" [5, 9]. That hackneyed remark is silly and thoughtless. If your study addressed a precise question and obtained valid results, then you should be able to present some kind of conclusion on that question, however tenuous, so "further research" should not be necessary. No one single study ever provides a final definitive answer on any question, nor does any study ever present information on everything we might want to know. So it goes without saying that "further research" would be needed for those reasons. If "further research" is truly needed to provide any kind of answer at all to the question your study addressed, then you are probably trying to publish your paper prematurely and should instead first go do that "further research" yourself.

The conclusion paragraph should instead present a clear "take-home message". No one is going to memorize your entire paper. In fact, a week later, most readers will barely remember anything from your paper. So what is the one point your want to really hammer home, so your readers will (hopefully) still remember it a week later? What is the one point that you want your readers to remember, so they will think and act differently than they did before they read your paper? Now write that point in one short, simple, memorable sentence, so readers can and will remember it a week later; (for example: "Drinking coffee reduces the risk of depression.") That short, simple, memorable sentence you wrote is your take-home message. Every paper should end with its take-home message. The rest of the paper should support that take-home message.

When readers reach the end of the Discussion, there is nothing much else in your paper for them to read. Some of them might glance briefly at the Acknowledgments and/or the References. Others might go back and look at some of the other sections of the paper, especially if they skipped over them before. But most people will feel that they are done reading your paper. If your Discussion section was dull or fragmented into multiple different directions, most people will probably just continue on with their other activities. So your Discussion section needs to give them something coherent and engaging to keep thinking about after they are done reading it. If your Discussion section succeeds in keeping the readers thinking, then oftentimes the readers will soon go back to other sections of the paper, to read them again and see if it all really adds up. Thus it is important that your Discussion section is also consistent with the other sections of the paper. If your Discussion section is consistent with the other sections of the paper and also gives the readers something engaging to think about, then your paper will probably be successful in influencing the thinking and/or behavior of your readers.

References

1. Elefteriades JA. Twelve Tips on Writing a Good Scientific Paper. Inter J Angiol. 2002; 11: 53-55.
2. Hess DR. How to Write an Effective Discussion. Respir Care. 2004; 49: 1238-1241.
3. Branson RD. Anatomy of a Research Paper. Respir Care. 2004; 49: 1222-1228.
4. Moher D, Hopewell S, Schulz KF, Montori V, Gøtzsche PC, Devereaux PJ, Elbourne D, Egger M, Altman DG. CONSORT 2010 Explanation and Elaboration: updated guidelines for reporting parallel group randomised trials. BMJ. 2010; 340: c869.
5. Vandenbroucke JP, von Elm E, Altman DG, Gøtzsche PC, Mulrow CD, Pocock SJ, Poole C, Schlesselman JJ, Egger M, for STROBE Initiative. Strengthening the Reporting of Observational Studies in Epidemiology (STROBE): Explanation and Elaboration. PLoS Med. 2007; 10: e297.
6. Saper CB. Academic Publishing, Part III: How to Write a Research Paper (So That It Will Be Accepted) in a High-Quality Journal. Ann Neurol. 2015; 77: 8-12.
7. Clarke M, Chalmers I. Discussion Sections in Reports of Controlled Trials Published in General Medical Journals: Islands in Search of Continents? JAMA. 1998; 280: 280-282.
8. Horton R. The rhetoric of research. BMJ. 1995; 310: 985-988.
9. Foote MA. The Proof of the Pudding: How to Report Results and Write a Good Discussion. Chest. 2009; 135: 866-868.

Chapter 26
Aligning the IMRD

All four sections of your paper (Introduction, Methods, Results, Discussion) need to work together as one coherent paper. Unfortunately, some researchers never look at their overall paper. First, they bring up three different issues in the Introduction. Next, they describe Methods that are poorly suited to addressing any of the issues they mention in the Introduction. Then they present Results that only partially correspond to the Methods they just described and do not really answer any of the issues raised in the Introduction. Finally, they write a rambling Discussion that brings up new issues not mentioned in the Introduction and spends less time discussing their current Results than they do talking about results from other researchers or their own clinical observations not from the present study. Probably the most common cause of this kind of mess is failure to write an outline prior to writing the paper. Lack of coordination between multiple co-authors drafting the paper may also sometimes be a contributing factor. But regardless of how this discordance between the four sections comes about, it does not work, and the paper will not make much sense.

So when you write your outline and now again after your have drafted your paper, look at the overall composition of the paper. Compare each section to each of the other three, and examine how well they are working together. Even more importantly, ask yourself what is the one single *story*, *message*, or *argument* of the paper as a whole? Write that down in one clear sentence. Now take a close look at each section of your paper. Do all the sections support that one story, message, or argument? Are all four sections on the same single track? If each section of your paper goes off in a different direction, the readers will not understand where your paper is going and will only get lost in your labyrinth of unrelated thoughts and numbers. If all four sections of your paper are on the same track, your readers will travel smoothly from the starting point of your investigation, through your research process and findings, to your final conclusion.

You should also streamline your paper to stay focused on that one single track. Do not try to cover too many different subtopics. Stay on topic; stay focused; stick to your main message. If your paper starts to bring up something else that veers off

© Springer Nature Switzerland AG 2019
M. Hanna, *How to Write Better Medical Papers*,
https://doi.org/10.1007/978-3-030-02955-5_26

in another direction, cut it out. A journal paper is like a train ride: you do not want to be making stops at every little tiny town along the way; you want to be on an express train that rockets forward to one major destination. So cut out all the other side-points, interesting little observations, etc. that do not advance the main line of your paper. If you have too much data or too many different ideas, try cutting it up into two (or more) smaller, more tightly focused papers, (while still taking care to avoid falling into "salami" publication). This will enable each paper to have a single, sharp focus, which is how research papers should be written. A journal paper is not a doctoral dissertation or reference book. Every research paper should be tightly focused on one single research question. Two (or more) short sharply-focused publications are usually better than one long and wide-ranging paper. Within each paper, all four sections of the paper – Introduction, Methods, Results, Discussion – should be on the same track, working together.

Chapter 27
Citing the Literature

Science is not scientific unless it is based on the scientific literature. Regrettably, many authors make all kinds of vague assertions without supplying references [1–3]. Consequently, these assertions are often misinformed or outright wrong, thus weakening the papers' positions and the authors' credibility. So look at each single sentence of your paper (especially in the Introduction and Discussion) to identify any such assertions without supporting references. Whenever you make an assertion about something, you should verify it against the scientific literature and provide adequate citations to back up that assertion [4 (pp. 110–112)]. For major points in your paper, provide more than one reference, if possible. Yet you should not cite numerous references at any one point [5]. If many papers are available as possible citations, choose the few that are the best (i.e. are the highest quality evidence, most recent, most relevant, etc.)

Thus the question arises, "What can be considered a scientifically valid reference?" This question can be answered by first mentioning all the kinds of documents that people sometimes try to cite that are not scientific and not acceptable as citations. Any kind of unpublished research manuscript is unacceptable, regardless of whether it is marked as "under review", "in preparation", "personal communication" etc. These manuscripts have not yet passed peer-review and are not available to readers to examine, so they cannot be used to support assertions. Conference abstracts and posters are also not acceptable as scientific citations [5, 6], because they have never really undergone peer review and revision (and therefore are not scientifically reliable) and because they are generally unavailable to your readers anyway. Newspaper and magazine articles are not acceptable as citations, because they have never undergone peer-review and thus are not scientific. (They are acceptable as citations when they provide the source for information on some news event or opinion statement.) Websites are also unacceptable to support facts or assertions, because they have not undergone peer review and because they are not permanently archived anywhere, so there is no guarantee that readers will still be able to find them even 2 months later. (Official websites of established groups are fine as a reference when this is used to provide the source of opinions or claims from those groups,

© Springer Nature Switzerland AG 2019
M. Hanna, *How to Write Better Medical Papers*,
https://doi.org/10.1007/978-3-030-02955-5_27

such as a position statement from a medical society or a country report from a non-governmental health organization.) There are other kinds of sources that people sometimes try to cite as references that are also not scientific. Of course, if you drew information directly from any of these subscientific sources, you must cite it, in order to avoid plagiarism. But you should either find further acceptable scientific citations for that assertion, or remove that assertion from your paper as unsupported subscientific speculation.

The only truly acceptable scientific citation – the "gold standard" so to speak – is another paper already published in a peer-reviewed journal. And even these journal papers are not really acceptable as citations unless you have actually read them in full and double-verified that they do in fact provide valid evidence for the point for which you are citing them. Journal papers are also unacceptable as citations if they have been retracted (unless you are citing them precisely to discuss that retraction). So just prior to submitting your manuscript, you should always double-check that none of your references has been retracted [5].

The main criteria for judging any source is whether it has undergone peer review, (or if not, what else, if anything, assures its credibility). With that in mind, you should also always be careful to not cite papers in journals produced by "predatory publishers". "Predatory publishers" are publishers that produce journals that look quite similar to scientific journals but that will publish anything (or virtually anything) for a fee, without using peer review and editorial judgment to assess its quality [7–10]. Consequently, articles produced by predatory publishers are no more reliable than a webpage posted directly by the authors.

Established textbooks, reference books, and scholarly books are also entirely acceptable as citations, but they are cited much less often in medical research. In medicine and health care, books usually present knowledge that is already well-established, not emerging new evidence, current debates, or highly specialized information. If your paper is stating something that is already well-established or has been reviewed well in a book, then it is appropriate to cite that book. But most of the assertions made in journal papers that are most in need of supporting citations will require citations to other journal papers, not to books, because journals are where that emerging information and debate in being published. Books are entirely acceptable as citations, but in medicine they serve mostly for the transmission of established knowledge.

Official government publications, either on the internet or in print, are usually (but not always) acceptable as a source of statistics, information, or government positions. (Exceptions arise if there are public doubts about the willingness of that government agency to publish accurate and reliable information on the topic in question.)

Citations should only be made if they are warranted for scientific/scholarly reasons. Do not cite papers for the primary sake of manipulating citation metrics or courting favor with other people [11, 12]. This includes especially citing your own papers, your colleagues' papers, specific papers recommended by anonymous peer reviewers, or papers published in your target journal [5, 13].

Finally, you (or your co-authors) should always read every reference you cite, in full, and verify that it actually says what you claim it says. Sometimes papers say something in the Abstract that they do not really say in the full paper, or they say something in both the Abstract and full text that is not really supported by the data they present [14–18]. It is the responsibility of every scientist to verify that the literature cited truly provides evidence for the claims it is cited to support [19]. Not doing this is how unfounded claims become received wisdom that is actually erroneous. So always read the papers you cite, and – as a rigorous and responsible scientist – decide for yourself whether or not those papers provide adequate evidence for the statements you want to support.

References

1. Jones R, Scouller J, Grainger F, Lachlan M, Evans S, Torrance N. The scandal of poor medical research: Sloppy use of literature often to blame. BMJ. 1994; 308: 591.
2. Altman DG. The scandal of poor medical research. BMJ. 1994; 308: 283-284.
3. Smith AJ, Goodman NW. The hypertensive response to intubation. Do researchers acknowledge previous work? Can J Anaesth. 1997; 44: 9-13.
4. Booth WC, Colomb GC, Williams JM. The Craft of Research, 3rd ed. Chicago: University of Chicago Press; 1995, 2008.
5. International Committee of Medical Journal Editors. Recommendations for the Conduct, Reporting, Editing, and Publication of Scholarly Work in Medical Journals. Philadelphia: American College of Physicians; 1978, 2017. Accessed on 12 January 2018 at: www.icmje. org/icmje-recommendations.pdf
6. DeMaria AN. Of Abstracts and Manuscripts. J Am Coll Cardiol. 2006; 47: 1224-1225.
7. Beall J. Ban predators from the scientific record. Nature. 2016; 534: 326.
8. Bartholomew RE. Science for sale: the rise of predatory journals. J R Soc Med. 2014; 107: 384-385.
9. Bohannon J. Who's Afraid of Peer Review? Science. 2013; 342: 60-65.
10. Cals JWL, Kotz D. Literature review in biomedical research: useful search engines beyond PubMed. J Clin Epidemiol. 2016; 71: 115-116.
11. Council of Science Editors. CSE's White Paper on Promoting Integrity in Scientific Journal Publications, 2012 Update, 3rd Revised Edition. Wheat Ridge, CO: Council of Scientific Editors; 2012.
12. ALLEA – All European Academies. The European Code of Conduct for Research Integrity, Revised Edition. Berlin: ALLEA; 2017. Accessed on 5 November 2017 at: www.allea.org/wp-content/uploads/2017/04/ALLEA-European-Code-of-Conduct-for-Research-Integrity-2017.pdf
13. Graf C, Deakin L, Docking M, Jones J, Joshua S, McKerahan T, Ottmar M, Stevens A, Wates E, Wyatt D. Best practice guidelines on publishing ethics: a publisher's perspective, 2nd edition. Int J Clin Pract. 2014; 68: 1410-1428.
14. Fontelo P, Gavino A, Sarmiento RF. Comparing data accuracy between structured abstracts and full-text journal articles: implications in their use for informing clinical decisions. Evid Based Med. 2013; 18: 207-211.
15. Pitkin RM, Branagan MA, Burmeister LF. Accuracy of Data in Abstracts of Published Research Articles. JAMA. 1999; 281: 1110-1111.
16. Bernal-Delgado E, Fisher ES. Abstracts in high profile journals often fail to report harm. BMC Med Res Methodol. 2008; 8: 14.
17. Chiu K, Grundy Q, Bero L. 'Spin' in published biomedical literature: A methodological systematic review. PLoS Biol. 2017; 15: e2002173.
18. Lazarus C, Haneef R, Ravaud P, Boutron I. Classification and prevalence of spin in abstracts of non-randomized studies evaluating an intervention. BMC Med Res Methodol. 2015; 15: 85.
19. Accurately reporting research. Nat Cell Biol. 2009; 11: 1045.

Chapter 28
The Abstract

The Abstract is the most important part of a journal paper, because most people will never read the rest of the paper. Often, there is no reason why they should. People read the abstract to determine whether or not that particular paper is applicable to the clinical or scientific issues they want to learn more about. If the full paper is not relevant to a reader's needs and the abstract makes this clear, then the abstract has successfully fulfilled its main purpose: preventing a reader from squandering time and effort reading the wrong paper [1]. If a reader of an abstract decides that this publication *is* relevant to his or her needs, then he or she should always read the full article, because an abstract is never long enough to provide all the information a clinician or scientist should understand before applying the paper to his or her work. Regrettably, many readers either cannot or will not retrieve the full article, so the abstract must accurately summarize all the most important information from the full paper. In some cases (especially readers in low-resource parts of the world or clinicians in private practice), people would like to read the full paper but do not, because they do not have immediate free access to it. In other cases, there are readers who judge the paper relevant to their questions and have access to the full paper, but very regrettably, they simply do not bother to read the full paper (often with the illusion that they are "too busy"). Even the journal Editors to whom you submit your manuscript may never read further than the abstract [2–7], especially if the abstract is poorly written. Because most people will never read the full paper, it is crucial to spend several hours, even days, perfecting every aspect, word, and number of the abstract. The abstract should make it clear to readers whether or not the paper is relevant to the issues they want to know more about. It should also provide a complete and accurate summary of the full paper, in case a reader relies on the abstract without ever reading the rest of the paper [8, 9].

Before discussing the abstract further, it must be clarified that this chapter refers only to the abstracts of journal papers, not also to abstracts for scientific conferences. Even though they are both called "abstracts", there are several meaningful differences between these two types of documents. The most important difference is that abstracts for scientific conferences are usually stand-alone documents with

© Springer Nature Switzerland AG 2019
M. Hanna, *How to Write Better Medical Papers*,
https://doi.org/10.1007/978-3-030-02955-5_28

no further information available to the readers; whereas, abstracts in journal papers are always accompanied by a full paper providing more numbers and explanations. Because conference abstracts are stand-alone documents, they are better understood as (very brief) Brief Reports. (In fact, it would be better to call them "Conference Reports"; "abstracts" is usually a misnomer.) So if you need to write a conference abstract, the chapter on Brief Reports will be of more help than this chapter on Abstracts. Abstracts for scientific conferences are just outside the scope of this book about journal papers, so they are not discussed specifically here. There are numerous papers in the literature providing advice on how to prepare a successful abstract for a scientific conference [10–12]; search online for possible additional papers providing guidance for your specific field or conference.

When it is time to write up a journal paper, many authors start by writing the abstract first. But this is wrong and inefficient, and it often leads to substantial problems. By definition, an abstract is a summary of the main points of the full paper. But how can anyone know exactly what the main points of a paper are, much less how to summarize them, if the paper has not yet been written? As you and your many co-authors write and rewrite the paper again and again, the contents and focus of the paper will evolve substantially. If the abstract is written before the main paper, the abstract will not accurately reflect the final paper [6, 9]. Several studies have documented and criticized the fact that there are substantial discrepancies between published abstracts and the full papers [1, 13–19]. The main explanation for these discrepancies is surely that the authors of these papers wrote the abstract before the main paper, and then never seriously compared the two at the end. Many researchers make the mistake of writing the abstract first, so they have a brief overview of what their paper will be about [20, 21]. But this is the not the right approach. You should write the *outline* first (see chapter 9) to serve as your blueprint for the paper, and you should get your co-authors to agree to that outline before starting to write the paper. Because the outline serves as the blueprint for your paper, there is no reason to write the abstract before writing the full paper. (If you already have an abstract from a scientific conference, just forget about it and start over with a new outline, new full paper, and new abstract. Ultimately, you will not save any time or effort by trying to recycle the material from a conference abstract, and doing so will probably only lower the quality of your journal paper.) When you and your co-authors are finally done writing the main manuscript, it will be easy to draft an abstract that accurately reflects the final paper. You simply go through the main manuscript, subsection by subsection, copying and then condensing the main points from each subsection. The abstract should be an accurate summary of the paper, so it should only be a very short version of exactly what you wrote in the paper. The abstract should not say anything different from the main paper. Do not worry about sounding repetitive. Repetitiveness is good. It makes things sink in. (And remember, many people will never read the full paper anyway.)

Abstracts should be as informative as possible, within the word limit allowed. To help reach this goal, most journals converted to structured abstracts with subheadings (instead of unstructured summaries) a couple decades ago, at least for research papers, and often for other types of papers as well [22, 23]. Although some journals use a highly structured format with eight subheadings, the majority of journals today prefer just four subheadings [24] – Background, Methods, Results, and Conclusions – which correspond approximately to the Introduction, Methods, Results, and Discussion subsections of the main paper. Check your target journal's "Instructions to Authors" for their required format for Abstracts, and follow their instructions exactly. The amount of words devoted to each of these four subsections should not be grossly imbalanced. Some authors write abstracts consisting of mostly Background and Methods, with little or no specifics about the Results and Conclusions. This occurs most often in unstructured summaries, which were more common in the past. These authors mistakenly believe that the readers are less likely to read the full paper, if the authors give away their findings and conclusions in the abstract. But these kinds of "teaser" or "movie trailer" type of abstracts are inappropriate, because they do not summarize all the most important information from the paper [25, 26]. Many readers will have no reason to read the full paper or will not have access to it, so the abstract must be an accurate and complete summary. And most readers today are more likely to read a full paper if the abstract already tells them the main findings and conclusion, because they become curious to learn more; whereas, abstracts lacking this vital information fail to engage the interest of the readers and provide the information necessary to decide if the full paper is worth retrieving or not. Conversely, some authors write abstracts that are heavy on the Results or Conclusions. Abstracts that are disproportionately long in the Results subsection come across as an unselective data-dump, the meaning of which remains foggy to the readers (and probably to the authors as well). Abstracts with disproportionately long Conclusions subsections are rare, but they usually seem like unscientific editorializing. So the amount of material in the four subsections of the abstract should not be grossly imbalanced.

Abstracts should be *more informative* than they usually are. Indeed, the abstract should pack as much of the most important information as possible into the space available. The problem is that most authors do not really know which types of information are "*the* most important" for inclusion in the abstract. Fortunately, an expert working group has already devoted substantial time and effort to developing guidelines – "More Informative Abstracts" – which describe and justify which kinds of information should be included in the abstracts [27–30]. Most medical journals have endorsed these guidelines and encourage authors to follow them. The "More Informative Abstracts" guidelines are one of the most important publications for medical scientific communication. Every researcher should read them and use their checklists each time he or she writes an abstract. There may sometimes be legitimate reasons to deviate from these guidelines, but there is no excuse for never reading them or ignoring their advice altogether. The next few paragraphs attempt to summarize which kinds of material should appear in each subsection of the Abstract, based largely on the "More Informative Abstracts" guidelines and more recent discussions in the literature.

The Background subsection of the Abstract should start with one or two sentences on the issues that motivated the research and why it is important. This serves to orient the readers to the topic, clarify the rationale for the research, and provide a framework for understanding the rest of the information in the abstract. The Background subsection should end with a sentence that precisely states the main study aim, question, hypothesis, or objective. The three sentences of the Background subsection of the Abstract correspond roughly to the three paragraphs of the Introduction; (see chapter 22 for further guidance on the kinds of contents to write). But three short sentences is not much, so you really need to think long and hard about how best to summarize the issue you studied and why.

The Methods subsection of the Abstract should simply make it clear to the readers which type of study this was, what was done, where, on which kind of subjects, and what was measured. There is no need to go further into unnecessary details. For a clinical study, it should start with the study design (e.g. "prospective crossover active-comparison trial", see "More Informative Abstracts Revisited" [29] for a list of common terms to use). If the kind of study performed could conceivably be either prospective or retrospective, then it is essential to state which one it was, because this is a major determinant of the data quality and level of evidence. The Methods subsection should continue with the setting (e.g. "outpatient referral clinic at a large urban university hospital"). Authors often forget or skip this item, but it is thought to be important for helping clinicians decide whether the study applies to their practice [29, 31]. Research is still needed on whether this is always truly essential information that affects the interpretation, selection, and/or use of abstracts. Next, the Methods subsection should name the study population from which the subjects were drawn. This includes the clinical disorder (e.g. "diagnosed with type 2 diabetes", "reporting chronic low back pain"), key eligibility criteria (e.g. "non-smoking", "receiving disability payments"), and how they were sampled (e.g. "consecutive convenience sample", "chosen at random within pregiven quotas for age blocks"). Demographic data on the subjects that were actually enrolled is usually not important enough to justify space in the Abstract, but when it is, it should be in the Results subsection, not the Methods subsection (contrary to the advice in "More Informative Abstracts" [29]; for further explanation why, see chapter 23). Then, the Methods subsection should state the intervention, in enough numerical detail that a clinician would know precisely what was done. For clinical studies of medication for example, this would include the generic drug name, dosage, administrative route, frequency, and duration [29, 31]. Finally, the Methods subsection should state what the main outcome was, including both its timepoint and means of measurement. The duration of follow-up should also be stated, if it differs from the main outcome's measurement timepoint [32]. Beyond all these items, you do not need to go further into details in the Abstract Methods subsection, and the word limit will probably prevent it anyway. If readers really want to know any details about the methods, they will look them up in the full paper. In the Abstract Methods, you just need to give readers brief clear descriptions of these points, so they can judge whether this study meets their search criteria and will know how the results were obtained.

The Results subsection of the Abstract should present all the key findings using exact numbers. It should start with a description of the patients actually enrolled, including the exact number in each study group and the rate of follow-up completion [31]. If a post hoc power analysis was performed (as it often should be), the

Abstract Results should state how much power the study had, with the given sample size, to detect what magnitude of clinically meaningful effect. (If only an a priori power analysis was performed, it could be stated in the Abstract Methods.) The "More Informative Abstracts" guidelines do not mention power analyses, probably because the issue of statistical power was less well recognized at the era those guidelines were written. But this is surely key information worthy of the Abstract, because it clarifies what a relevant outcome would be, and whether the study was large enough to detect it. Thus it also clarifies whether negative findings are reliable or not. If the main outcome was negative, it is essential that a post hoc power analysis be performed and reported in the Abstract Results. The Abstract Results subsection should continue with the main outcome, in exact numbers, including the 95% confidence interval. Space permitting, further secondary results may be mentioned, but avoid trying to pack in many secondary results at the expense of other important information elsewhere. Any quantitative results reported in the abstract (especially p-values) should be reported using exact numbers; (see chapters 13 and 14 on Statistics and 24 on The Results for further guidance on the optimal ways to report statistical results). If there were any major or frequent treatment-related harms, they absolutely *must* be reported in the abstract. Although it is poor practice, many clinicians will make treatment decisions based in part on reading only the abstract of a study, without ever reading the full paper, sometimes because they cannot access the full paper [33–35]. If a study finds treatment-related harms but does not report them clearly in the abstract, then patients will be exposed to risks of harm that neither the patients nor the treating clinicians are aware of. Thus, it is unethical and unacceptable to omit such data on harms from the abstract. Regrettably, many abstracts are deficient in this regards [36–39]. On the other hand however, if no treatment-related harms were observed, this should not be stated in the abstract, because it gives a false impression of safety. The sample size of any one study is almost never anywhere near large enough to draw any kind of statistically reliable inferences about safety from the absence of observed harms. Also, harms may not have been observed simply because the method of collecting data on them may have been suboptimal or inadequate. But most readers will mistakenly infer that a treatment is safe, if they read a statement that no harms were observed. (For further elaboration of this point, see chapter 24.) So reporting the absence of observed harms should be reserved for only the full paper, where it can be accompanied by caveats on the sample size and methodology of recording harms.

The Conclusion subsection of the Abstract should be scientifically rigorous and sober. It should start with the main conclusion of the study, whether positive or negative or inconclusive. It should be kept in mind that firm conclusions and recommendations cannot be made on the basis of a single study (except for metaanalyses and systematic reviews with a good base of primary research evidence), so you should word your conclusions with appropriate restraint. Studies and commentaries have complained about conclusions in Abstracts being unsupported by the results of the full paper [40, 41]. Do not contribute to this problem. Critically assess whether the wording of your conclusion is really supported by the main outcome of the full paper. Do not overgeneralize your findings to other patient populations (e.g. a study only on young adults may not apply to geriatric patients), and do not pretend that your study is the first or last word on the subject. The Abstract Conclusion subsection may continue with the main limitations or a statement of what further work is first needed before clinical implementation. It should end with a succinct and memorable take-home message, which must however be supported by the paper's findings and the body of previous scientific literature. If the study was a clinical trial, then the Abstract should provide the trial registration number at the end [42]. If the raw data is publicly available, its location should be indicated at the end of the Abstract [42].

Although you should not go into non-essential details, your abstract should be as *informative* as possible, meaning you should pack in all the key information that people need to quickly comprehend and assess your study. The best way to ensure this density of information is to start with a draft that goes well over the word limit: at least 300 words for an abstract with a limit of 250 words. Then stare at each sentence, and find ways to boil it down, by saying things more succinctly, or cutting out information that is not really essential. (However, you should still use standard English grammar. Do not try to accommodate the word limit by using an abnormal writing style, unless this is consistent with the journal format (e.g. "Study Design: Prospective double-blind randomized comparative trial.")) This process of exceeding the word limit and then distilling the abstract to get back under the limit will help ensure that the abstract contains as much of the most important information as possible.

Middle co-authors are often unsure what they should do with a manuscript that has already been completely drafted by someone else. There are many things co-authors should do, but the most important activity is to scrutinize the abstract. In particular, co-authors should examine the abstract closely for the kinds of commonplace problems that studies have documented and criticized [13, 15, 36, 38, 40]. They should verify that every sentence – and especially every number – in the abstract matches the information and numbers in the main paper. Co-authors should also double-check that the abstract contains all the key information called for in the "More Informative Abstracts" guidelines [29], especially treatment-related harms. They should verify that the conclusions are supported by the results and do not exceed the study scope and level of evidence. Each co-author should spend at least one hour reading and revising just the abstract. By scrutinizing the abstract, co-authors help ensure that readers will receive all the information they require to determine if the full paper is relevant to their needs.

References

1. Estrada CA, Bloch RM, Antonacci D, Basnight LL, Patel SR, Patel SC, Wiese W. Reporting and Concordance of Methodologic Criteria Between Abstracts and Articles in Diagnostic Test Studies. J Gen Intern Med. 2000; 15: 183-187.
2. Groves T, Abbasi K. Screening research papers by reading abstracts. BMJ. 2004; 329: 470-471.
3. Ketcham CM, Hardy RW, Rubin B, Siegal GP. What editors want in an abstract. Lab Invest. 2010; 90: 4-5.

4. Groves T. Why submit your research to the BMJ. BMJ. 2007; 334: 4-5.
5. Cals JWL, Kotz D. Effective writing and publishing scientific papers, part II: title and abstract. J Clin Epidemiol. 2013; 66: 585.
6. Annesley TM. The Abstract and the Elevator Talk: A Tale of Two Summaries. Clin Chem. 2010; 56: 521-524.
7. Langdon-Neuner E. Hangings at the *bmj*: What editors discuss when deciding to accept or reject research papers. The Write Stuff. 2008; 17: 84-85.
8. Berk RN. Preparation of Manuscripts for Radiology Journals: Advice to First-Time Authors. AJR. 1992; 158: 203-208.
9. Branson RD. Anatomy of a Research Paper. Respir Care. 2004; 49: 1222-1228.
10. Pierson DJ. How to Write an Abstract That Will Be Accepted for Presentation at a National Meeting. Respir Care. 2004; 49: 1206-1212.
11. Japiassú AM. How to prepare and submit abstracts for scientific meetings. Rev Bras Ter Intensiva. 2013; 25: 77-80.
12. Taboulet P. Advice on writing an abstract for a scientific meeting and on the evaluation of abstracts by selection committees. Eur J Emerg Med. 2000; 7: 67-72.
13. Pitkin RM, Branagan MA, Burmeister LF. Accuracy of Data in Abstracts of Published Research Articles. JAMA. 1999; 281: 1110-1111.
14. Pitkin RM, Branagan MA. Can the accuracy of abstracts be improved by providing specific instructions? A randomized controlled trial. JAMA. 1998; 280: 267-269.
15. Winker MA. The need for concrete improvement in abstract quality. JAMA. 1999; 281: 1129-1130.
16. Altwairgi AK, Booth CM, Hopman WM, Baetz TD. Discordance Between Conclusions Stated in the Abstract and Conclusions in the Article: Analysis of Published Randomized Controlled Trials of Systemic Therapy in Lung Cancer. J Clin Oncol. 2012; 30: 3552-3557.
17. Ward LG, Kendrach MG, Price SO. Accuracy of abstracts for original research articles in pharmacy journals. Ann Pharmacother. 2004; 38: 1173-1177.
18. Harris AHS, Standard S, Brunning JL, Casey SL, Goldberg JH, Oliver L, Ito K, Marshall JM. The Accuracy of Abstracts in Psychology Journals. J Psychol. 2002; 136: 141-148.
19. Fontelo P, Gavino A, Sarmiento RF. Comparing data accuracy between structured abstracts and full-text journal articles: implications in their use for informing clinical decisions. Evid Based Med. 2013; 18: 207-211.
20. Baille J. On Writing: Write the Abstract, and a Manuscript Will Emerge From It! Endoscopy. 2004; 36: 648-650.
21. Langdorf MI, Hayden SR. Turning Your Abstract into a Paper: Academic Writing Made Simpler. West J Emerg Med. 2009; 10: 120-123.
22. Hartley J. Current findings from research about structured abstracts. J Med Libr Assoc. 2004; 92: 368-371.
23. Ripple AM, Mork JG, Knecht LS, Humphreys BL. A retrospective cohort study of structured abstracts in MEDLINE, 1992-2006. J Med Libr Assoc. 2011; 99: 160-163.
24. Nakayama T, Hirai N, Yamazaki S, Naito M. Adoption of structured abstracts by general medical journals and format for a structured abstract. J Med Lib Assoc. 2005; 93: 237-242.
25. Tuddenham WJ. On the Art of the Abstract. Radiographics. 1989; 9: 583-584.
26. Howie JW. How I read. BMJ. 1976; 2 (6044): 1113-1114.
27. Ad Hoc Working Group for Critical Appraisal of the Medical Literature. A Proposal for More Informative Abstracts of Clinical Articles. Ann Intern Med. 1987; 106: 598-604.
28. Altman DG, Gardner MJ. More Informative Abstracts. Ann Intern Med. 1987; 107: 790-791.
29. Haynes RB, Mulrow CD, Huth EJ, Altman DG, Gardner MJ. More Informative Abstracts Revisited. Ann Intern Med. 1990; 113: 69-76.
30. Haynes RB. More informative abstracts: current status and evaluation. J Clin Epidemiol. 1993; 46: 595-599.
31. Hopewell S, Clarke M, Moher D, Wagner E, Middleton P, Altman DG, Schulz KF; and CONSORT Group. CONSORT for Reporting Randomized Controlled Trials in Journal and Conference Abstracts: Explanation and Elaboration. PLoS Med. 2008; 5: e20.

32. Moher D, Hopewell S, Schulz KF, Montori V, Gøtzsche PC, Devereaux PJ, Elbourne D, Egger M, Altman DG. CONSORT 2010 Explanation and Elaboration: updated guidelines for reporting parallel group randomised trials. BMJ. 2010; 340: c869.
33. Marcelo A, Gavino A, Isip-Tan IT, Apostol-Nicodemus L, Mesa-Gaerlan FJ, Firaza PN, Faustorilla JF Jr, Callaghan FM, Fontelo P. A comparison of the accuracy of clinical decisions based on full-text articles and on journal abstracts alone: a study among residents in a tertiary care hospital. Evid Based Med. 2013; 18: 48-53.
34. Barry HC, Ebell MH, Shaughnessy AF, Slawson DC, Nietzke F. Family Physicians' Use of Medical Abstracts to Guide Decision Making: Style or Substance? J Am Board Fam Pract. 2001; 14: 437-442.
35. Lock S. Structured abstracts: Now required for all papers reporting clinical trials. BMJ. 1988; 297: 156.
36. Bernal-Delgado E, Fisher ES. Abstracts in high profile journals often fail to report harm. BMC Med Res Methodol. 2008; 8: 14.
37. Ioannidis JPA, Evans SJW, Gøtzsche PC, O'Neill RT, Altman DG, Schulz K, Moher D, for CONSORT Group. Better Reporting of Harms in Randomized Trials: An Extension of the CONSORT Statement. Ann Intern Med. 2004; 141: 781-788.
38. Berwanger O, Ribeiro RA, Finkelsztejn A, Watanabe M, Suzumura EA, Duncan BB, Devereaux PJ, Cook D. The quality of reporting of trial abstracts is suboptimal: survey of major general medical journals. J Clin Epidemiol. 2009; 62: 387-392.
39. Pitrou I, Boutron I, Ahmad N, Ravaud P. Reporting of Safety Results in Published Reports of Randomized Controlled Trials. Arch Intern Med. 2009; 169: 1756-1761.
40. Mathieu S, Giraudeau B, Soubrier M, Ravaud P. Misleading abstract conclusions in randomized controlled trials in rheumatology: comparison of the abstract conclusions and the results section. Joint Bone Spine. 2012; 79: 262-267.
41. Alasbali T, Smith M, Geffen N, Trope GE, Flanagan JG, Jin Y, Buys YM. Discrepancy between Results and Abstract Conclusions in Industry- vs Nonindustry-Funded Studies Comparing Topical Prostaglandins. Am J Ophthalmol. 2009; 147: 33-38.
42. International Committee of Medical Journal Editors. Recommendations for the Conduct, Reporting, Editing, and Publication of Scholarly Work in Medical Journals. Philadelphia: American College of Physicians; 1978, 2017. Accessed on 12 January 2018 at: www.icmje.org/icmje-recommendations.pdf

Chapter 29
The Capsule Summary

Some journals use capsule summaries in the table of contents, to help readers select papers to look at [1, 2]. A capsule summary can also be used in other contexts to quickly present your work, such as the cover letter for submission to the journal, a grant proposal, or a CV. Even if your target journal does not require a capsule summary, it is usually helpful to write one, to see clearly the essence of your paper.

Unless the journal specifies otherwise, a capsule summary should have 50 words or less; otherwise, it is not really a capsule summary. With those 50 words, it should be possible to summarize: A) the study aim, B) the study design and sample, C) the main result, and D) the take-home message. And conversely, there is probably never any need to say anything more than that in the capsule summary of a standard research paper. The use of numbers is generally avoided in the capsule summary, because capsule summaries are only intended to quickly tell people what the paper is about, not to serve as a substitute for reading the report (or at least the Abstract). The capsule summary should be consistent with the paper's Abstract (which should in turn be consistent with the full paper). The capsule summary is written precisely by summarizing the Abstract to hit those four elements listed above in under 50 words.

Here is a fictitious example of a capsule summary:

A double-blind randomized crossover trial was conducted to determine if NewDrug is better than OldDrug as treatment for chronic brainfog in overworked scientific researchers. NewDrug provided more rapid alleviation of symptoms but also more side-effects, so OldDrug remains the preferable first-line treatment for brainfog.

Notice how that example succinctly covers the four points listed above, in a mere 44 words. In less than one minute, the readers have a snapshot picture of what the paper is about, so they can decide if the paper is one that they need to read.

You might compare your capsule summary to the elevator speech you wrote earlier, but in most cases, you should not alter your capsule summary just to match the elevator speech more. If the two texts are different, it is probably because your

© Springer Nature Switzerland AG 2019
M. Hanna, *How to Write Better Medical Papers*,
https://doi.org/10.1007/978-3-030-02955-5_29

understanding of the study has evolved through the process of writing up your paper. Differences may also exist because the two texts serve somewhat different purposes: the elevator speech is more about "what we are doing and why it matters"; whereas the capsule summary is more strictly about "what this paper reports". Moreover, the capsule summary is written for people who might read the full paper; whereas, the elevator speech is usually spoken to a broader audience with no access to the paper.

The capsule summary should always be clear and engaging. If your capsule summary is confusing or boring, there are only two possible explanations: either your capsule summary is not well written or your research itself is confusing or boring. In either case, further reflection is needed.

References

1. Callaham ML. A New Feature for Readers: Capsule Summaries. Ann Emerg Med. 2003; 42: 609-610.
2. Callaham ML. Whole Bowel Irrigation and the Capsule Summary. Ann Emerg Med. 2004; 44: 667.

Chapter 30
The Title

It is absolutely crucial to get your title exactly right, because most people will never read anything more than your paper's title. Researchers look at dozens of titles to find just one paper that interests them. Looking only at your title, they will make a snap judgment about whether or not your paper is sufficiently relevant and interesting to them to go look at the Abstract. Your title should make it crystal clear what your paper is about.

The title should descriptively state your research topic and study design. Typically this is done by first naming the topic of the paper (e.g. "Use of High-Dose Arsenic in the Treatment of Migraine Headaches"), followed by a colon (":"), and then ending with a description of the study design (e.g. "A Double-Blind Randomized Controlled Trial".) All your main keywords should appear in your title, so people will find your paper when searching databases (such as PubMed) for papers on your topic. Your title should be sufficiently specific that someone who sees only the title will know whether or not this is the kind of paper he or she is searching for [1]. So for example, do not write "Treatment of Migraine Headaches", because that is too vague and there are hundreds of different papers on that broad theme. Instead write, "Treatment of Migraine Headaches with High-Dose Arsenic in Outpatient Geriatric General Practice: A Retrospective Multicenter Chart Review". This high specificity of the title will help potential readers decide more quickly whether your paper matches their reading needs.

Titles should not use verbs, abbreviations, or numbers. Some researchers use verbs in their titles to broadcast their conclusion (e.g. "High-Dose Arsenic Cures Tension Headaches"), but this is uncollegial and unscientific. It expects readers to believe the conclusion before they have read anything else about the study. Further, the assertions of such titles with verbs are almost never justified, because no one single study can provide a definitive answer about anything. Several studies must provide consistent results to achieve a sufficient body of evidence to make firm conclusions. The title should also avoid using abbreviations (unless they are better known then the words they stand for, such as "DNA"), because many readers will not know what the abbreviation means. Numbers should be avoided in the title

© Springer Nature Switzerland AG 2019
M. Hanna, *How to Write Better Medical Papers*,
https://doi.org/10.1007/978-3-030-02955-5_30

because such precision in the title is unnecessary, less readable, and unhelpful in understanding the paper's topic. For example, the title may describe the study magnitude (e.g. "Large"), but it should not state the study sample size numerically (e.g. "…in 2,158 Patients").

Sometimes authors write a title that aims to be catchy, usually by being colloquial or witty. Done successfully, there is nothing wrong with this, especially for editorials, narrative literature reviews, qualitative research, or small studies making some interesting and unusual point. These kinds of catchy titles implicitly alert readers that this paper will give them something insightful to think about. Catchy titles are not really appropriate though for regular research studies, which rely upon a more formal and serious tone to ensure their credibility. Catchy titles also have the pitfall that people will not find them if they search for keywords in a database, such as PubMed. For this reason, catchy titles should only be used for less formal papers aimed at the regular readership of that journal, not for formal research reports.

Reference

1. Berk RN. Preparation of Manuscripts for Radiology Journals: Advice to First-Time Authors. AJR. 1992; 158: 203-208.

Part IV
Special Types of Articles

Chapter 31
Brief Reports

Paradoxically, brief reports can take even more time to write than a full report. Why? Because the only way to write a good brief report is to first write the full report and then boil that down to a brief report. If you try to simply write a brief report directly, it will never come out right. The contents will seem thin or diluted. A brief report is so short that it only works if the authors really make full use of every sentence and every word. The only way to do that is to write twice as much material as you are allowed (so you can see everything you might possibly say if you were allowed more journal space) and then to cut out all the fluff that is not essential for the readers to know. You may be disappointed to hear that a brief report actually requires more work than the longer full report. The compensation is that brief reports, when written that way, usually come out much better and people are more likely to actually read them.

The exact form of the brief report may vary some, depending on the target journal's style guidelines. Generally though, it still consists of the same four sections – Introduction, Methods, Results, and Discussion – which are all written in a similar way to full reports, but denser.

The Introduction normally consists of one well-developed paragraph, which condenses the three paragraphs of a full report (general topic, specific issue, aims of the study). It should make it clear why there is a need for this study or paper.

The Methods is written as one unified section without subheadings. It covers the same information as in a full report, in the same order, but in much less detail. If the study methodology is relatively routine (e.g. a standard retrospective clinical study), then the Methods might be written as one long unified paragraph. If the methodology was more unusual, the Methods might be written as several short paragraphs, going into more detail wherever the methodology was unusual.

The Results of a brief report takes a somewhat different approach to condensation. Instead of simply saying everything from the Results of a full report but in fewer words, a brief report focuses on the main outcomes and drops most everything else (except treatment-related harms). If you feel that you cannot delete your other secondary results, then you should stick to a full paper, not a brief report. You should use however many figures and tables the journal will allow, so you can conserve your allotted word count for other parts of the paper.

There is more flexibility about how to reduce the Discussion for a brief report. It depends mostly on how many words the journal will allow you and what you have to say. Generally, one well-developed paragraph should suffice, because the Discussion section will be streamlined to make one single point. Yet you could write three short paragraphs, if you have more space. The Discussion should start by stating the issue that justifies doing the study at all, citing only essential past literature. It should continue by providing your interpretation of the meaning of your results. It should wrap up by drawing a conclusion about the issue you raised, in light of the results you found. The last sentence should be your take-home message.

This process of distilling a long research paper down to a brief report is also the key to getting papers published in top-tier journals. Chapter 41 looks more closely at how to say more with fewer words. In some sense, only the main report from a major study truly justifies a full report. Most other research papers in the medical literature could probably be written better as brief reports.

Chapter 32
Letters

There are essentially two kinds of letters in the medical literature: 1) original research, 2) responses to previous publications. They are written quite differently from each other.

Original research letters may be thought of as ultrashort Brief Reports. Indeed, some research letters are originally written as brief reports (or even full reports), but then the journal Editor offers to publish it (only) as a letter, (with the corresponding word limit). Other times, the authors themselves already realize that anything longer than a letter would not be justified, either because the topic is too obscure or minor or because the research quality is not adequate for anything more. In either situation, a research letter is written like a brief report, condensed down to one essential point, expressed within the journal's given word limits. If the word limit allows, the letter is typically written in four paragraphs – background, methods, results, conclusion. Even without subheadings, readers will quickly comprehend this four paragraph structure, and it enables them to make sense of the letter quickly and easily. Thus, the three paragraphs of a full report's Introduction are often condensed down to three sentences: general topic, specific issue, aim of the study. Methods are boiled down to only the absolute essential information: study design, intervention, outcome measures. The results quickly characterize the sample (e.g. number, sex, age, medical condition) and then present the one or two essential findings that the authors want to convey. If the journal allows it (as they usually do), a figure or a table is the fastest and clearest way to present the main results. The discussion is then often drastically reduced to a quick and simple conclusion, based on the results. If the word limits are very tight, the letter is written with the same four components but altogether in one single paragraph. In short, a research letter is written much like an Abstract. Therefore, the best way to write a research letter is to first write a longer report (ca. twice the word limit permitted for a letter), and then to boil it down under the word limit. This process of condensation is quite similar to the way that Abstracts are condensed versions of the full paper and quite similar to the advice given in the chapter on Brief Reports.

© Springer Nature Switzerland AG 2019
M. Hanna, *How to Write Better Medical Papers*,
https://doi.org/10.1007/978-3-030-02955-5_32

Letters responding to previous publications can be composed any way the authors want; there is no pregiven form. Nonetheless, it is important to understand why Editors devote journal space to such letters, which are often nothing more than personal opinions. Editors want their readers to have the feeling that there is a community of other people who are intently reading that journal and stirred up enough by its articles to spend time writing response letters. This makes all readers feel that the journal is something important and exciting to read and that they can participate in a public debate. So Editors have an implicit preference that such response letters are composed in four passages. First, the letter should make it clear which earlier article it is responding to, and very briefly, what that article was about. Many people reading a letter never saw the original article, and even those who did read it (a month or two ago) may not remember it well. So the first one or two sentences of a response letter should summarize and cite the original article to which the letter responds. Second, the response letter should praise the original article for something it did well in regards to the specific point to which the present letter is responding. This serves two purposes: it focuses the readers' attention on the specific issue that is relevant to the present letter and it demonstrates collegial diplomacy toward the original authors. Third, the response letter should state and support its counterpoint. This can be done, for example, by stating your opposing thesis, and then providing three short reasons for your viewpoint. Alternately, it is possible to simply add more information on another aspect that the original authors did not consider, but generally this is not as interesting as a counterargument type rebuttal letter. Fourth, the letter should state its conclusion, often in just one crisp sentence. Finally, it is important to understand that a response letter must be written extremely succinctly. For a response letter is little more than personal opinion (i.e. it does not contain any new research), and no one wants to read a long-winded opinion. Above all journal Editors prefer letters that are pithy. So keep it brief.

Chapter 33
Case Reports

Here is the best advice there is about case reports: *do not waste your time writing them.* Case reports are viewed as very low quality research (level 4 evidence) [1–5], barely worth more than personal opinion. Moreover, every medical doctor sees dozens of patients every week. By mere statistical chance, every doctor will have "a really interesting case" sooner or later. But it is extremely rare that anyone has a single patient whose condition or treatment truly constitutes new and important medical knowledge. Furthermore, unless the patient's treatment was deliberately designed and conducted to be published as a case report, it is rather unlikely that the data available will be sufficiently comprehensive and rigorous to pass the skeptical standards of peer-review. Instead, the case report manuscript will be dismissed as poorly documented occupational gossip. For these reasons, journal Editors generally dislike case report submissions [6–9], and most good journals no longer print them at all [10–14]. Indeed, because case reports are almost never cited by other papers, they sink the impact factor of any journal that still publishes them. So almost by definition, a "good journal" is a journal that rarely to never publishes any case reports. But if you are still undeterred and want to write a case report anyway, then read on.

The first step in writing a case report is to obtain the patient's written consent to publish his or her case. If the patient will not provide that written consent, it will be quite difficult to find a journal to publish it, and unethical and legally hazardous if you do. So if the patient will not provide written consent to publish his or her medical information, you can spare yourself the time and effort of writing that manuscript.

A case report generally consists of three parts: the case history, the discussion, and the conclusion. The case history attempts to recreate the "detective story" that the clinician went through to diagnose the patient and/or the "drama" of progressively treating the patient. It descriptively presents information about the patient in roughly the same order that the clinician originally learned it. The case history does not jump ahead to the diagnosis before it was actually made, nor does it make hindsight comments on the case with knowledge only gained later. Yet the information

© Springer Nature Switzerland AG 2019
M. Hanna, *How to Write Better Medical Papers*,
https://doi.org/10.1007/978-3-030-02955-5_33

must also be written in an thematically organized way; it should not jumble together unrelated information merely to adhere to a strict minute-by-minute chronology of what happened. So the case history starts with the simplest facts about the patient (sex, age, occupation, and the patient's reason for presenting). It continues with the relevant history and exams. The case history then proceeds to presenting results from the laboratory and other diagnostic tests. The diagnosis can be stated at the point the clinician became sure of it. If the main interest of the case is the therapy, rather than the disease and diagnosis, then the case history section continues with the therapy that was given, and the state of symptoms at subsequent follow-up visits. Case reports should continue up through the most recent information available. To write a more sophisticated case history, "narrative medicine" can be used to give the readers a better sense of what this specific human patient was like as a person [15, 16].

The discussion section aims to provide a lesson to the readers, based on the case material, analytic reasoning, and the relevant scientific literature. If the main interest of the case is a new or unusual medical condition, then the discussion often focuses on what was novel, what differentiates this case from similar known diagnoses, and especially the underlying biological mechanisms of this novel pathology. If the main interest of the case is a new therapy, then the discussion often focuses on why this treatment was better than conventional treatments and the supposed mechanisms of its action. Whatever the nature of the case may be, you should identify what is the novel and important knowledge to be gained from this case, and you should then streamline the discussion to focus on that novel important knowledge. The discussion should not comment on every routine secondary aspect of the case. A case report should not be written as if the readers are residents who have only just begun to see patients; it should be written as if the readers are experienced specialists who already know everything they need to know, except what is novel in this particular case. A case report should cite the relevant scientific literature as appropriate, but it should not switch or slide into a literature review [17]. If you want to write a literature review, then write a literature review and drop the case history entirely.

The conclusion should be one short paragraph. It must be kept in mind that case reports are idiosyncratic level 4 evidence, so the conclusion should generally be restrained and not make any firm clinical recommendations. Yet it should state the lesson to be learned by other clinicians from this specific case. Implicitly, the conclusion should make it clear why this case merits publication. If you are unsure why a particular case merits publication, reread the first paragraph of this chapter.

References

1. Howick J, Chalmers I, Glasziou P, Greenhalgh T, Henghan C, Liberati A, Moschetti I, Phillips B, Thornton H. The 2011 Oxford CEBM Levels of Evidence: Introductory Document. Accessed on 18 February 2018 at: https://www.cebm.net/wp-content/uploads/2014/06/CEBM-Levels-of-Evidence-Introduction-2.1.pdf
2. Oxford Centre for Evidence-Based Medicine, Levels of Evidence Working Group. Oxford Centre for Evidence-Based Medicine 2011 Levels of Evidence. Accessed on 18 February 2018 at: https://www.cebm.net/wp-content/uploads/2014/06/CEBM-Levels-of-Evidence-2.1.pdf

3. Wright JG, Swiontkowski MF, Heckman JD. Introducing Levels of Evidence to *The Journal*. J Bone Joint Surg Am. 2003; 85-A: 1-3.

4. Balshem H, Helfand M, Schünemann HJ, Oxman AD, Kunz R, Brozek J, Vist GE, Falck-Ytter Y, Meerpohl J, Norris S, Guyatt GH. GRADE guidelines: 3. Rating the quality of evidence. J Clin Epidemiol. 2011; 64: 401-406.

5. Gross RA, Johnston KC. Levels of evidence. Neurology. 2009; 72: 8-10.

6. Richardson JD. Case Reports: Boon or Bane for the Medical Editor? Am Surg. 2006; 72: 663-664.

7. Ehara S. Assessing the scientific and educational value of case reports: an editor's view. Jpn J Radiol. 2011; 29: 1-2.

8. Mahajan RP, Hunter JM. Case reports: should they be confined to the dustbin? Br J Anaesth. 2008; 100: 744-746.

9. Garcia-Doval I, Ingram JR, Naldi L, Anstey A. Case reports in dermatology: loved by clinicians, loathed by editors, and occasionally important. Br J Dermatol. 2016; 175: 449-451.

10. Boiselle PM. A Fond Farewell to *JTI* Case Reports. J Thorac Imaging. 2012; 27: 337-338.

11. Leopold SS. Case Closed—Discontinuing Case Reports in *Clinical Orthopaedics and Related Research*. Clin Orthop Relat Res. 2015; 473: 3074-3075.

12. Why not to publish Case Reports? Clin Transl Oncol. 2010; 12: 157.

13. Abdulla R. Conveying Science: Original Studies Versus Case Reports. Pediatr Cardiol. 2013; 34: 1761.

14. Eisenach JC. Case Reports Are Leaving Anesthesiology, but Not the Specialty. Anesthesiology. 2013; 118: 479-480.

15. Charon R. Narrative and Medicine. NEJM. 2004; 350: 862-864.

16. Charon R. Narrative Medicine: A Model for Empathy, Reflection, Profession, and Trust. JAMA. 2001; 286: 1897-1902.

17. Pascal RP. Case Reports—Desideratum or Rubbish? Hum Pathol. 1985; 16: 759.

Chapter 34
Literature Reviews

Literature reviews are extremely useful these days, because most people do not have enough time to read, evaluate, and synthesize all the medical scientific literature on every topic they might want to know about. So literature reviews serve the crucial function of providing an overview guide about what is currently known on some specific topic. They should be performed and published much more often than they currently are. Also, most journal Editors would like to publish more literature reviews, because generally they are read and cited much more often than original research papers. Unfortunately, despite all this, literature reviews can often be more difficult to publish (especially by inexperienced authors), probably because they do not really present any new and original data. And if they are not done well, literature reviews are actually quite unhelpful.

Although the majority of researchers will never try to publish a literature review in a journal, literature reviews (more broadly considered) are an essential part of every study and every paper. Prior to starting any new research study, every researcher should conduct a thorough literature review (for his or her own use, and maybe even for later publication), in order to get a clear overview of what is already known and what still needs to be studied [1, 2]. Failure to conduct such a literature review often leads to performing new research on a question that has already been answered several times by other people [2–4]. When it comes time to write up a paper, the authors should again perform an informal literature review, so everything is fresh in their minds and up-to-date. When drafting the Introduction and Discussion of a research paper, the authors should be drawing upon their literature review. (The Introduction and Discussion of research papers should never be written as literature reviews – if you want to write a literature review, then write a literature review paper. But for brief moments, the Introduction and Discussion may resemble a literature review in some aspects.) So even if you are not planning to write a literature review, it is very useful to know how they should be written. Literature reviews cannot simply be written up any old way one pleases. They have a certain methodology for how they should be conducted and how they should be written. The methods for conducting a literature review are beyond the scope of this book, so anyone wishing

© Springer Nature Switzerland AG 2019
M. Hanna, *How to Write Better Medical Papers*,
https://doi.org/10.1007/978-3-030-02955-5_34

to publish a literature review should learn more about how they are done. Here, we will only cover some of the essentials about how to *write* one, especially the points that are most applicable when literature is informally reviewed in a normal research paper.

There are two kinds of literature reviews: narrative literature reviews and systematic literature reviews. Systematic literature reviews follow a fixed set of protocols to gather all the available papers, grade each study's methodological quality, and evaluate the overall strength of evidence for the therapy or procedure under consideration [5–9]. The four parts of a systematic review paper (Introduction, Methods, Results, Discussion) follow the same general considerations as for a regular research paper. The Introduction identifies an issue that justifies a review of the literature. The Methods must clearly describe the search procedures used to gather all the literature. It should also spell out the criteria used to grade the studies and then to weigh the strength of evidence. The Results section often centers on a table that lists all the studies included and extracts their key characteristics (year, sample size, study population, main results, conclusion, grade of methodological quality, etc.) The Discussion puts the findings of the literature review into the larger context, draws a conclusion on the issue, and suggests what new research needs to be undertaken (if any). One key difference between a systematic review and a regular research paper is that a systematic review really must sound as scientifically unbiased as possible. The Introduction and Discussion should avoid saying anything that sounds like personal opinion, and they should avoid arguing for or against anything, beyond simply stating what the body of evidence in the literature supports or fails to support. A systematic literature review that sounds slanted will rapidly lose validity in the eyes of its readers.

Narrative literature reviews are more informal. Often they amount to little more than summaries of many papers with a commentary on the state of knowledge. Narrative literature reviews are still used when: A) the literature available is sparse, difficult to compare, and/or low quality, or B) the author is trying to reinvigorate research on some question and therefore wants to synthesize what is known and discuss what needs more scientific attention. Thus, in a narrative literature review, the main interest is not really the literature itself, but rather the main interest is the thinking of the author(s) when looking over the body of literature available – i.e. the "narrative" the authors tell about the literature. A narrative literature review is typically written as one unified essay without structural sections (Introduction, Methods, etc.) If the review is long, it might use topical subheadings on the different aspects, just to break up the paper and organize it all better. How much is said about each paper depends on how many papers are available and how long the literature review is. Up to an entire paragraph can be spent on a single paper if that seems sensible, but often it is not necessary to spend more than a few sentences on each paper. The key features of each paper, including its conclusion, can always be summarized in as little as one single sentence, albeit a long one. Next, the unique strength or critical flaws of the study can be highlighted. Finally, the meaning of that study can be commented upon. Although a narrative literature review relies on summarizing and commenting on many papers, what holds it all together and gives it life is the new meaning and message imparted to the literature by the author(s) writing the literature review. In other words, a narrative literature review can never be merely one summary after another. A narrative literature review depends upon having something new and important to say about the literature: the narrative the authors tell. Narrative literature reviews should not make recommendations for clinical practice; any such recommendations should be based on a systematic review of the literature.

Although many people reading this book will never write a literature review paper, it is very useful to know how to write one. The techniques used in writing a literature review can and should be applied in any paper you write, whenever you summarize or comment on someone else's paper. For example, the methods used in a systematic literature review to search and grade the papers available should be used whenever you need to find and select literature for a research paper you are writing. Similarly, the manner of summarizing and commenting on papers that is used in narrative literature reviews should be emulated when you summarize and comment on past studies in your research papers. So it is quite helpful to read many literature reviews on whatever topics, to acquire a sense of the right way to write about other papers. Indeed, you should always conduct a literature review on your topic before beginning your research, to verify whether there is even any need for a study on your topic.

References

1. Chalmers TC, Frank CS, Reitman D. Minimizing the Three Stages of Publication Bias. JAMA. 1990; 263: 1392-1395.
2. Chalmers I, Glasziou P. Avoidable waste in the production and reporting of research evidence. Lancet. 2009; 374: 86-89.
3. Jones R, Scouller J, Grainger F, Lachlan M, Evans S, Torrance N. The scandal of poor medical research: Sloppy use of literature often to blame. BMJ. 1994; 308: 591.
4. Smith AJ, Goodman NW. The hypertensive response to intubation. Do researchers acknowledge previous work? Can J Anaesth. 1997; 44: 9-13.
5. Oxman AD, Guyatt GH. The Science of Reviewing Research. Ann N Y Acad Sci. 1993; 703: 125-133.
6. Guyatt G, Oxman AD, Akl EA, Kunz R, Vist G, Brozek J, Norris S, Falck-Ytter Y, Glasziou P, deBeer H, Jaeschke R, Rind D, Meerpohl J, Dahm P, Schünemann HJ. GRADE guidelines: 1. Introduction—GRADE evidence profiles and summary of findings tables. J Clin Epidemiol. 2011; 64: 383-394.
7. Oxman AD, Guyatt GH. Guidelines for reading literature reviews. CMAJ. 1988; 138: 697-703.
8. Ressing M, Blettner M, Klug SJ. Systematische Übersichtsarbeiten und Metaanalysen. Dtsch Arztebl Int. 2009; 106: 456-463.
9. Moher D, Liberati A, Tetzlaff J, Altman DG; and PRISMA Group. Preferred Reporting Items for Systematic Reviews and Meta-Analyses: The PRISMA Statement. PLoS Med. 2009; 6: e1000097.

Chapter 35
Editorials

Editorials are of course written by the journal Editors themselves, so you will probably not be publishing an Editorial, strictly defined, anytime soon. But if we think about "editorials" a bit more broadly, we will see that they occur quite frequently in medical journals, simply under other names. An "editorial", broadly defined, is simply an essay that presents the author's thinking rather than new data. Besides research papers, most journals allow for other kinds of essay publications, which they give various names, such as "Perspectives" or "Viewpoint". Furthermore, many journals allow for "Special Reports" or other scholarly essays that, although different from mere "Editorials" or "Viewpoints", usually still involve some degree of editorializing. Besides all these kinds of editorial-like essay publications, the Discussion section of a research paper often resembles an editorial, especially when the thoughts of the authors are more interesting than their data. Therefore, it is useful to know how to write editorials, even if you are not yet the Editor-in-Chief of a journal.

An editorial is simply a well-written one-page essay. There is nothing especially different about such essays in scientific medical journals than in other scholarly or even non-scholarly fields. An editorial might typically consist of 4–6 paragraphs. The first paragraph is an introduction, presenting what the issue is that this editorial is addressing. The next several paragraphs then develop a discussion on this issue. The author normally has a viewpoint to present, and lays out a line of thinking about the topic or even a clear argument for or against something. As discussed below (in the chapter, "Build Good Paragraphs"), each paragraph is a coherent block of thought or step in the argument. The paragraphs are presented in a logical order. Finally, the last paragraph is a conclusion paragraph, as discussed above (in the chapter, "The Discussion"). It ends on a "take-home message".

An editorial may consider opposing viewpoints or other ways of thinking about the subject, but the author is not obliged to do so. If the author believes there is some validity in the alternative perspectives and wants to make them known, that is fine. If he or she wants to rebut opposing viewpoints, that is also fine. But no author is obliged to argue both sides of the issue, simply to appear "objective" or "scientific".

© Springer Nature Switzerland AG 2019
M. Hanna, *How to Write Better Medical Papers*,
https://doi.org/10.1007/978-3-030-02955-5_35

For example, an editorial against smoking, does not need to be "fair" and also discuss the advantages of smoking. An editorial simply states the author's position (e.g. smoking is toxic and deadly and should be banned) and then lays out his or her line of argument for that position. The readers achieve "objectivity" and "scientific knowledge" by reading many papers and thinking critically about them. Even if the author's position would be widely debated in the medical community, he or she is not obliged to argue both sides of the coin. (That is why many journals publish two opposing viewpoints back-to-back, as "Point" and "Counterpoint" essays.) The only obligation for the author of an editorial is to truthfully state his or her own viewpoint and then support it with valid reasoning and evidence. Nonetheless, editorials are always stronger if the author has actually thought about the opposing viewpoints and arguments.

Part V
Revising

Chapter 36
The Need for Revision

You have finished drafting your title page, Abstract, Introduction, Methods, Results, and Discussion, including all your tables, figures, and references. So now you are ready to send your manuscript in to the journal, right?

Wrong. At this point, you have only finished your first draft. Now your manuscript needs to go through several rounds of extensive revision. If you are lucky, your first draft will already be about half-way to the point where your manuscript is ready to submit to some journal. In other words, revision of the first draft is at least half the work involved in preparing a manuscript for publication. Revision is an essential part of all writing [1 (p. 72)].

Revision is the process where you closely reread what you wrote, delete passages that are low quality, reflect on how the paper could be better, and then rewrite the paper. Rewriting is the secret key to good writing [2]. In the following chapters, we will look more closely at some of the ways you can actually revise your paper. Altogether, this process of revision is the way you improve the quality of your manuscript, in terms of the scientific contents, the thinking, and the writing style – all three of which are closely intertwined [3 (pp. 230–231, 233, 248)].

Whenever you have a complete first draft, you might think to yourself, "Oh, but is it really necessary to do that extra work of rereading the paper again and tinkering with it? It seems good already. Can't I send it to the journal now, just to see what they think?" Well what happens if you do not do this revision (or do not do enough of it) and instead simply send your first draft to the journal, ("just to see what they think")? The answer is simple: the journal will reject your manuscript with a long list of basic criticisms from the peer reviewers. In particular, they will point out obvious typographical errors, as evidence that you are a sloppy researcher who does not pay any attention to what you are doing or writing. Or more likely, the Editors will just reject your manuscript without a long list of criticisms. They will simply send you a standardized reply that they receive N manuscripts per year and only publish 17% of them, and your manuscript did not seem to merit further review. So if you send your manuscript in before it is truly ready for review, you will only be wasting your time and the journal's goodwill. As mentioned in chapter 2, laziness is

© Springer Nature Switzerland AG 2019
M. Hanna, *How to Write Better Medical Papers*,
https://doi.org/10.1007/978-3-030-02955-5_36

one of the three vices that leads to low-quality (and erroneous) scientific reports; whereas, diligence is a virtue that leads to better scientific papers. At no point in the entire research process is this more applicable than the phase of revising manuscripts for submission to the journal.

Whenever you write a paper, plan to spend as much time revising your manuscript as you originally spent writing the first draft. For it is unrealistic (even absurd) to assume that the first way you wrote something is the best possible way to write it. You need to invest time in improving the quality of your manuscript. Once you make that mental commitment – to invest time in making your paper as good as you possibly can, rather than rushing to get it off your desk as soon as possible – you will find that revising a paper is actually quite enjoyable. It is the opportunity to look closely at the fruit of your research and reflect deeply about what you really want to say to everyone. It is the opportunity to take pride in doing high quality work that people will read and remember.

Revision is the difference between a bad first draft and a good publishable paper.

Revision is the difference between a manuscript that will be rejected and a submission that will be accepted.

Revision is the difference between a good paper that will be published in a good journal versus a better paper that will be published in a better journal.

References
1. Strunk W Jr., White EB. The Elements of Style. Boston: Allyn & Bacon; 1959, 1979.
2. Berk RN. Preparation of Manuscripts for Radiology Journals: Advice to First-Time Authors. AJR. 1992; 158: 203-208.
3. Nietzsche F. Der Wanderer und sein Schatten. In: Colli G, Montinari M, eds. Nietzsche Werke. Berlin: Walter de Gruyter & Co; 1880, 1967, vol. IV (3), pp. 173-342.

Chapter 37
Build Good Paragraphs

When you are writing the first draft, the most important goal is to get the scientific contents onto the page. During the initial drafting, it is usually a bad idea to worry much about *how* you actually write, because this can lead to writer's-block, and then nothing gets done. It is better to start by getting all the information and ideas onto the page, and then to go back and revise it all afterwards for better writing style.

The first step in revision is to look at the structure of each paragraph. In fact, if you can, you should try to write your first draft already in good paragraphs. In either case, building good paragraphs is the first step in editing your manuscript.

In English, the paragraph is the basic building-block of any text [1 (pp. 15–17)]. It represents a coherent and developed unit of thought. It is composed of several related sentences that work together to develop that thought or subtopic. The series of paragraphs then build upon one another to develop the line of thinking or discussion of the overall text.

Because the paragraph serves as a building-block of thought in any text, there are certain rules or guidelines about how to write a good paragraph in English. A paragraph is normally composed of a "main sentence" and several supporting sentences. The main sentence expresses the topic or key idea of the paragraph. It is usually the first sentence in the paragraph, but it may appear elsewhere. The other sentences then support or develop the topic or idea presented in the main sentence. All other sentences in a paragraph relate to the main sentence somehow; they do not drift off onto other topics.

Normally, a paragraph has about 5–7 sentences. A paragraph should never have less than three sentences. There is in theory no upper limit on the number of sentences in a paragraph, but most paragraphs with 10 or more sentences can be broken into two paragraphs and will then seem more conceptually coherent. Start each paragraph with its main sentence, which simply makes it clear what the whole paragraph is about. The last sentence (and/or sometimes the first sentence) of a paragraph may serve as a "transition" sentence", to improve the flow between paragraphs or to make the relation between the two paragraphs' topics more clear.

© Springer Nature Switzerland AG 2019
M. Hanna, *How to Write Better Medical Papers*,
https://doi.org/10.1007/978-3-030-02955-5_37

Here is a simple example of a fictitious paragraph (and the beginning of the subsequent paragraph), to illustrate the guidance just presented.

There are a few reasons why surgery is better than medication for treating Schmerzmeister's disease. First and foremost, surgery has higher one-year clinical success rates. Second, there is no risk of systemic toxicity. Third, surgical treatment is effective immediately; whereas, medications can take up to a month to show meaningful improvement in symptoms. For these reasons, surgery is usually the recommended treatment for Schmerzmeister's disease.

Nonetheless, there are a couple advantages of pharmacological treatment that lead some patients to prefer it. [...]

What makes this a paragraph is that all the sentences work together on one unified idea: the advantages of surgery for Schmerzmeister's disease. When the author starts a new idea (here: some patients' preference for pharmacological treatment), the author starts a new paragraph. Structuring a text into paragraphs in this way enables readers to move more easily from one block of thought to the next.

When writing a medical paper, it is important to look closely at the construction of the paragraphs. The outline you write for your paper should list each paragraph in the paper. When you are actually writing, each paragraph in your paper should be conceptually unified. It should consist of a main sentence and several related supporting sentences. Then the series of paragraphs should be presented in a logical order that builds up a line of thinking, rather than jumping around from one idea or subtopic to some other unrelated idea or subtopic. It is especially important to examine the construction of paragraphs in the Introduction and Discussion, where there are no subheadings to guide the readers. If your paper has well-constructed paragraphs, the readers should be able to follow the thinking that your paper builds, block by block, step by step.

Reference
1. Strunk W Jr., White EB. The Elements of Style. Boston: Allyn & Bacon; 1959, 1979.

Chapter 38
Edit Each Sentence

Long, complicated sentences are the bane of good scientific writing. Long sentences pack more words into the readers' heads than they can hold in one thought. Complicated sentences are difficult for the readers to understand the first time. So good medical scientific writing uses short, direct sentences. "Short" sentences have less than 20 words, in only one or two clauses. "Direct" sentences reveal the most important information early and then proceed straight to their point. They do not start with inessential information first or make unnecessary detours during the sentence.

You need to go through your entire manuscript, sentence by sentence, and make each sentence as short and direct as possible. Look at each sentence in your manuscript, and identify the main subject, the main verb, and any secondary verbs (in any form). That should give you a good sense of the structure of the sentence. In English, the main subject and verb should appear early in the sentence, and there should be no more than one or two other verbs, if any. Sentences should not be too long. They should be easy to read aloud [1 (p. 208)]. If you see long or complicated sentences in your manuscript, find some way to simplify them. Cut them into two short sentences. Delete unnecessary clauses. Rearrange them into a better sequence of words. Simplify the wording. Make the sentence clear and direct, by any means necessary.

The worst offense of sentence structure is a so-called "run-on" sentence. These are sentences that seem fine at the outset, but they never come to an end. Just when you feel it is time for a period to finally end the sentence, the author adds something more and keeps going. Eventually the sentence no longer makes any sense. Here is an example of a "run-on sentence", and a few possible ways to correct it:

Original: On a stack of short axis views covering the entire left ventricle, endocardial and epicardial contours were drawn in each slice, using commercially available software (CAAS, Pie Medical, Maastricht, the Netherlands), in order to analyze functional parameters, such as ejection

© Springer Nature Switzerland AG 2019
M. Hanna, *How to Write Better Medical Papers*,
https://doi.org/10.1007/978-3-030-02955-5_38

fraction (EF), end-diastolic volume (EDV), end-systolic volume (ESV), and stroke volume (SV) by multiplying the area with slice thickness according to Simpson's method.

Comment: This sentence is quite long in any case, but when it adds "by multiplying…" it undeniably crosses the limit between a sentence that is merely "long" (but still grammatically defensible) and a "run-on" sentence that is unacceptably wrong. (Moreover, it is probably unnecessary to explain how stroke volume was calculated – that is simply too detailed for a journal paper.)

Minimal Correction: On a stack of short axis views covering the entire left ventricle, endocardial and epicardial contours were drawn in each slice, using commercially available software (CAAS, Pie Medical, Maastricht, the Netherlands), in order to analyze functional parameters such as ejection fraction (EF), end-diastolic volume (EDV), end-systolic volume (ESV), and stroke volume (SV). SV was calculated by multiplying the area times slice thickness, according to Simpson's method.

Better: On a stack of short axis views covering the entire left ventricle, endocardial and epicardial contours were drawn in each slice, using commercially available software (CAAS, Pie Medical, Maastricht, the Netherlands). These contours were used to analyze functional parameters, such as ejection fraction (EF), end-diastolic volume (EDV), end-systolic volume (ESV), and stroke volume (SV) according to Simpson's method.

That sentence could (and should) be edited even further for other reasons, but this example is limited to editing the "run-on" aspect.

A long subordinate clause at the beginning of the sentence is a much more frequent problem. The main subject and verb should appear early in the sentence, so the readers know from the start what the sentence is about. Need be, it is acceptable to place a few words before the main subject and verb. But the use of long clauses or secondary verbs or nouns before the main subject and verb is only rarely preferable in medical scientific texts. Most often, the sentence should be edited to move the main subject and verb closer to the front. Here is an example of how to improve poor use of a subordinate clause at the start of a sentence:

Original: As the real position of the anterior rectum wall cannot be characterized after removal of the ultrasound probe, the potential rectum and prostate locations under this condition were evaluated.

Better: The potential rectum and prostate locations were evaluated under this condition, because the real position of the anterior rectum wall cannot be characterized after removal of the ultrasound probe.

Comment: Here the subordinate clause ("the real position…") has been moved to the second half of the sentence. Notice also how the phrase "under this condition" has been moved back, so the main verb ("were evaluated") appears sooner.

Here is another example of how to improve poor use of a subordinate clause at the start of a sentence:

Original: Besides taking a look at dose coverage in the target volume, we focused on doses for organs at risk and the establishment of a fast and feasible quality assurance system, which has the potential to be universally adopted in other brachytherapy departments.

Better: We studied both the dose coverage in the target volume and the doses for at-risk organs. We aimed to establish a fast and feasible quality-assurance system that can be implemented at any brachytherapy department.

Comment: The original version opens somewhat paradoxically. On the one hand, it gives prominence to "dose coverage in the target volume" by placing it early in the sentence. On the other hand, that same content is made to seem less relevant by constructing it as a subordinate clause starting with "Besides". In the revised version, that content ("dose coverage in the target volume") is both elevated up into the main sentence but also moved back after the main verb ("studied"). Also, notice how the original sentence actually contains two distinct sets of content: A) what they studied and B) what they aimed to do. Thus it is simpler and more logical to cut the sentence in two.

There are many other ways to edit sentences with cumbersome subordinate clauses.

Starting a sentence with a subordinate clause is acceptable under a few circumstances: A) the subordinate clause is only four words or less, B) the authors need to give special emphasis to the information in the subordinate clause, in order to convey the right meaning to the main clause, or C) the logical relation between the subordinate clause and the main clause would change if their order was changed. Nonetheless, there should never ever be more than one subordinate clause before the main subject. That is too confusing for the readers.

Sentences can also have too many subordinate or relative clauses in places that break the flow of the sentence. Remember: every sentence should be easy to read aloud. Each sentence should flow smoothly. Here is an example of how to fix a sentence that has too many clauses:

Original: By providing for a temporal resolution of 83 ms under use of two X-ray tubes and two corresponding detector units mounted onto a single gantry, DSCT allows visualization of coronary arteries at elevated heart rates and therefore a significant decrease of coronary segments unassessable due to motion.

Better: DSCT uses two X-ray tubes and detector units mounted onto a single gantry. The higher resolution of this set-up makes it possible to visualize coronary arteries at elevated heart rates. DSCT thus reduces the number of coronary segments that cannot be assessed due to motion.

Comment: In the original sentence in this example, "DSCT" is the main subject, but it appears far too late. The revised version cuts the sentence into three short simple sentences. Moreover, it rearranges the ideas into a more logical order. First, it describes the device itself. Next, it explains the advantage of that device. Finally, it presents the clinical benefit resulting from the technical advantage. In the original sentence, the readers are expected to absorb these three ideas all at once, but that is too much. (The original also thoughtlessly used the word "significant" without any intended reference to statistical testing.)

Whenever you see a sentence with multiple clauses, try to find some way to simplify that sentence. Sometimes one of the clauses contains unimportant information that can be deleted. Sometimes the sentence needs to be rewritten as two separate sentences. Sometimes the clauses merely need to be rearranged, or information in one sentence needs to be moved to some other nearby sentence.

The difference between a clause and a full sentence is that a clause cannot be written alone on its own. Thus a "compound sentence" may look like a multi-clause sentence, but it actually consists of two "simple sentences" joined together into one sentence. Compound sentences are acceptable in medical scientific writing, if: A) there is some logical reason for joining the two simple sentences into one compound sentence, B) each simple sentence has no more than one additional subordinate or relative clause, and C) each of the two simple sentences is relatively short and clear. If a compound sentence does not meet all three of these criteria, then it is probably too long and complicated for medical scientific writing. In that case, it is preferable to just break the compound sentence into two separate simple sentences. (One exception is sentences with item lists, where numbering or lettering can enable readers to comprehend multiple clauses.)

Finally, some special guidance is needed for sentences in the Results section, because they often must report numerical data. First, if you are putting data in a sentence, try to write a sentence that summarizes the finding and then move all the numbers to the end in parentheses [2 (p. 178)]. This enables the readers to comprehend the meaning first and then examine the numbers, instead of jumbling those two mental activities together. Here is an example:

Original: Mean recipient wait time was 1.8 ± 0.5 years for transplant recipients versus 4.1 ± 1.4 years for historical controls (p<0.001).
Better: Transplant recipients waited less than half as long as historical controls (mean (SD): 1.8 (0.5) vs. 4.1 (1.4) years, p<0.001).
Comment: Despite being one word shorter, the improved version gives a more meaningful account of the results and also makes it easier to compare the numbers for the two groups. (Notice also how the ± sign has been replaced [3 (p. 103), 4 (pp. 42, 488)], and the numbers 0.5 and 1.4 have been clearly identified as the SD.)

Second, if you have a sentence with many numbers or many sentences with related numbers, consider making a table or figure for that data instead. It keeps everything neater, and makes your paper easier to read. Third, avoid using the words "table" or "figure" as the subject of a sentence [5]. Instead, put the figure or table number in parentheses at the end of the sentence, and use the sentence to summarize what is found in the figure or table. Here is an example:

Original: Table 1 shows the demographic characteristics of the study sample.

Better: The study sample consisted mainly of elderly women (table 1).

Comment: In this example, either sentence will make the readers look at the table. But the poor way of writing the sentence puts the emphasis on the table itself and adds nothing more to the readers' understanding beyond what is already in the table itself. By contrast, the improved sentence puts the emphasis on the scientific information being presented in the table and adds a meaningful summary of the main numbers in the table.

Editing each sentence is an essential part of revising the first draft. This process enables the readers to focus on the scientific contents of your paper, rather than spending all their mental energy trying to make sense of convoluted writing. Just look at the editorials in the top medical journals, and you will see that most sentences are simple and direct. That is how opinion leaders convey their message to as large an audience as possible.

References

1. Aristotle. On Rhetoric. [Translated from the Ancient Greek by Kennedy GA.] Oxford: Oxford University Press; (ca. 355 BCE), 2007.
2. Tufte ER. The Visual Display of Quantitative Information, 2nd ed. Cheshire, CT, USA: Graphics Press; 1983, 2001.
3. Bland M. An Introduction to Medical Statistics, 4th ed. Oxford: Oxford University Press; 2015.
4. Altman DG. Practical Statistics for Medical Research. Boca Raton, FL, USA: CRC Press; 1991, 1999.
5. Hamilton CW. On the Table. Chest. 2009; 135: 1087-1089.

Chapter 39
Choose the Right Words

Scientific research requires precision and accuracy in everything you do. This is also true in regards to writing up your papers. It is essential that you choose the words that mean exactly what you want to say. If instead you use words that are close to what you mean, but not exactly what you mean, your readers will think about the topic somewhat differently than you intended.

Most words have other words with similar but different meanings, as any thesaurus will show. Do not write the patient was "tired" (physically fatigued), if you mean that the patient was "sleepy" (somnolent). Do not describe an illness as "chronic" (has a long-lasting continuous duration), if you mean that the illness is "recurrent" (occurs repeatedly but disappears between episodes). Do not write "study patients" (receiving beneficial healthcare), if in fact you mean "study subjects" (receiving experimental treatment of unknown value or even placebos). Do not describe the subjects' mean blood-pressure as "increased" (higher than at a previous timepoint), if you mean that their blood pressure was "elevated" (high compared to normal levels of the population). Do not say that patients' mental status was "measured" (precisely quantified with an instrument), if you actually mean that it was "assessed" (clinically evaluated by categories). Further possible examples are endless.

After you are done writing your first draft, go back through it and look at each word, one by one. For each word, ask yourself: "Is this exactly what I mean? Or is there a better word, the meaning of which is closer to what I really want to say?" Here is an example of how your manuscript might be changed by this process:

Original: The patients were examined using several standard psychological measures.
Meant to Say: The subjects were assessed using three validated quality-of-life questionnaires.

© Springer Nature Switzerland AG 2019
M. Hanna, *How to Write Better Medical Papers*,
https://doi.org/10.1007/978-3-030-02955-5_39

Explanation: A) The term "psychological measures" is vague, and the instruments used in this study were actually all questionnaires designed to measure quality-of-life. B) The word "several" is also vague. How many is "several"? C) The word "standard" is meaningless here. There is nothing that makes a questionnaire either "standard" or "not standard".

Here is another example of how your manuscript might be changed by improving the precision of word choices:

Original: All the records of patients with DMH were then analyzed in detail for the patients' standard characteristics.

Meant to Say: The records of all patients with DMH were then reviewed for the patients' demographic and clinical characteristics.

Explanation: A) The term "standard characteristics" is vague and meaningless. These researchers were referring to variables such as age, sex, weight, blood pressure, etc., which are "demographic and clinical characteristics". B) Each patient would have a large file of medical records. We know that the researchers did not look at "all the records", which would include all kinds of laboratory results, intake questionnaires, referral forms, etc. Instead, they merely looked at a few main sheets to find the specific demographic and clinical information they needed. But they did this for every patient diagnosed with DMH at their hospital. Thus they mean, "The records of all patients with DMH", not "All the records of patients with DMH". C) Again, we know that these records were not "analyzed in detail". Instead, someone simply flipped through them as quickly as possible to find the information needed.

Two other general principles about proper word choices should also be observed. One, try to avoid using any abbreviations that are not part of the general English language (i.e. cannot be found in a normal college-level dictionary), unless the abbreviation is commonly used in other medical papers and your paper will use it several times. Otherwise, just write the words out in full every time. If you use an abbreviation, you must write it out in full the first time it appears in the Abstract and the first time it appears in the main body of the paper, putting the abbreviation in parentheses, so readers will know what it means. Thereafter, you should use just the abbreviation. Second, choose one single term to refer to any given thing, and then stick with that one term throughout the entire paper [1]. Do not use two or more different words to refer to the same single thing or process ("for the sake of variety"), because then the readers may become confused or start to wonder what the difference is between those two words/things or not even realize you are only referring to one single thing with both of those words. Similarly, avoid using general terms that conceivable refer to two or more different things or processes in the given context, because then the readers might not know which one you are referring to or might even assume you are referring to the other one. In so far as possible, you should use terms such that there is a one-to-one correspondence between the word you use and the thing or process to which it refers [2].

Taken one by one, these word choices may not seem so important sometimes. But poor word choices add up across a paper. If you are making poor word choices twice per sentence in every sentence, your paper will not be saying what you want to say. Readers will become confused about various aspects of your research, findings, and ideas. Instead, each word you use should be the best choice to express your exact thoughts, so your entire paper will be clear and precise. This kind of extra effort gives you a better chance of being published in higher quality journals. Medical journal papers have very short word limits, so you really want to make every word count. Using words with exact precision is an essential feature of good scientific writing.

References

1. Derish P, Eastwood S. A Clarity Clinic for Surgical Writing. J Surg Res. 2008; 147: 50-58.
2. Frege G. Über die wissenschaftliche Berechtigung einer Begriffsschrift. In: Frege G. Funktion, Begriff, Bedeutung: Fünf logische Studien. Göttingen, Germany: Vandenhoeck & Ruprecht; (1892), 1962, 2008, pp. 70-76.

Chapter 40
Use "Plain English"

Scientific research is inherently complex and difficult to understand. It talks about highly specialized topics that most people know nothing about and even specialists may not be entirely familiar with. Science involves methods and knowledge that require years of university education to learn. There is no need to make your paper even more complicated and difficult by writing in some obscure pedantic way. Instead, you should make every effort to write as simply as you can, in everyday plain English [1–5, 6 (pp. 76–78)]. Your goal is to make it as easy as possible for your readers to understand what you are saying.

So read through your first draft – slowly – word by word, and rewrite everything in plain English that any second-year medical student could understand. "Plain English" means that you write the same way you would talk in everyday life. Avoid using Latin (except when needed to specify anatomy or binomial nomenclature). Latin otherwise ceased to be a lingua franca of medicine and science about three centuries ago, and surely less than 1% of all medical doctors today have ever studied it. Writing phrases that no one else understands does not make you more intelligent. Similarly, avoid throwing in other foreign phrases [6 (p. 81)]; English is already foreign enough for most readers [7]. Do not use jargon (i.e. occupational slang terminology and convoluted expressions commonly repeated in a medical setting but not easily decipherable to anyone unfamiliar with it) [2, 5, 6 (pp. 81–84), 8–11]. Jargon will only restrict the number of people who can understand you, thus reducing your readership. Replace jargon with normal words.

Similarly, avoid using obscure specialist terms if simple everyday words can be used instead. Of course, every field of science has its own specialized terminology, and it is often useful or even necessary to use this terminology, in order to discuss a topic accurately. But more often the use of specialist terminology is merely the thoughtless habit of a specialist who spends too many hours talking only with other specialists. Your paper will be read by many people who are not specialists for your topic or even your field. So look through your paper and every time you see a specialist term, ask yourself if a plain everyday word could be used instead. If so, replace it. If not, you should consider explaining what it refers to, if the word is not

© Springer Nature Switzerland AG 2019
M. Hanna, *How to Write Better Medical Papers*,
https://doi.org/10.1007/978-3-030-02955-5_40

well known, so readers outside your field will understand what you mean. Here is an example:

Original: The patient complained of intermittent cephalgia in the occipital cranium.

Better: The patient reported periods of pain in the back of her head.

Comment: In this example, it is clear that a patient would not complain of "cephalgia", because patients never talk that technically. Also, there is no need to use medical anatomical terms here, because they imply more spatial precision than is likely to be the case for a patient report of a subjective sensation, (and moreover pain is not experienced in bones).

Now look at your draft again, sentence by sentence. Do not try to make things sound more complicated than they actually are. Do not try to sound like the world's most learned expert. And above all, do not use mumbo jumbo [4, 6 (pp. 81–84)]. "Mumbo jumbo" is when someone uses many big obscure words, and long convoluted sentences, in order to make their paper sound very sophisticated. Usually it is an attempt to cover up the fact that they do not really know what they are talking about. The problem with mumbo jumbo is that it makes it difficult for the readers to understand what is being said. A further consequence is that mumbo jumbo almost always makes the text somewhat illogical. Here is a mild instance of mumbo jumbo and how to correct it:

Original: The possibility of the development of recurrent respiratory papillomatosis in the child is determined by the ability of the mother to develop an immune response and to provide the child with an adequate amount of antibodies.

Better: Recurrent respiratory papillomatosis in the child can be averted if the mother has an immune response and passes enough antibodies to the fetus.

Comment: Notice how the general wordiness of the sentence (e.g. "The possibility of the development", "is determined by", "the ability of the", "adequate amount", etc.) makes everything sound more complicated and erudite, without adding anything substantial. But this rhetorical effect then disturbs the intended meaning. For the use of the words "ability" and "provide" also makes it sound as if this is something that the mother is actively and consciously involved in making happen, rather than something that merely occurs or not, regardless of her will. Also the original sentence makes it seem that if the mother develops an immune response, then the child will develop recurrent respiratory illness; the intended sense that one event prevents or negates the other is lost in the original but restored with the word "averted".

Exercise caution and restraint before using any abbreviations, because they can also hinder comprehension, much like jargon or mumbo jumbo. It is entirely acceptable to use an abbreviation, if that abbreviation is: 1) commonly used in general English (e.g. "Dr." or "et al."), 2) commonly used in medical science (e.g. "DNA" or "VAS"), 3) is a standard unit of measure (e.g. "mmol/L" or "mm Hg"), or 4) is a standard parameter of statistics (e.g. "p" or "r^2"). If a set of three or more words will be used as a single term several times in your paper, it should also be easier for the readers if you abbreviate it. But if you are going to use a term only a few times in your paper, or if the full term is only one or two words anyway, then it is not helpful to invent a new abbreviation for it. Just write the full word(s) out every instance. If you are going to use an abbreviation, it should be written out in full the first time it appears, followed by the abbreviation in parentheses. Thereafter, use only the abbreviation; do not switch back sometimes to using the full words instead. Abbreviations should not be used in the Abstract [12], except for the four acceptable uses of abbreviations listed earlier in this paragraph.

Many researchers have been trained to never say "I" or "We". Instead, they write sentences in "third-person" ("It is believable that….") or "passive voice" ("A further attempt to obtain missing data was not made by us, because…"). This avoidance of writing "I" or "We" is sometimes outdated and unjustified [13 (pp. 263–264)]. In the Methods and Results sections of a paper, it is usually appropriate and preferable to avoid writing "I" or "We", because the emphasis should be on the objects studied, the process of research, the outcomes, etc., rather than on you, the scientist doing the work. So for example, in a Methods section it is preferable to write "The samples were centrifuged…", rather than "We centrifuged the samples…". However, in the Introduction and Discussion, it is often preferable to write in "first person, active voice", i.e., to use "I" or "We", because the sentence will sound unnatural and cumbersome if these words are avoided, and because the emphasis of the sentence really is on the author(s). For example, in a Discussion, it is better to write, "We believe these results show…" rather than writing, "The belief is held by the present research group that these results show…" There is no need to avoid writing "I" or "We" in the Introduction or Discussion.

Medicine and science have their own writing styles, which are different from the ideal writing styles in other fields, such as Law, Government, Literature, History, Philosophy, etc. Medicine uses a clean, direct, modern writing style. As a patient, you would not want to go to a hospital that was dirty, cluttered with outdated junk, cold, and lifeless. You would want to be in a hospital that was clean, well-organized, modern, warm, and vital. In the same way, readers of medical science do not want to struggle through a paper that is messy, cluttered, old-fashioned, cold, and lifeless. So go through your paper and give it a good scrubbing – make sure every sentence is written in a clean, direct, modern style, using "plain English".

The reason medical researchers write in English is so that as many researchers and healthcare professionals as possible around the world can read the report [14]. But for many readers, English is not their first (or even second, or third) language. It requires extra effort for them to read English; some of them may even struggle considerably to read something in English. Do not make this process any more difficult for them than it already is [7]. Similarly, some readers may be patients with limited medical knowledge trying to learn more about their condition, so they can better understand what their doctors are telling them. Also, healthcare professionals and researchers in other specialties may also be reading your paper to learn more about a topic that is outside their field but nonetheless relevant to their work. And even if the readers are native English speaking medical doctors in your field, they may be trying to read your paper quickly because of time pressures. If you write in simple, clear, plain English, then everyone will have an easier time reading and understanding your paper [15, 16]. When revising your manuscript, always ask yourself for each and every sentence, "Will my colleagues in Japan understand what this says?" If you write something so complicated that even native English speakers struggle to decipher it, then your colleagues in Japan will probably not understand it either. And if your colleagues in Japan do not understand what you write, then they will not cite your paper in their papers. If you say what you mean in plain English, more people will understand and remember what you wrote.

References

1. Plain English. J Coll Gen Pract. 1958; 1: 311-313.
2. Ronai PM. A Bad Case of Medical Jargon. AJR Am J Roentgenol. 1993; 161: 592.
3. O'Donnell M. Evidence-based illiteracy: time to rescue "the literature". Lancet. 2000; 355: 489-491.
4. Asher R. Why are medical journals so dull? BMJ. 1958; 2 (5094): 502-503.
5. Langdorf MI, Hayden SR. Turning Your Abstract into a Paper: Academic Writing Made Simpler. West J Emerg Med. 2009; 10: 120-123.
6. Strunk W Jr., White EB. The Elements of Style. Boston: Allyn & Bacon; 1959, 1979.
7. Kirkman J. Confine yourself to forms of English that are easily understood. BMJ. 1996; 313: 1321-1322.
8. Knight J. Clear as mud. Nature. 2003; 423: 376-378.
9. Coates R, Sturgeon B, Bohannan J, Pasini E. Language and publication in *Cardiovascular Research* articles. Cardiovasc Res. 2002; 53: 279-285.
10. Derish P, Eastwood S. A Clarity Clinic for Surgical Writing. J Surg Res. 2008; 147: 50-58.
11. Sand-Jensen K. How to write consistently boring scientific literature. Oikos. 2007; 116: 723-727.
12. Annesley TM. The Abstract and the Elevator Talk: A Tale of Two Summaries. Clin Chem. 2010; 56: 521-524.
13. Booth WC, Colomb GC, Williams JM. The Craft of Research. 3rd ed. Chicago: University of Chicago Press; 1995, 2008.
14. Smith R. The rise of medical English. BMJ. 1986. 293: 1591-1592.
15. Davis AJ. Readers don't have to come from overseas to benefit from plain English. BMJ. 1997; 314: 753.
16. Collier L. Be clear, concise, and correct. BMJ. 1997; 314: 753-754.

Chapter 41
Cut It Down

The most widespread problem of medical writing is that authors write too much [1]. Either they use too many words to say something, or they write about more aspects of the subject than readers want to know. Often, both these problems co-exist. There is no need to write everything you can possibly think of. There is no need to use 20 words to say something, if you could say it with only 15 words. There is no need to express the same idea three different ways. Brevity is better [2 (pp. xi–xiv), 3 (pp. 23–25), 4].

So now that you have your first draft, go back through it line by line, and boil it all down to the minimum necessary. Delete unnecessary information that no one needs to know. Delete unnecessary words. Do not write something in 20 words, if you could say it better in 15. Do not write something in 15 words, if you could say it better in 12. Do not write something in 12 words if you could say it better in 10. No one has the time or patience to read something that goes on and on and on. Get to the point; say it concisely, and stop [5, 6].

Here are four examples:

Original: Therefore, TGM appears promising as a therapeutic intervention for the treatment of ALS.
Better: Therefore, TGM appears promising as therapy for ALS.

Original: It is clear that implementing an intervention before the deleterious insult has occurred affords the best opportunity for attenuating the course of DGF.
Better: Implementing an intervention before damage has occurred is the best way to attenuate DGF.
Comment: There is never any need to start by saying "It is clear that" or other similar such clauses. Those kinds of "...that..." clauses do not add anything. Also, "the course of" is unnecessarily wordy.
Even Better: Intervening before damage occurs is the best way to attenuate DGF.

© Springer Nature Switzerland AG 2019
M. Hanna, *How to Write Better Medical Papers*,
https://doi.org/10.1007/978-3-030-02955-5_41

Original: Therefore it is helpful to compare the given dose distribution with values for dose distributions of former patients to have a better basis for deciding whether the obtained results are within a normal range or reflect a significant deviation.

Better: Comparing the dose with values of former patients provides a better basis for determining where the results lie in relation to the normal range.

Comment: Clauses such as "it is helpful to" usually add several words without adding any meaning. So cutting them out rarely changes the essential meaning and usually increases the speed and clarity of communication. Notice also that the original thoughtlessly used the words "significant" and "deviation" without having a clear understanding of what the intended meaning of these statistical terms would be here.

Even Shorter, So Perhaps Even Better: Comparing the dose with values of former patients illuminates the results' relation to the normal range.

Original: The concentrations of Fel d 1 were high at the first sampling time point in spring with a significant difference to the second sampling time point in the summer (median: 1376 ng/g vs. 478 ng/g, p=0.03).

Better: The concentrations of Fel d 1 were statistically significantly higher in the spring than in the summer (median: 1376 ng/g vs. 478 ng/g, p=0.03).

Even Better: Fel d 1 concentrations were higher in the spring than in the summer (median: 1376 ng/g vs. 478 ng/g, p=0.03).

So print out your manuscript. Get a red pen. Cross out any unnecessary words.

However, be careful to not formulate a sentence in some way that sounds unusual or infringes on good grammar, merely to cut out more words. That is going too far, because the unusual style or bad grammar will distract readers away from the meaning of the sentence.

Most journals have specific word limits for the various types of papers they publish. If your manuscript is over the word limit for your target journal, you need to boil it down further. If you and your co-authors cannot shorten your manuscript under the given word limit, you are probably looking at the wrong journal for your manuscript (or need more formal training in scientific writing).

Watson and Crick once wrote a paper titled "A Structure for Deoxyribose Nucleic Acid" [7]. That paper described their double-helix model of DNA. The word count for that paper was a mere 941 words. They won the 1962 Nobel Prize in Medicine for those 941 words. So cut your manuscript down, and maybe you too will win the Nobel Prize.

References

1. Byrne DW. Common Reasons for Rejecting Manuscripts at Medical Journals: A Survey of Editors and Peer Reviewers. Sci Ed. 2000; 23 (2): 39-44.
2. White EB. Introduction. In: Strunk W Jr., White EB. The Elements of Style. Boston: Allyn & Bacon; 1959, 1979, pp. xi-xvii.
3. Strunk W Jr., White EB. The Elements of Style. Boston: Allyn & Bacon; 1959, 1979.

4. Asher R. Six Honest Serving Men for Medical Writers. JAMA. 1969; 208: 83-87.
5. Billings JS. An Address on Our Medical Literature. BMJ. 1881; 2: 262-268.
6. Lock S. How editors survive. BMJ. 1976; 2 (6044): 1118-1119.
7. Watson JD, Crick FHC. Molecular structure of nucleic acids: A structure for Deoxyribose Nucleic Acid. Nature. 1953; 171: 737-738.

Chapter 42
Revise the Abstract and the Title

The reason the abstract is the most important part of the paper is because most people will never read anything more than the abstract (unfortunately). Think about it: when you go looking for papers on a search engine or in a journal, how many times do you read the abstract and then quit and move on to the next paper? After reading the abstract, a reader often realizes that the paper is about some other topic that is not what he or she was looking for. But sometimes, even though the abstract seems to be on the topic a reader was looking for, he or she simply feels that that full paper would not be worth the time to read. This is usually because the abstract has been so poorly written that it fails to engage the readers' interest and even warns the readers that the full paper will be equally tedious or worse. If you want people to read your full paper, you really must write an excellent abstract that will convince them to spend the time reading the rest of the paper.

So when you are done revising your first draft, invest at least two hours in revising the abstract. First, make sure that the abstract still faithfully summarizes the rest of the paper, despite all the revisions of your paper. The abstract should not say something different from the main paper [1, 2]. If it does, revise to make the two consistent.

Next, trim out the fat. A frequent problem in almost all published abstracts is that they contain sentences or information that are not important enough to warrant writing in the abstract. How can you decide if a sentence or piece of information is important enough to mention in the abstract? Simple: look at each sentence and ask yourself whether or not readers will need to know that information, in order to understand what the article is about and to decide whether or not they should read the full paper. If the answer is "No", then that information is probably not important enough to be in the abstract and should be replaced with something else that is.

Make sure your abstract is as informative as possible [3]. It should state your study aim or question exactly. Its Methods subsection should tell the readers about the study design, the study setting, the kind of subjects, the interventions performed, and how the outcomes were measured and analyzed. The main outcomes should be presented in exact numbers, including the 95% CI and exact p-value. For clinical

© Springer Nature Switzerland AG 2019
M. Hanna, *How to Write Better Medical Papers*,
https://doi.org/10.1007/978-3-030-02955-5_42

studies, any major treatment-related harms should be stated clearly [4–6]. The abstract should end with a well-supported "take-home message". Do not write any conclusions that are not firmly supported by your data – that is completely unscientific. Rein in your conclusions until they are standing on solid ground.

Reflect on whether the abstract is compelling enough that readers will want to go read the full paper, (assuming its topic is relevant to their needs). Look again at each subsection of the abstract. Is the Background clear and convincing? Is the Methods subsection limited to the key features, rather than minor details? Is the Results subsection focused on the main findings that answer the study question? Does the Conclusion end with a clear take-home message?

Then look at each and every word. Are they all essential? Or could some of them be cut out or replaced? Because your abstract is usually limited to 250 words, you need to make every word count. The best way to ensure that every word is essential is to start by writing about 300–350 words and then boil it down until you are under the limit of 250 words, (see chapter 41, "Cut It Down"). For normal articles, your Abstract should always use 95–100% of its maximum word allowance (thus 238–250 words if the limit is the standard 250). There should also be some balance between the four subsections. In general, no one subsection should be less than 50 words or more than 75. Do not waste those 250 words saying something extra that the readers do not need to know already in the abstract. But also do not write in ungrammatical or abnormal ways to fit the word limit; that is never necessary. Finally, double-check that each and every number in the abstract is the same as the corresponding number in the full paper [7–9].

For similar reasons, the title is even more important than the abstract. When people search for literature, the first set of results they see on most search engines is a list of citations with the titles but no abstracts. Many people will choose which abstracts to look at, using only the title to judge whether the paper is on their topic and looks interesting. Similarly, when people look at the table of contents of each journal issue, they use the titles to judge which abstracts to read. Also, whenever someone looks at the reference list of a paper, the title is all they can read. If the title does not make it clear what the paper is truly about, then people will not go though the effort of retrieving the abstract and full paper [10]. So you really need to get your title exactly right. It should be precise, accurate, and written in plain English [11]. The title is the absolute most important line of your entire paper. That is why journals write the title in big bold letters.

This process of revising the abstract and the title should take you at least two hours. If you invest less than two hours in this revision, then you are not really doing the work. You are doing a sloppy rush job. If you "finish" in an hour, and you feel that there is nothing more to do, just commit yourself to staring at the abstract for another hour. If you know you cannot leave early anyway, and you sit still staring at it long enough, you will find more ways to improve the abstract, because every piece of writing can always be made even better. Remember: most people will read the abstract and then quit right there, unless it looks really good. Put extra time into perfecting the abstract and making maximum use of the allotted 250 words, so people will be excited to go read the full paper. Your abstract should be a masterpiece of writing that clearly communicates all the essential knowledge from your paper.

References

1. Estrada CA, Bloch RM, Antonacci D, Basnight LL, Patel SR, Patel SC, Wiese W. Reporting and Concordance of Methodologic Criteria Between Abstracts and Articles in Diagnostic Test Studies. J Gen Intern Med. 2000; 15: 183-187.
2. Altwairgi AK, Booth CM, Hopman WM, Baetz TD. Discordance Between Conclusions Stated in the Abstract and Conclusions in the Article: Analysis of Published Randomized Controlled Trials of Systemic Therapy in Lung Cancer. J Clin Oncol. 2012; 30: 3552-3557.
3. Haynes RB, Mulrow CD, Huth EJ, Altman DG, Gardner MJ. More Informative Abstracts Revisited. Ann Intern Med. 1990; 113: 69-76.
4. Hopewell S, Clarke M, Moher D, Wagner E, Middleton P, Altman DG, Schulz KF; and CONSORT Group. CONSORT for Reporting Randomized Controlled Trials in Journal and Conference Abstracts: Explanation and Elaboration. PLoS Med. 2008; 5: e20.
5. Bernal-Delgado E, Fisher ES. Abstracts in high profile journals often fail to report harm. BMC Med Res Methodol. 2008; 8: 14.
6. Ioannidis JPA, Evans SJW, Gøtzsche PC, O'Neill RT, Altman DG, Schulz K, Moher D; for CONSORT Group. Better Reporting of Harms in Randomized Trials: An Extension of the CONSORT Statement. Ann Intern Med. 2004; 141: 781-788.
7. Pitkin RM, Branagan MA, Burmeister LF. Accuracy of Data in Abstracts of Published Research Articles. JAMA. 1999; 281: 1110-1111.
8. Pitkin RM, Branagan MA. Can the accuracy of abstracts be improved by providing specific instructions? A randomized controlled trial. JAMA. 1998; 280: 267-269.
9. Fontelo P, Gavino A, Sarmiento RF. Comparing data accuracy between structured abstracts and full-text journal articles: implications in their use for informing clinical decisions. Evid Based Med. 2013; 18: 207-211.
10. Howie JW. How I read. BMJ. 1976; 2 (6044): 1113-1114.
11. Asher R. Why are medical journals so dull? BMJ. 1958; 2 (5094): 502-503.

Chapter 43
Do a Two-Week Follow-Up

Now you and your co-authors have spent countless hours revising your first draft. You have read through the paper dozens of times, replacing and reducing the material there. You have rewritten every sentence a few times each. You have stared at every word and replaced many of them. Finally you feel "done" revising your first draft for good writing style. Now you may say that you have finished your "second draft".

Never rush to send your second draft off to the journal [1]. But are you not done yet? No, not quite yet. Put your second draft away for a couple weeks, and do not think about it [2]. Go do something else. Ideally, take a vacation. If you cannot take a vacation, go catch up on all the other activities you neglected while writing and revising your paper – lab work, reading, hobbies, social life, etc. – anything but that manuscript.

A few weeks later, take a new look at your second draft. It looks different than you remember, doesn't it? It is not quite what you thought you said, nor is it quite what you wanted to say. So now that you have a fresh perspective, it is time to revise your paper again. Discuss it again with your co-authors. Mark up the parts that were not quite what you wanted to say. Insert notes on other important points you overlooked. Then start rewriting those passages. In particular, look at your Introduction and Discussion. Your Methods and Results probably have not changed much, (though you might now realize that you did not present some aspects in the optimal way). But your Introduction and Discussion may not have been quite on target the first time you wrote them. Think again about what exactly you really want to say, and revise accordingly.

Never submit your second draft without "sleeping on it" a few weeks. If you wait a few weeks, you will see your paper in a different light, and you will want to improve it. If instead you rush to submit your second draft to the journal, you will see it again in a different light a few weeks later after the journal sends it back for major revision. So just put it away, take a break for a few weeks, and then read and revise it again.

© Springer Nature Switzerland AG 2019
M. Hanna, *How to Write Better Medical Papers*,
https://doi.org/10.1007/978-3-030-02955-5_43

References

1. Bauchner H. The Rush to Publication: An Editorial and Scientific Mistake. JAMA. 2017; 318: 1109-1110.
2. Asher R. Six Honest Serving Men for Medical Writers. JAMA. 1969; 208: 83-87.

Chapter 44
Get Internal Peer Review

After taking a vacation and revising your paper again, but before sending it into the journal, you should ask three colleagues to read the manuscript and provide feedback on it. These can be any three people who were not involved in the study. (Needless to say, all your co-authors should have read and substantially revised the manuscript already [1]). The three new people can be other researchers at your institute, a colleague you used to work with somewhere else, someone you met at a conference once, or whomever. Most people, even if they are really busy, will be flattered that you are asking them for their candid opinion about your paper, and they will agree to tell you what they think of it. Ideally, you should try to get detailed written feedback from them, or at least some comments and edits typed in the manuscript itself. In any case, it is important to get these people to say more than, "Oh yeah, I liked it; it's really good." You want them to tell you what is wrong with it and to make recommendations on how to improve it. If they are not forthcoming, ask them directly: "Please give me three specific suggestions about how to make the paper even better than it already is." Most importantly, when they do tell you what is wrong with the paper and how to make it better, take that advice seriously. Do not simply brush it off or forget it. You do not have to make the changes they suggest, but you should give serious thought to why they are making those specific suggestions.

Think of this process as "internal peer review". When you submit your paper to a journal, they will (hopefully) send it to three other anonymous researchers at other institutions for *external* peer review. Before you ask total strangers to criticize your paper from behind a shield of anonymity and one-way communication, it is a prudent and wise idea to ask your colleagues to suggest improvements, face-to-face. This has four advantages. First, the internal peer review will, hopefully, remove all of the most obvious "stupid" mistakes in you paper. Many peer reviewers love to point out these kinds of stupid little mistakes because it helps prove that the paper is low quality, so they must be right about other more substantial points as well.

© Springer Nature Switzerland AG 2019
M. Hanna, *How to Write Better Medical Papers*,
https://doi.org/10.1007/978-3-030-02955-5_44

Second, no matter how well-polished your paper is, there will always be some small aspects that other people do not quite understand well in your paper, simply because they are not familiar with what you have been doing in your clinic or lab. So internal peer review can help you improve those areas of the paper that are not so clear to unfamiliar readers. Third, internal peer reviewers will hopefully point out some of the limitations of your work or present counterarguments to your conclusions. Hearing those criticisms will enable you to revise your paper accordingly, to modify or better justify your methods and arguments. Fourth, internal peer reviewers will tell you what they thought was most valuable about the paper. Oftentimes, they will be drawing attention to aspects that you thought were relatively minor. Depending on the ensuing discussion, you may realize that you want to develop or emphasize certain aspects of the paper more, so readers will see its full value. Altogether, getting internal peer review will strengthen your paper and spare you some of the most painful criticism from the journal. Internal peer review will improve your chances for positive journal review and swift acceptance.

Unfortunately, when deficiencies or shortcomings of a manuscript are pointed out to researchers, they often take this position: "Well let's just submit it to the journal and see what they say," especially if improving the manuscript for those deficiencies would involve substantial work or change the conclusions of the paper. The implicit belief behind this attitude is that if their manuscript passes peer review and is published in the journal, then everything they wrote must be acceptable the way it is. That belief is terribly mistaken. Systematic reviews often grade original research papers as deficient in substantial ways. Also, research papers routinely point out the deficiencies of past studies on the same subject to explain why past results differed or could not be confirmed. The fact is that most peer reviewers do not have the time and expertise to see every deficiency in a manuscript, and even major errors can slip by them [2–7]. Peer reviewers are volunteering their time, and providing what expertise they do have, so they cannot be blamed for this in any way. This attitude of researchers (of just submitting questionable manuscripts to journals) has two troubling aspects. First, this attitude exhibits a fundamental laziness – an unwillingness to make extra efforts to do better quality work, even if the current work might be invalid. Second, by taking this attitude, researchers are essentially abdicating their responsibility to determine what is the best way to perform and report the study and then to take responsibility for it. Instead, they leave these judgments to the peer reviewers and/or journal Editors and displace the final responsibility to them. Fortunately, the consequence is often that the journals just reject the manuscript as shoddy, often without even wasting the reviewers' time. Unfortunately, as mentioned above, shoddy manuscript do often snake their way past peer reviewers and get published. Researchers should make every effort possible to improve their manuscripts themselves, prior to submitting them to the journals. Getting internal peer review is one key way to do that.

References

1. International Committee of Medical Journal Editors. Recommendations for the Conduct, Reporting, Editing, and Publication of Scholarly Work in Medical Journals. Philadelphia: American College of Physicians; 1978, 2017. Accessed on 12 January 2018 at: www.icmje.org/icmje-recommendations.pdf
2. Kassirer JP, Campion EW. Peer Review: Crude and Understudied, but Indispensable. JAMA. 1994; 272: 96-97.
3. Lock S. Peer review weighed in the balance. BMJ. 1982; 285: 1224-126.
4. Goodman SN, Berlin J, Fletcher SW, Fletcher RH. Manuscript Quality before and after Peer Review and Editing at *Annals of Internal Medicine*. Ann Intern Med. 1994; 121: 11-21.
5. Hopewell S, Collins GS, Boutron I, Yu L-M, Cook J, Shanyinde M, Wharton R, Shamseer L, Altman DG. Impact of peer review on reports of randomised trials published in open peer review journals: retrospective before and after study. BMJ. 2014; 349: g4145.
6. Baxt WG, Waeckerle JF, Berlin JA, Callaham ML. Who Reviews the Reviewers? Feasibility of Using a Fictitious Manuscript to Evaluate Peer Reviewer Performance. Ann Emerg Med. 1998; 32: 310-317.
7. Schroter S, Black N, Evans S, Godlee F, Osorio L, Smith R. What errors do peer reviewers detect, and does training improve their ability to detect them? J R Soc Med. 2008; 101: 507-514.

Chapter 45
Proof-Read the Manuscript

Many researchers believe that grammar and spelling is not really so important. But when journal Editors or peer reviewers see a manuscript with numerous errors of grammar, punctuation, or spelling, they quickly come to the conclusion that the manuscript is not ready to be published, regardless of what the contents are. These kinds of errors prove that the authors have not spent much time trying to write a good paper. These errors also suggest that the research itself was not done well either, because the authors appear to be the kind of people who do sloppy work without ever double-checking anything they do [1, 2]. If an Editor or reviewer is having a hectic day and has too many other things to do, numerous spelling and grammar errors will be sufficient reason for him or her to stop reading the manuscript and send it back to the authors. Reviewers may sometimes be more understanding if none of the authors is a native speaker of English (or if the review himself or herself is not), but nonetheless they never accept that as an excuse, (and sometimes they become even more critical, regrettably).

So before you submit your manuscript to the journal, you (or someone else) really should proof-read it, to ensure that all the grammar, punctuation, and spelling are correct, according to the established rules and norms of the English language. A scientific paper is a very formal piece of writing, so it must be written correctly. Most people make numerous errors of grammar, punctuation, and spelling when they write, regardless of whether or not English is their native language. So it is crucial to spend time focused only on searching out these errors and correcting them.

There are essentially two aspects of the basic language proof-reading. First, the manuscript should use correct standard grammar, including appropriate punctuation. There are already many other comprehensive guidebooks on English grammar, syntax, punctuation, usage, style, and so on [3–6]. So the present book will not try to repeat or summarize all the detailed grammar rules of the English language. Anyone with a university level education doing scientific research should take the time, once in their life, to read at least one of those fundamental books about the English language itself. Further good books on the English language and grammar

© Springer Nature Switzerland AG 2019
M. Hanna, *How to Write Better Medical Papers*,
https://doi.org/10.1007/978-3-030-02955-5_45

are listed in the bibliography at the end of this book. Second, a manuscript should not contain spelling or typographical errors. Any dictionary will provide the necessary guidance on spelling. The manuscript should use either American English or British English, not a mixture of both.

There are basically three steps to doing the proof-reading of a manuscript for correct grammar, punctuation, and spelling. First, simply re-read the paper without thinking about the scientific contents. Just look at everything slowly to confirm that it is typed correctly and – to the best of your abilities and awareness – seems to use correct grammar. Manuscripts often contain obvious errors, especially when numerous co-authors have been hastily revising a messy manuscript in all different directions. Even if you have little knowledge of English grammar rules, you should be able to see major typographical errors. Second, check the spelling. Every computer word-processing program has a built in spell-check function that will identify 95% of your misspelled words. It is amazing how many people never bother to use this simple, nearly automatic tool to clean up their manuscripts. Nonetheless, the automatic "spelling check" feature of software, although helpful, will not identify spelling errors that create another word, (e.g. writing "their" instead of "there" or "DAN" instead of "DNA"). So the manuscript should always also be read, sentence by sentence, by a human being. Third, have someone else proof-read your paper [7], preferably someone who has the special skills to do such work. Proof-reading requires both acquired knowledge of the formal rules of grammar and the ability to read texts in a certain unusual way to see any errors of grammar or punctuation. Most people – even most native speakers of English – do not have either of these capabilities, nor do they have much experience proof-reading. A professional proof-reader can help ensure that your manuscript is properly polished and sparkling clean.

References

1. Berk RN. Preparation of Manuscripts for Radiology Journals: Advice to First-Time Authors. AJR. 1992; 158: 203-208.
2. Making the most of peer review. Nat Neurosci. 2000; 3: 629.
3. Strunk W Jr., White EB. The Elements of Style. Boston: Allyn & Bacon; 1959, 1979.
4. Greenbaum S, Nelson G. An Introduction to English Grammar, 3rd ed. Harlow, England: Pearson; 1999, 2009.
5. Stilman A. Grammatically Correct, 2nd ed. Cincinnati, OH, USA: Writer's Digest Books; 1997, 2010.
6. Iverson C, Christianse S, Flanagin A, Fontanarosa PB, Glass RM, Gregoline B, Lurie SJ, Meyer HS, Winker MA, Young RK, eds. AMA Manual of Style: A Guide for Authors and Editors, 10th ed. Oxford: Oxford University Press; 2007.
7. Elefteriades JA. Twelve Tips on Writing a Good Scientific Paper. Inter J Angiol. 2002; 11: 53-55.

Part VI
Publishing

Chapter 46
Ethics of Scientific Publishing

Introduction

Publishing is simply the process of making a paper available to the public. Today there are many ways to publish and disseminate reports, but most of them would not be considered scientific. In the present era, publication in a peer-reviewed journal is really the only form of scientific publication. (Publishing a book or conference abstract would also be scientific, when peer-review is involved, but usually it is not really. Academic theses are normally also scientific, but they are only rarely published). Publications in peer-reviewed journals can be considered scientific, precisely because they have undergone a process of peer review and journal selection. This process weeds out much of the material that does not meet the prevailing standards of the scientific community for reliable knowledge. Compared to the ethical issues arising during the conduct, analysis, and write-up of medical research, the ethical issues of the publishing phase are rather minor. The ethical issues of publishing all revolve around communicating honestly and transparently with the journal Editors and peer-reviewers, so they can evaluate the manuscript appropriately. Ethical scientific publishing mainly involves four different issues: 1) avoiding redundant publications, 2) being honest about who are the authors, 3) disclosing all potential conflicts of interest and sources of funding, and 4) notifying the journal of any errors or problems discovered after publication. Despite their names, the ethical problems of "salami publication" and "non-publication" are actually a consequence of writing too much or too little about a research study, and thus arise almost entirely prior to the phase of submitting and publishing the paper. Accordingly, they were discussed in chapter 21, "Ethics of Scientific Writing".

© Springer Nature Switzerland AG 2019
M. Hanna, *How to Write Better Medical Papers*,
https://doi.org/10.1007/978-3-030-02955-5_46

No Redundant Publications

Redundant publication is the publishing of the same paper in two or more different journals or the reusing of substantial portions of a paper or database in another subsequent publication. Redundant publication is a waste of the journals' resources and the reviews' volunteer efforts [1–3]. If the redundancy is not recognized as such, it will also bias the outcomes of any metaanalysis or systematic review [4]. Redundant publication is also in many cases a violation of copyright laws. Such conduct was already considered unethical before the internet era; the existence of internet search engines now also nullifies the excuse that some readers might not find the paper if it were not published in multiple journals. Redundant publication reveals the authors' laziness and greed to obtain more readers or more credit than their work actually merits; it is a form of misconduct. So you should not publish the same material more than once: neither publishing the same paper in two different journals, nor reusing substantial portions of the data or results in further papers [1–3, 5–10]. It is entirely permissible to publish translations of a paper into other languages, but the translations should always clearly state that they are translations and cite the original paper. If portions of a paper need to be republished for some legitimate reason, the original source should be cited and the journal Editor should be informed of the reuse at the time of submission. It may also be necessary to obtain permission from the original journal or their publisher, if they hold the copyright. Reuse of material from a conference abstract in a subsequent journal publication is normally permitted, but the journal paper should cite the original conference and/or the publication of the conference abstract.

Honest Authorship Claims

One of the most widespread and serious ethical problems at the publishing phase is falsification of the list of authors and acknowledged contributors. Nearly all journals in medicine and related subjects follow the recommendations of the International Committee of Medical Journal Editors (ICMJE) about the criteria for authorship [5]. The ICMJE states:

The ICMJE recommends that authorship be based on the following 4 criteria:

1. Substantial contributions to the conception or design of the work; or the acquisition, analysis, or interpretation of data for the work; AND
2. Drafting the work or revising it critically for important intellectual content; AND
3. Final approval of the version to be published; AND
4. Agreement to be accountable for all aspects of the work in ensuring that questions related to the accuracy or integrity of any part of the work are appropriately investigated and resolved.

[...]

All those designated as authors should meet all four criteria of authorship, and all who meet the four criteria should be identified as authors [5].

The technical aspects of determining the authorship of a paper according to these criteria are discussed in the next chapter on authorship. This chapter focuses on the larger ethical dimension of why it is so important to be honest about the listing of authors and contributors.

Listing someone as a co-author who clearly does not meet all four criteria of authorship is called "guest authorship" (or "gift authorship") [11, 12]; it is unethical, and many journal Editors have denounced it [1, 10, 12–19]. Leaving out someone who did meet all four criteria of authorship makes that person into a ghost and amounts to stealing credit for their contributions [11, 20]; again, journal Editors have repeatedly denounced this as being unethical [1, 15, 17, 19]. (And as the ICMJE states, anyone who fulfilled criteria 1 should be given the opportunity to fulfill the other three criteria [5].)

Falsification of the list of co-authors of a paper is essentially a serious form of lying and theft. It is lying, because readers assume that the people listed as authors are in fact the people who did the research, wrote the paper, and take responsibility for it. Readers may often interpret the paper in light of who are listed as the authors. Falsification of the list of co-authors is also theft, because anyone falsely listed as a co-author takes unearned credit for the publication and anyone falsely excluded from the list of co-authors loses the credit they deserved for the work they did. If the list of co-authors becomes shorter or longer as a consequence, or if the position of names in the list changes, then the amount of credit conferred to the co-authors listed will also change, inappropriately.

Some people might view such "changes" of the authorship list as relatively harmless exchanges among only the people involved, with no wider ramifications. That viewpoint is seriously mistaken. Society's allocation of research funding, academic appointments, and so on is based to a substantial degree on the publication track records of the people in question. The net macrosocial consequence of the widespread falsification of authorship lists is that the socially precious resources of research funding, employment opportunities, and so on become misallocated. People who did the research and writing but received less credit than they deserved will receive fewer resources in the future to do further research or other related work. Instead, resources will be directed disproportionately to people who have less capability than their list of publications implies. The ultimate result is that society will receive less scientific progress for the amount of funding it directs toward research. That partial loss of progress then undermines society's willingness to invest in research.

Disclosures

Every co-author should report any potential conflicts of interest that he or she has in regards to the research publication. Primarily this means any financial relations they might have to any products studied in the research. But conflicts of interest can also refer to other non-financial issues that might have influenced what a co-author wrote. Most journals require that potential conflicts of interest be disclosed at the time of submitting the manuscript [5]. Authors should not feel any hesitation to provide full disclosures [21–23]. The current best way to properly disclose all potential conflicts of interest is to just fill out and submit the "ICMJE Form for Disclosure of Potential Conflicts of Interest" [5, 24], which is freely available on the internet. Nonetheless, disclosure of potential conflicts of interest does not absolve authors from the responsibility to make every effort to write a scientifically rigorous paper free of bias [25].

Furthermore, every paper should clearly state the source(s) of any funding (including donated supplies or services) and what involvement, if any, the funder(s) had in the study planning, conduct, analysis, and/or reporting [26]. If there was no funding at all, this should be stated explicitly, but it is rarely the case that there is truly no funding of a research study, unless everyone did the work as volunteers. When researchers state that there was no funding, what they usually mean is that no additional external funding was received. But if the researchers are receiving salary from their employer (e.g. a university or hospital) to do the research, or are using the employer's facilities or materials, then effectively the employer is funding that research. Although it is not yet common practice, such funding should be explicitly stated, so readers can see clearly who actually paid for the research and what involvement they may have had in it. Only in some very rare situations (e.g. a physician recently retired from private practice writing up a case report) is there truly no funding of a research publication.

Post-Publication Corrections

Finally, if you discover (or even suspect) errors or other problems in the paper after publication, you have a scientific and ethical obligation to inform the journal Editor about those errors or problems, so the Editor can correct the scientific literature. Depending on the extent of the errors and the reason for them, the journal will publish one of various types of correction notices or take whatever other steps may be needed to rectify the published literature [5, 27–30]. If the error was an innocent mistake, then you certainly want to fix your paper, so your readers have correct and clean information. If the "error" was not innocent, readers will notice it sooner or later, so you should notify the Editor before they do. The goal of corrections is to improve the quality of current scientific knowledge available to the research community, healthcare professionals, policy makers, and the general public.

Conclusion

The four ethical issues discussed in this chapter all arise primarily during the phase of submitting and publishing papers with the journals. Despite the apparent diversity of these four issues, they all have something quite specific in common: honesty with the Editors of the journals. And actually, their common feature is something even more specific than just honesty in general with the Editors. For the most part, these ethical aspects during the publishing phase are not about not telling lies to the Editors; instead, they are about eliminating deceptive silences and omissions when communicating with the Editors. Thus we can posit one general golden rule of ethics for the publishing phase: tell the Editors everything they need to know to make the right decisions about your manuscripts; do not keep silent about anything for the purpose of trying to boost your chances of publication. That golden rule should provide you sufficient guidance for any other issues that arise during the publication phase that have not been explicitly discussed here.

References

1. Huth EJ. Irresponsible Authorship and Wasteful Publication. Ann Intern Med. 1986; 104: 257-259.
2. Lock S. Repetitive publication: a waste that must stop. BMJ. 1984; 288: 661-662.
3. Fye WB. Medical Authorship: Traditions, Trends, and Tribulations. Ann Intern Med. 1990; 113: 317-325.
4. Tramèr MR, Reynolds DJM, Moore RA, McQuay HJ. Impact of covert duplicate publication on metaanalysis: a case study. BMJ. 1997; 315: 635-640.
5. International Committee of Medical Journal Editors. Recommendations for the Conduct, Reporting, Editing, and Publication of Scholarly Work in Medical Journals. Philadelphia: American College of Physicians; 1978, 2017. Accessed on 12 January 2018 at: www.icmje.org/icmje-recommendations.pdf
6. Asher SL, Iserson KV, Merck LH, for the Society for Academic Emergency Medicine Ethics Committee. Society for Academic Emergency Medicine Statement on Plagiarism. Acad Emerg Med. 2017; 24: 1290-1292.
7. Graf C, Deakin L, Docking M, Jones J, Joshua S, McKerahan T, Ottmar M, Stevens A, Wates E, Wyatt D. Best practice guidelines on publishing ethics: a publisher's perspective, 2nd edition. Int J Clin Pract. 2014; 68: 1410-1428.
8. DeAngelis CD. The Roman Article: Read It Again – in the Same Journal. JAMA. 2009; 301: 1382-1383.
9. Neill US. Publish or perish, but at what cost? J Clin Invest. 2008; 118: 2368.
10. Asher R. Six Honest Serving Men for Medical Writers. JAMA. 1969; 208: 83-87.
11. Flanagin A, Carey LA, Fontanaros PB, Phillips SG, Pace BP, Lundberg GD, Rennie D. Prevalence of Articles With Honorary Authors and Ghost Authors in Peer-Reviewed Medical Journals. JAMA. 1998; 280: 222-224.
12. Greenland P, Fontanarosa PB. Ending Honorary Authorship. Science. 2012; 337: 1019.
13. Glass RM. Guest authors: no place in any journal. Nature. 2010; 468; 765.
14. McKneally M. Put my name on that paper: Reflections on the ethics of authorship. J Thorac Cardiovasc Surg. 2006; 131: 517-519.
15. Marco CA, Schmidt TA. Who Wrote This Paper? Basics of Authorship and Ethical Issues. Acad Emerg Med. 2004; 11: 76-77.
16. Riesenberg D, Lundberg GD. The Order of Authorship: Who's on First? JAMA. 1990; 264: 1857.
17. Rennie D, Flanagin A, Yank V. The Contributions of Authors. JAMA. 2000; 284: 89-91.
18. Authorship without authorization. Nat Mater. 2004; 3: 743.
19. Scientific Integrity Committee of the Swiss Academies of Arts and Sciences. Authorship in scientific publications: analysis and recommendations. Swiss Med Wkly. 2015; 145: w14108.
20. Gøtzsche PC, Kassirer JP, Woolley KL, Wager E, Jacobs A, Gertel A, Hamilton C. What Should Be Done To Tackle Ghostwriting in the Medical Literature? PLoS Med. 2009; 6: 0122-0125.
21. Lippert S, Callaham ML, Lo B. Perceptions of Conflict of Interest Disclosures among Peer Reviewers. PLoS One. 2011; 6: e26900.

22. Welch SJ. Conflict of Interest and Financial Disclosure: Judge the Science, Not the Author. Chest. 1997; 112: 865-867.
23. Buffel du Vaure C, Boutron I, Perrodeau E, Ravaud P. Reporting funding source or conflict of interest in abstracts of randomized controlled trials, no evidence of a large impact on general practitioners' confidence in conclusions, a three-arm randomized controlled trial. BMC Med. 2014; 12: 69.
24. Drazen JM, de Leeuw PW, Laine C, Mulrow C, DeAngelis CD, Frizelle FA, Godlee F, Haug C, Hébert PC, James A, Kotzin S, Marušić A, Reyes H, Rosenberg J, Sahni P, Van Der Weyden M, Zhaori G. Toward More Uniform Conflict Disclosures—The Updated ICMJE Conflict of Interest Reporting Form. NEJM. 2010; 363: 188-189.
25. The *PLoS Medicine* Editors. An Unbiased Scientific Record Should Be Everyone's Agenda. PLoS Med. 2009; 6: 0119-0121.
26. Hakoum MB, Jouni N, Abou-Jaoude EA, Hasbani DJ, Abou-Jaoude EA, Lopes LC, Khaldieh M, Hammoud MZ, Al-Gibbawi M, Anouti S, Guyatt G, Akl EA. Characteristics of funding clinical trials: cross-sectional survey and proposed guidance. BMJ Open. 2017; 7: e015997.
27. Christiansen S, Flanagin A. Correcting the Medical Literature: "To Err is Human, to Correct Divine". JAMA. 2017; 318: 804-805.
28. Scarlat MM. Erratum, corrigenda et emendatio or "mistake, correction and amendment". Int Orthop. 2017; 41: 1071-1072.
29. Pulverer B. When things go wrong: correcting the scientific record. EMBO J. 2015; 34: 2483-2485.
30. The *PLoS Medicine* Editors. Getting Closer to a Fully Correctable and Connected Research Literature. PLoS Med. 2013; 10: e1001408.

Chapter 47
Authorship

One thorny issue that often comes up with medical papers is deciding who to list as the authors. The larger ethical issues about authorship were discussed in the previous chapter; this chapter focuses more on the practicalities of determining authorship. The rules on authorship are quite clear-cut, so it should always be simple to figure out who is or is not a co-author of a journal paper.

The "Recommendations for the Conduct, Reporting, Editing, and Publication of Scholarly Work in Medical Journals", written by the International Committee of Medical Journal Editors, states:

The ICMJE recommends that authorship be based on the following 4 criteria:
1. Substantial contributions to the conception or design of the work; or the acquisition, analysis, or interpretation of data for the work; AND
2. Drafting the work or revising it critically for important intellectual content; AND
3. Final approval of the version to be published; AND
4. Agreement to be accountable for all aspects of the work in ensuring that questions related to the accuracy or integrity of any part of the work are appropriately investigated and resolved.
[…]
All those designated as authors should meet all four criteria of authorship, and all who meet the four criteria should be identified as authors [1].

These guidelines from the ICMJE leave little uncertainty about who really is or is not a co-author on a paper. Each co-author must somehow have had a substantial influence on the results being reported and must also have had meaningful involvement in the write-up of the manuscript. If there are any genuine doubts about whether or not someone met both of those criteria, then he or she probably did not do enough to be considered a co-author. He or she should either do more work on the research or manuscript or should be moved to the Acknowledgments section. If an objective outside observer was familiar with the ICMJE guidelines and knew which persons made which contributions to a particular manuscript, then that

© Springer Nature Switzerland AG 2019
M. Hanna, *How to Write Better Medical Papers*,
https://doi.org/10.1007/978-3-030-02955-5_47

outside observer could always quickly and reliably decide who does or does not meet the ICMJE criteria for authorship. There is rarely or never any real ambiguity or uncertainty about that assessment. When this decision is made by the potential co-authors of the paper themselves, two different types of problems can arise: either they all reach tacit consensus among themselves to falsify the authorship list in a particular way (usually by adding people who did not truly meet the authorship criteria, but sometimes by excluding people who did) or they get into disputes among themselves about who should or should not be listed as the co-authors.

The first type of authorship problem – consensus to falsify the list of co-authors – is regrettably widespread in medical science. Shamefully, many people in academia frequently add the names of their co-workers to the list of co-authors even though those people did not really fulfill all the ICMJE criteria of authorship [2–10]. Sometimes this is based on pure fabrication of those persons' involvement, but much more often it is based on exaggerating the relevance of their contributions. "Substantial contributions" in ICMJE criteria 1 means that if anyone else had done that work instead, the final published paper would probably be meaningfully different [11]. Work that would have been done essentially the same by anyone else or work that was too scant to have an influence on the final paper would not qualify for co-authorship and should be mentioned in the Acknowledgments instead. The growing tendency to inflate the list of co-authors should be rigorously avoided [8–10, 12–17].

For each person listed as a co-author, it should also be possible to identify substantial portions of the final manuscript that were written by that co-author. If no substantial portion of the final text was written by someone listed as a co-author, then that person does not meet criteria 2 for authorship. Simply reading the manuscript and changing a few words does not equate to "revising it critically for important intellectual content". If someone does meet criteria 1, then he or she should be given the opportunity to add substantial content to the writing of the manuscript [1]. If he or she does not do that, then he or she should be moved from the list of co-authors to the list of acknowledged contributors. As a rough general guideline, there should probably be a maximum of one co-author for each 250 words in the manuscript, because there simply is not enough text there to say that more than that number of people contributed substantially to the writing. One expert even made a good case for a limit of three co-authors [10].

The second type of authorship problem – disputes among the potential co-authors about whom to credit as a co-author or not – is less common but much more acrimonious. Generally, the main reason such disputes ever arise is because people ignore the ICMJE guidelines and instead follow their own internal power politics [2–7, 10, 18–26]. It is quite rare that such disputes involve genuine protracted difficulties interpreting and applying these criteria and nothing more. In many cases, disputes can be resolved by reminding everyone about these guidelines developed by the ICMJE and endorsed by nearly all reputable journals. Journals generally refuse to arbitrate such disputes and leave the responsibility for such decisions to the authors themselves [14, 27–31]. So if you find yourself in an irresolvable authorship dispute, your institution/employer – or a lawyer – is your only recourse.

As with health and many other aspects of life, taking measures to prevent authorship disputes from ever arising is better than passively waiting for problems to arise and then trying to fix them. One good way to prevent authorship disputes is to establish an informal written agreement about what each person will contribute to a project and who will or will not be the co-authors of the paper; this document should be written up and signed by everyone before the research ever begins and again before drafting the manuscript begins [26, 28, 31–35]. Such an authorship agreement may need some revisions or updates as the research project or manuscript evolves, but it is much easier to fairly negotiate those kinds of updates than it is to try to decide authorship for the first time at the last minute before submission to the journal, after everyone has already done their work or not.

The list of authors should honestly reflect who did the work for the paper. The authors should be listed in the order of descending amount of contributions to that specific paper [26, 28, 36–40]. Thus the main researchers/writers are listed toward the beginning, specialists and assistants making contributions to specific aspects come in the middle, and senior authors who supervised the study and reviewed that paper come toward the end – *if and only if they truly meet the ICMJE criteria for authorship*, something which is often not the case [2–4, 6, 18, 21, 22, 24–26], disappointingly. In order to better illuminate who did what, the paper should always include a section at the end "Author Contributions", which describes the contributions of each co-author. These descriptions should be much more specific and detailed than they currently are: e.g. not "revised the manuscript for critical content", but instead "substantially rewrote the Questionnaires subsection of the Methods, redesigned figures 2 and 3, substantially revised the Discussion paragraphs on study limitations and conclusions, and provided minor edits throughout the rest of the paper." It is always possible to determine who contributed more or less to a given paper, so there should never be a footnote claiming that two or more authors contributed equally. That is untrue, illogical, and unethical.

The ICMJE criteria for authorship should always be followed for the ethical reasons mentioned in the previous chapter. But there is another strong reason for rigorously enforcing the authorship criteria: it will make the contents of the paper much better. When people can claim authorship credit without contributing much to a paper, then often they will not actually contribute much. Similarly, when people know that they will not get authorship credit for their contributions anyway, then they also will not contribute much. When instead the authorship criteria are rigorously enforced, then most people start investing more time, effort, and brainpower into doing and discussing that research and writing and revising the manuscript. The ultimate outcome of that increased effort of all the co-authors is a better paper that will be published in a better journal.

References

1. International Committee of Medical Journal Editors. Recommendations for the Conduct, Reporting, Editing, and Publication of Scholarly Work in Medical Journals. Philadelphia: American College of Physicians; 1978, 2017. Accessed on 12 January 2018 at: www.icmje.org/icmje-recommendations.pdf
2. Bhopal R, Rankin J, McColl E, Thomas L, Kaner E, Stacy R, Pearson P, Vernon B, Rodgers H. The vexed question of authorship: views of researchers in a British medical faculty. BMJ. 1997; 314: 1009-1012.

3. Hoen WP, Walvoort HC, Overbeke AJPM. What Are the Factors Determining Authorship and the Order of the Authors' Names? A Study Among Authors of the *Nederlands Tijdschrift voor Geneeeskunde* (Dutch Journal of Medicine). JAMA. 1998; 280: 217-218.

4. Pignatelli B, Maisonneuve H, Chapuis F. Authorship ignorance: views of researchers in French clinical settings. J Med Ethics. 2005; 31: 578-581.

5. Maisonneuve H. Guest Authorship, Mortality Reporting, and Integrity in Rofecoxib Studies. JAMA. 2008; 300: 902.

6. Goodman NW. Survey of fulfillment of criteria for authorship in published medical research. BMJ. 1994; 309: 1482.

7. Boerma T. New authorship practices are needed in developing countries. BMJ. 1997; 315: 745-746.

8. Fye WB. Medical Authorship: Traditions, Trends, and Tribulations. Ann Intern Med. 1990; 113: 317-325.

9. McKneally M. Put my name on that paper: Reflections on the ethics of authorship. J Thorac Cardiovasc Surg. 2006; 131: 517-519.

10. Asher R. Six Honest Serving Men for Medical Writers. JAMA. 1969; 208: 83-87.

11. Branson RD. Anatomy of a Research Paper. Respir Care. 2004; 49: 1222-1228.

12. Parker GB. On the breeding of coauthors: just call me Al. MJA. 2007; 187: 650-651.

13. Kapoor VK. Polyauthoritis giftosa. Lancet. 1994; 346: 1039.

14. Marco CA, Schmidt TA. Who Wrote This Paper? Basics of Authorship and Ethical Issues. Acad Emerg Med. 2004; 11: 76-77.

15. van Loon AJ. Pseudo-authorship. Nature. 1997; 389: 11.

16. Asher R. Why are medical journals so dull? BMJ. 1958; 2 (5094): 502-503.

17. Sigma Xi. Honor in Science. Research Triangle Park, NC, USA: Sigma Xi; 2000.

18. Jain SH. Negotiating Authorship. J Gen Intern Med. 2011; 26: 1513-1514.

19. Scott T. Changing authorship system might be counterproductive. BMJ. 1997; 315: 744.

20. Ezsias A. Authorship is influenced by power and departmental politics. BMJ. 1997; 315: 746.

21. Kwok LS. The White Bull effect: abusive coauthorship and publication parasitism. J Med Ethics. 2005; 31: 554-556.

22. Wagena EJ. The scandal of unfair behaviour of senior faculty. J Med Ethics. 2005; 31: 308.

23. Wilcox LJ. Authorship: The Coin of the Realm, The Source of Complaints. JAMA. 1998; 280: 216-217.

24. Lawrence PA. Rank injustice. Nature. 2002; 415: 835-836.

25. Greenland P, Fontanarosa PB. Ending Honorary Authorship. Science. 2012; 337: 1019.

26. Scientific Integrity Committee of the Swiss Academies of Arts and Sciences. Authorship in scientific publications: analysis and recommendations. Swiss Med Wkly. 2015; 145: w14108.

27. Drazen JM. Authorship Limits. NEJM. 2002; 347: 1118.

28. Riesenberg D, Lundberg GD. The Order of Authorship: Who's on First? JAMA. 1990; 264: 1857.

29. Yentis SM. Another kind of ethics: from corrections to retractions. Anaesthesia. 2010; 65: 1163-1166.

30. Kennedy D. Multiple Authors, Multiple Problems. Science. 2003; 301: 733.

31. Neill US. Stop misbehaving! J Clin Invest. 2006; 116: 1740-1741.

32. Primack RB, Cigliano JA, Parsons ECM. Coauthors gone bad; how to avoid publishing conflict and a proposed agreement for co-author teams. Biol Conserv. 2014; 176: 277-280.

33. Cals JWL, Kotz D. Effective writing and publishing scientific papers, part IX: authorship. J Clin Epidemiol. 2013; 66: 1319.

34. Albert T, Wager E. How to handle authorship disputes: a guide for new researchers. In: Committee on Publication Ethics. The COPE Report 2003. Norfolk, England: Committee on Publication Ethics; 2003, pp. 32-34.

35. Chakravarty K. Excluding authors may be impossible. BMJ. 1997; 315: 748.

36. Bhandari M, Einhorn TA, Swiontkowski MF, Heckman JD. Who Did What? (Mis)Perceptions About Authors' Contributions to Scientific Articles Based on Order of Authorship. J Bone Joint Surg Am. 2003; 85-A: 1605-1609.
37. Tscharntke T, Hochberg ME, Rand TA, Resh VH, Kraus J. Author Sequence and Credit for Contributions in Multiauthored Publications. PLoS Biol. 2007; 5: e18.
38. Bhopal RS, Rankin JM, McColl E, Stacy R, Pearson PH, Kaner EFS, Thomas LH, Vernon BG, Rodgers H. Team approach to assigning authorship order is recommended. BMJ. 1997; 314: 1046.
39. de Sa P. Bhopal and colleagues' suggested method of ordering authors wouldn't work. BMJ. 1997; 315: 745.
40. Rennie D, Flanagin A, Yank V. The Contributions of Authors. JAMA. 2000; 284: 89-91.

Chapter 48
Acknowledgments

At the end of every manuscript (just before the References), there should be an "Acknowledgments" section. This section allows the authors to give credit to all the people who contributed in various ways to generating the research paper without qualifying for authorship [1–3]. It is not the appropriate occasion for the authors to thank their families, former teachers, co-workers uninvolved in the research, patients who participated in the study, etc. For the Acknowledgments section has a very specific and important underlying function: to inform the readers about all the other people who influenced the research paper in various ways.

Foremost, the Acknowledgments section should name all the people who met one or more criteria of authorship but not all four [1]. This might include for example: a clinician who delivered study treatment to the patients but did not participate substantially in writing this particular paper, a statistician who performed some data analysis but declined to get involved in writing the paper, a medical writer who edited the paper for better writing style but was not involved in data interpretation or developing substantial content of the paper, or a department chair who read and approved the final paper for submission but was not involved in the research or writing.

The Acknowledgments section should also mention people who contributed to the research or paper in other meaningful ways that do not match the authorship criteria. This might include a nurse who administered study questionnaires, lab technicians, a research assistant who did data entry, a department chair who helped acquire study funding, colleagues or anonymous peer reviewers whose advice led to substantial changes in the contents of the manuscript, a proof-reader at the journal, and so on. The litmus test to determine whether or not to mention someone in the Acknowledgments section is the following question: if that person made a mistake or did or said something differently, could that have changed some detail in the paper that people could point to and say, "This detail of the paper appears this way because so-and-so did such-and-such"? If so, then that person should be acknowledged [3]. The acknowledgment should state as specifically as possible what the person actually contributed, for example not "help preparing the manuscript" but

© Springer Nature Switzerland AG 2019
M. Hanna, *How to Write Better Medical Papers*,
https://doi.org/10.1007/978-3-030-02955-5_48

"proof-reading the final manuscript and formatting the references", or for another example, not "technical assistance" but "providing technical support for the EKG data collection and performing all data entry".

If you would like to thank other people who had no real direct influence on the paper itself – such as your friends, family, patients, and cafeteria staff – thank them in person, not in the Acknowledgments section of the paper.

Finally, any and all sources of financial support for the research and paper should be clearly stated. Most journals list this under a separate heading ("Funding Sources"), but if not, the study sponsors must be named in the Acknowledgments section [4].

References
1. International Committee of Medical Journal Editors. Recommendations for the Conduct, Reporting, Editing, and Publication of Scholarly Work in Medical Journals. Philadelphia: American College of Physicians; 1978, 2017. Accessed on 12 January 2018 at: www.icmje. org/icmje-recommendations.pdf
2. Hare D. Giving credit where credit is due—Authorship versus acknowledgment. Can Vet J. 2001; 42: 249-250.
3. Hall T. Without a putative contributor, would the integrity of the work change? BMJ. 1997; 315: 746-747.
4. Graf C, Deakin L, Docking M, Jones J, Joshua S, McKerahan T, Ottmar M, Stevens A, Wates E, Wyatt D. Best practice guidelines on publishing ethics: a publisher's perspective, 2nd edition. Int J Clin Pract. 2014; 68: 1410-1428.

Chapter 49
The References

The reference list provides the bibliographic information on all the works you cited. It enables readers to retrieve further literature supporting the assertions of your paper. No other works should appear in the reference list that you did not cite in your paper. Items that a librarian would be unable to retrieve (e.g. an email from a colleague or a poster presented at a conference but not otherwise published) should be cited directly in the text but never in the reference list. Above all, you should never cite something that neither you nor any of your co-authors have actually read in full. Always read your references, in full, to verify that they actually say what you claim they do.

In nearly all medical journals, the references are listed in the order they first appear in the paper, (not in alphabetical order). For the formatting of the references, most medical journals use the "Vancouver" style. Vancouver style for a few of the most common types of citations are illustrated here.

This is an example of how to format the reference for a journal paper, in Vancouver style:

Haynes RB, Mulrow CD, Huth EJ, Altman DG, Gardner MJ. More Informative Abstracts Revisited. Ann Intern Med. 1990; 113: 69–76.

The reference starts with the list of author names (last name, then the initials of the first and middle names), with each author separated by a comma, yet no other punctuation until a period at the end. Journals vary in policies about the maximum number of authors to list, but one standard recommendation is that if there are more than 6 authors, the reference should list the first 3, followed by "et al." [1 (pp. 44–45)]. Then the reference shows the title of the article (including the subtitle if there was one), followed by a period. If the work cited was written in a language other than English, it is best to just write that title in that other original language in which you read it; translating the title into English may lead someone to try to track down a citation that they are then unable to read. Next, the reference gives the title of the journal, using its standard abbreviation (the "MedAbbr" according to the "PubMed journal list" from the U.S. National Library of Medicine), followed by a period.

© Springer Nature Switzerland AG 2019
M. Hanna, *How to Write Better Medical Papers*,
https://doi.org/10.1007/978-3-030-02955-5_49

Finally the reference provides the year of publication, semi-colon, the volume number of the journal, colon, the page range, period. If you are citing a journal that restarts the page numbering at "1" for each issue, then the issue number should also be given, in parentheses, after the volume number. Otherwise, it is optional, because it is unnecessary but sometimes helpful.

Here is how to format the reference for a book chapter in Vancouver style:

> DeAngelis CD. Foreword. In: Iverson C, Christianse S, Flanagin A, Fontanarosa PB, Glass RM, Gregoline B, Lurie SJ, Meyer HS, Winker MA, Young RK, eds. AMA Manual of Style: A Guide for Authors and Editors, 10th ed. Oxford: Oxford University Press; 2007, pp. v–vi.

The reference starts with the name of the author of the chapter, and the title of the chapter (here, "Foreword"). It continues with "In:", followed by the list of names of the editors of the book followed by "ed" (editor) or "eds" (editors), and then the title of the book. Finally, the reference provides the main city in which the book was published, colon, the name of the press that published the book, semi-colon, the year of publication, comma, "pp." (for "pages"), and the page numbers of the chapter (here, "v–vi" (the pages used Roman numbering, because it was a foreword)). There is lack of consensus about the exact formatting between the year and the page numbers, but the approach shown here should be acceptable and clear to readers.

Most webpages should be avoided as citations because the material they contain is usually neither scientific nor reliable (see chapter 27, "Citing the Literature"). But there are some instances when it is necessary and acceptable to cite webpages. For the reference, it is insufficient and unacceptable to simply write the webaddress; your readers need more complete information. Yet the recommendations from the US National Library of Medicine [2] and the American Medical Association [1 (pp. 68–69)] on how to write the reference for a standard webpage differ in many details and are both somewhat outdated, senseless, or cumbersome in other aspects, especially those from the NLM. Blending them together and revising a bit further, it should be acceptable to write the reference for a standard webpage as follows:

> U.S. National Library of Medicine. Samples of Formatted References for Authors of Journal Articles. Published: 09 July 2003. Updated: 02 May 2018. Accessed on 21 May 2018 at: https://www.nlm.nih.gov/bsd/uniform_requirements.html

The reference starts with the name of the author(s) of the webpage; (if no specific person is credited as the author, provide the name of the organization that "authors" the website, as in the example above). Next, the reference provides the title of the webpage; (if there is nothing resembling a title on that webpage, provide the name of the website overall). If available, the reference continues with: "Published:" and the date the page was published; (if such information is not available on the webpage, this part is omitted). If available, the reference continues with: "Updated:" and the date it was last updated; (again, if such information is not available, this part is omitted). Finally, the reference says: "Accessed on:", the date you last looked at it, "at:", and then the internet address of that specific page.

(It is best to check it again when you are writing up your reference list and then use that date.) The internet address should be dumped to the end of the reference as shown in the example above (in contrast to the AMA recommendation but consistent with the NLM recommendation), because the internet address is often long and incomprehensible, and therefore disrupts the page layout and reading if it is placed anywhere else within the reference. It is preferable to omit the period that is usually placed at the end of a reference, so it will not accidentally become part of the internet address. Whenever you cite a webpage, you should save or print a copy, in case it disappears from the internet later [1 (p. 63)]. Indeed, this is why the recommendation from the NLM (to end the reference with "Available from" and then the web address) is wrong. The web-address can change, so there is no way to ensure that readers will find the document still "available from" the address provided in the reference.

The bibliography of this book is written in Vancouver style, so the references there serve as further examples of how to format references. The AMA's *Manual of Style* [1 (pp. 39–79)], the NLM's, "Samples of Formatted References for Authors of Journal Articles" [2], and most journals' "Instructions to Authors" webpages also provide extensive reliable examples and explanations for all different kinds of sources that one might ever possibly cite.

Although most medical journals use the Vancouver style, it is sensible to double-check your target journal's "Instructions to Authors". Some journals use other styles or have their own quirky house rules for various details. If a journal has variant house rules or uses some other style instead of Vancouver style, their "Instructions to Authors" will provide examples of references in that style and/or point you to the reference book where that citation style is presented.

References should always be written in the citation style of your target journal according to their "Instructions for Authors". In principle, medical journals are supposed to always accept reference lists formatted in Vancouver style, and make any formatting changes for other styles or house style themselves [3]. But submitting a manuscript to a journal with references that are not formatted in that journal's style implies that you wrote the manuscript for some other journal (which already rejected it) and you do not believe the current journal is actually going to accept and publish your manuscript. Therefore, it is preferable to format your references in the style of your target journal prior to ever submitting the manuscript to them. Various software programs can convert references from one formatting style to another and also keep your references properly numbered while you add and delete citations in the paper. Submitting a manuscript with references that are already formatted according to the journal's instructions eliminates that work and brings your manuscript that much closer to publication.

It is important to proof-read your references carefully, especially for proper punctuation. Numerous errors in the references are a giveaway sign that the authors: A) do sloppy research, B) may not have actually read the references, and C) did not spend much time and care in writing the manuscript. Erroneous references are also irritating to readers who want to find and read those other articles [4]. A neatly referenced manuscript is a reassuring sign of careful, high-quality work.

References

1. Iverson C, Christianse S, Flanagin A, Fontanarosa PB, Glass RM, Gregoline B, Lurie SJ, Meyer HS, Winker MA, Young RK, eds. AMA Manual of Style: A Guide for Authors and Editors, 10th ed. Oxford: Oxford University Press; 2007.
2. U.S. National Library of Medicine. Samples of Formatted References for Authors of Journal Articles. Published: 09 July 2003. Updated: 02 May 2018. Accessed on 21 May 2018 at: https://www.nlm.nih.gov/bsd/uniform_requirements.html
3. Lock S. Authors of the world, unite... BMJ. 1982; 284: 1726-1727.
4. Berk RN. Preparation of Manuscripts for Radiology Journals: Advice to First-Time Authors. AJR. 1992; 158: 203-208.

Chapter 50
Selecting the Target Journal(s)

Most journals accept only about one-third or fewer of the manuscripts they receive, so it is important to carefully choose an appropriate target journal. Usually it is preferable to choose your target journal early in the writing process, so you can custom-tailor your paper to the specific style of that journal [1, 2]. Yet manuscripts can evolve substantially during the write-up (or get rejected from the initial journal). Regardless of whether you are planning ahead or ready to submit, you will get your paper published much sooner and with less effort, if you invest some time reviewing all your options and carefully selecting the most appropriate target journal.

Instead of simply sending your manuscript to the first journal that comes to mind, give careful consideration to a half dozen journals or more, and then choose the journal that you believe will be best matched to your paper. First, look at the ranking lists for journals in the field(s) of your paper, based on impact factor, normalized Eigenfactor, or source-normalized impact per paper, for examples. But do not simply send your manuscript to the top-ranked journals, especially if you have not already published several papers [3]. Instead, use the list to identify other appropriate journals that you might not have thought about already. Also, look through all the citations in your reference list, and notice which journals published them. Journals that have already published papers of similar caliber to your own and on the same (or similar) topics are more likely to be receptive to your manuscript. Look at recent issues of the journal to get a clear sense of what they publish. Think twice before sending a clinical paper to a journal that predominantly publishes basic science papers, or vice versa [1, 4].

Generally speaking, unless you have already published several papers, it is probably preferable to select a modest journal in your field and get your paper published soon, rather than squandering a lot of time pitching your paper to several high caliber journals [5]. Ultimately, the choice of journal is not really yours – it is the journal Editor's choice. If you submit your manuscript to a journal that is mismatched, the decision from the journal Editor will be terse. Your goal should be to divine which journal will be eager to at least send your manuscript out for peer review. If the journal does not send your paper out for peer review at all, then in nearly all

© Springer Nature Switzerland AG 2019
M. Hanna, *How to Write Better Medical Papers*,
https://doi.org/10.1007/978-3-030-02955-5_50

cases you have simply wasted your time and theirs. If a journal sends your manuscript out for peer review, then your choice of journal was plausible, and you will benefit from the submission, even if the journal rejects your paper. The most appropriate target journal is the one that eventually publishes the manuscript after meaningful peer review and revision, not the journal with the highest impact factor or the quickest acceptance.

Regrettably, a few words of warning about dubious journals are necessary. In the past few years there has been a proliferation of "predatory journals": websites imitating the appearance of scientific journals and publishing papers on the internet – usually for a fee – without exerting any quality control over the scientific contents [6–12]. Always be very careful to not send your manuscripts to any such predatory journal. Publishing with these predatory journals is worse than just posting the manuscript on your own personal website. If you publish your paper with a predatory journal, you will usually pay a fee and probably lose the copyright, yet very few people will ever see your paper, and almost no one in the scientific community will consider it a valid scientific publication. If you are unsure about a journal's legitimacy, search online for current lists of predatory publishers and journals. Similarly, be cautious about sending your manuscript to new journals, even if they are being produced by a legitimate medical or scientific society. Specifically, you should avoid any journal that is not yet indexed in databases such as PubMed, does not yet have established journal metrics (such as an impact factor), or has not yet been in existence for at least five years. (Many predatory journals make false claims about being indexed and having journal metrics [13], so such information should always be verified elsewhere.) Until journals meet these criteria, it is difficult to know how good they will be, or even whether they will still be in existence next year. There are already so many well-established journals that there should never be any need to turn to any of these kinds of dubious journals.

References

1. Saper CB. Academic Publishing, Part III: How to Write a Research Paper (So That It Will Be Accepted) in a High-Quality Journal. Ann Neurol. 2015; 77: 8-12.
2. Bourne PE. Ten Simple Rules for Getting Published. PLoS Comput Biol. 2005; 1: e57.
3. Erren TC. The Long and Thorny Road to Publication in Quality Journals. PLoS Comput Bio. 2007; 3: e251.
4. Thompson PJ. How To Choose the Right Journal for Your Manuscript. Chest. 2007; 132: 1073-1076.
5. Berk RN. Preparation of Manuscripts for Radiology Journals: Advice to First-Time Authors. AJR. 1992; 158: 203-208.
6. Beall J. Ban predators from the scientific record. Nature. 2016; 534: 326.
7. Beall J. Predatory publishers are corrupting open access. Nature. 2012; 489: 179.
8. Bartholomew RE. Science for sale: the rise of predatory journals. J R Soc Med. 2014; 107: 384-385.
9. Cals JWL, Kotz D. Literature review in biomedical research: useful search engines beyond PubMed. J Clin Epidemiol. 2016; 71: 115-116.
10. Berger M, Cirasella J. Beyond Beall's List: Better understanding predatory publishers. College & Research Libraries News. 2015; 76: 132-135.

11. Bohannon J. Who's Afraid of Peer Review? Science. 2013; 342: 60-65.
12. International Committee of Medical Journal Editors. Recommendations for the Conduct, Reporting, Editing, and Publication of Scholarly Work in Medical Journals. Philadelphia: American College of Physicians; 1978, 2017. Accessed on 12 January 2018 at: www.icmje. org/icmje-recommendations.pdf
13. Beall J. Medical Publishing Triage – Chronicling Predatory Open Access Publishers. Ann Med Surg. 2013; 2: 47-49.

Chapter 51
Submission to the Journal

Publishing your manuscript is an extremely important stage of writing a paper, because publication is what makes your work available to everyone else. There may sometimes be legitimate reasons to withhold or defer publication of research work. But studies on the further fate of conference abstracts and rejected journal papers seem to indicate that most often authors simply stop making efforts to publish a study that merits (or could merit) publication [1–3]. So it is important to keep making efforts for any manuscript until it actually gets published. Getting papers published involves an arduous process of submitting the manuscripts to journals and then diligently following through on the revisions they require. Fortunately, if you have done sensible research, written your paper carefully, and chosen your target journal appropriately, it usually should not be too difficult to get the paper published. Just do not give up on the manuscript before it is published.

Before submitting your manuscript to the journal, read the "Recommendations for the Conduct, Reporting, Editing, and Publication of Scholarly Work in Medical Journals" from the International Committee of Medical Journal Editors, available on the internet [4]. It contains valuable guidance on the formalities of manuscript preparation and publication. You should also look at your target journal's "Instructions to Authors", which explains the formal details of how they want manuscripts to be prepared. Although most journals follow all the recommendations from the ICMJE, most journals provide substantial information about their own specific publishing formats and expectations, beyond what the ICMJE provides for journals in general. It is important that you follow your target journal's "Instructions to Authors" meticulously in all details [5, 6]. If you do not prepare your manuscript exactly the way the journal has asked you to, there is a good chance that it will be sent back by the Managing Editor for corrections, thus delaying the review of your manuscript by however many days or weeks it takes him or her to check submitted manuscripts. If your manuscript was not formatted according to the journal's instructions yet does not get rejected by the Managing Editor, then surely the Editor and/or peer reviewers will notice that you manuscript is not formatted correctly. They will then assume that the formatting is not correct because you previously

© Springer Nature Switzerland AG 2019
M. Hanna, *How to Write Better Medical Papers*,
https://doi.org/10.1007/978-3-030-02955-5_51

submitted it to another journal, which rejected your manuscript, and then you did not bother to change the formatting for the current journal [7]. Remember, journals only accept about 10–30% of the manuscripts they receive, so try not to give them one more reason to reject yours.

Normally, the "Corresponding Author" is responsible for actually submitting the manuscript to the journal. If that is you, be sure to get all your co-authors to reread and approve the final manuscript before you actually submit it to the journal. The best way to do this is to hold a mandatory meeting of all co-authors, read the manuscript aloud, and discuss or revise it until everyone is ready to approve it [8].

Never submit a manuscript to more than one journal at a time [4, 5, 9]. In the end, only one journal can publish the manuscript. If more than one journal is reviewing your manuscript at the same time, you are wasting the time and efforts of the journals and their peer reviewers [5].

References

1. Weber EJ, Callaham ML, Wears RL, Barton C, Young G. Unpublished Research from a Medical Specialty Meeting: Why Investigators Fail to Publish. JAMA. 1998; 280: 257-259.
2. Sprague S, Bhandari M, Devereaux PJ, Swiontkowski MF, Tornetta P III, Cook DJ, Dirschl D, Schemitsch EH, Guyatt GH. Barriers to Full-Text Publication Following Presentation of Abstracts at Annual Orthopaedic Meetings. J Bone Joint Surg Am. 2003; 85-A: 158-163.
3. Smith MA, Barry HC, Williamson J, Keefe CW, Anderson WA. Factors Related to Publication Success Among Faculty Development Fellowship Graduates. Fam Med. 2009; 41: 120-125.
4. International Committee of Medical Journal Editors. Recommendations for the Conduct, Reporting, Editing, and Publication of Scholarly Work in Medical Journals. Philadelphia: American College of Physicians; 1978, 2017. Accessed on 12 January 2018 at: www.icmje.org/icmje-recommendations.pdf
5. Berk RN. Preparation of Manuscripts for Radiology Journals: Advice to First-Time Authors. AJR. 1992; 158: 203-208.
6. Whalen E. An Author's Guide to the Guidelines for Authors. AJR Am J Roentgenol. 1989; 152: 195-198.
7. Roberts WC. Revising Manuscripts After Studying Reviewers' Comments. Am J Cardiol. 2006; 98: 989.
8. McQuay HJ, Moore RA. Work done by junior researchers gives rise to problems. BMJ. 1997; 315: 745.
9. Rogers LF. Salami Slicing, Shotgunning, and the Ethics of Authorship. Am J Roentgenol. 1999; 173: 265.

Chapter 52
The Cover Letter

Many researchers make the mistake of submitting their manuscripts without a cover letter or with a useless one. When you submit a manuscript to a journal, the Editor will only read two pages before making a decision to either reject your manuscript or send it out for review: 1) the Abstract and 2) the cover letter [1–4]. If you write an inappropriate cover letter or none at all, then you lose half your chance to convince the Editor to send your manuscript out for review.

There are three common ways of writing a cover letter that are wrong. 1) Do not write more than one single page (single-spaced, 12 point font, 1″ margins). The Editor does not want to spend that much time reading supplemental information from you. 2) Do not write a cover letter that repeats the Abstract in other words [3]. The Editor will read your Abstract, so there is no need to state anything more than the title (and maybe the capsule summary) in the cover letter. 3) Do not write a generic cover letter that could be sent to any journal. Your cover letter should always address the Editor by name (spelled correctly) [3], and the body of your cover letter should be obviously custom-written for that specific journal.

Instead of those wrong approaches, the cover letter should tell the Editor why you are sending your manuscript to his or her journal rather than to some other journal [3], and therefore why the Editor should publish your manuscript rather than someone else's. The best way to do this is to tell the Editor that you read a recent editorial in his or her journal, calling for more research precisely on the topic your current manuscript addresses. If that is not possible, another way to explain why your manuscript is a good match to this journal is to briefly compare it to the various other papers this journal recently published on the same topic. Alternately, you could try to explain why your manuscript is more suited to the readership of this particular journal, rather than to the readership of other plausible target journals.

There are three other pieces of information that authors often wonder whether or not they should include in their cover letter: 1) the history of which journals reviewed it previously and why they did not accept it; 2) statements that the manuscript has not been previously published, is not simultaneously under review elsewhere, and was approved by all co-authors; 3) the names of anyone you want or do not want to

© Springer Nature Switzerland AG 2019
M. Hanna, *How to Write Better Medical Papers*,
https://doi.org/10.1007/978-3-030-02955-5_52

be a reviewer. If the journal's "Instructions to Authors" requests any of that information, or if you believe it will increase the likelihood that your manuscript will be sent out for review, then include it. Otherwise, just skip it.

One final tip: always put your cover letter on official letterhead from your institute, so it looks like the manuscript is being submitted by someone credible. If you have no such electronic stationary, arrange to have some made.

Whatever you write in the cover letter, imagine yourself in the shoes of the Editor for a moment. Does the cover letter give you the feeling that the manuscript has been carefully prepared specifically for this journal? If not, the chances are high that you will receive a generic decision letter from the Editor as soon as he or she gets around to it.

References

1. Groves T, Abbasi K. Screening research papers by reading abstracts. BMJ. 2004; 329: 470-471.
2. Annesley TM. The Abstract and the Elevator Talk: A Tale of Two Summaries. Clin Chem. 2010; 56: 521-524.
3. Brice J, Bligh J. 'Dear Editor…': advice on writing a covering letter. Med Educ. 2005; 39: 876.
4. Langdon-Neuner E. Hangings at the *bmj*: What editors discuss when deciding to accept or reject research papers. The Write Stuff. 2008; 17: 84-85.

Chapter 53
The Journal Decision-Making Process

Top-tier journals receive several thousand manuscripts per year and publish less than 10% of them [1]. Even run-of-the-mill journals receive at least several manuscripts per day and publish less than one-third of them. So journals start by triaging the manuscripts they receive. Each incoming manuscript will be assigned to an Associate Editor or Section Editor. That Editor will not read the entire manuscript. He or she will only read the manuscript's title page, the Abstract, and maybe the cover letter. Based on just those two or three pages, that Editor will then make a decision either to send the manuscript out for peer review or (more often) to reject it without peer review [1–5]. The supply of peer reviewers' volunteered time for a journal is not unlimited, so Editors try to avoid soliciting reviews for manuscripts that they know they will never publish anyway [6]. Some common reasons for rejection without peer review include: 1) the manuscript does not fit the scope of the journal, 2) the topic appears to be of low interest for the readership, 3) the quality of evidence (in terms of study design, sample size, etc.) appears clearly below the usual standards of the journal, 4) the manuscript itself is very poorly prepared [1, 7, 8]. Any journal Editor who has been on the job for more than a month has already read hundreds of papers submitted to that journal, so his or her judgments about which manuscripts have no chance of ever being published at their journal are rarely to never wrong, especially if he or she is the Editor who actually makes that decision. So if your manuscript is rejected from a journal without peer review, just consult your co-authors and move on to the next journal; do not waste your time and energy feeling dejected or trying to dispute the journal's decision [6, 9–14].

If the journal does send your paper out for peer review, then eventually they will send you a decision letter (along with the reviewer comments). Although the wording of those letters is often a bit cryptic, the journal decision normally has one of four levels: 1) accept the manuscript as is without further revision, 2) offer to probably publish it if minor revisions are made, 3) offer to possibly publish or reconsider it if major revisions are made, 4) reject it. Legitimate scientific journals virtually never offer to accept a manuscript as is without further revision upon the first submission [7, 10, 11, 14–18]; that decision usually comes only after revision. On the

© Springer Nature Switzerland AG 2019
M. Hanna, *How to Write Better Medical Papers*,
https://doi.org/10.1007/978-3-030-02955-5_53

other end of the scale, rejection letters can be identified as such because the Editor never expresses any interest in seeing a revised version of the manuscript and/or wishes you better success at another journal or with a future manuscript [9, 10]. Between those two ends of the decision scale is a broad gray zone where the Editor expresses a willingness to consider a revised version of the manuscript, without making any promises that revision will lead to publication. These letters can be worded in a variety of ambiguous ways, and journals usually exaggerate how much revision is needed while remaining aloof about your prospects. However unencouraging such a decision letter might seem, if the journal is leaving the door open for you, you should revise your manuscript and resubmit it to that journal, as explained in subsequent chapters. Do not give up and switch to another journal.

The peer reviewers will provide an assessment of your manuscript, but ultimately the decision to accept or reject your manuscript for publication is made, not by the peer reviewers, but by the Editor-in-Chief of the journal [1, 5, 18–20]. Editors rely upon the reviewers to get outside expert perspectives about the relevance and quality of the paper, especially if it is outside the Editor's own personal areas of expertise. Although Editors often base their decisions mainly on the feedback of the reviewers, their decisions are not always consistent with the contents and tone of the reviewers' assessments. Editors always have more plausible manuscripts available than they can actually publish. If an Editor feels that your manuscript is not making the cut, there will always be at least some criticism in the reviews that the Editor can point to as justification for rejecting your manuscript, even if the reviews were quite positive overall. In any case, Editors have no obligation to justify their decisions – publishing of scientific work currently remains autocratic, not democratic. On the other hand, if the Editor wants to publish your manuscript, he or she can overlook the criticisms of the reviewers. The Editor can even orchestrate the peer review to reach a desired outcome. If an Editor would like to publish your paper but is not fully satisfied with your manuscript, all he or she has to do is send it out to (yet another) peer reviewer,... or two, or three. And if the Editor wants to see an especially supportive or critical review of your manuscript, he or she knows exactly which reviewers to contact to obtain such a review [18, 19]. In any case, even though the peer reviewers usually provide 95+% of the written feedback on your manuscript, the Editor is indeed the only person who makes the decision about publication [1, 18–20].

It is important to have a realistic sense of the timeframe for this entire decision-making process, because inexperienced authors are sometimes a bit impatient, but more often because many journals are too slow and disorganized. Within one or two weeks after submitting your manuscript to a journal, that journal should have completed its initial triage and reached a decision to either reject the manuscript outright without peer review or send it out for peer review. If the journal does send the manuscript out for peer review, the process can take much longer, because the journal staff has only limited influence on how quickly they can get feedback from the peer reviewers, most of whom are quite busy with many other responsibilities. Furthermore, a journal may have to go through a few rounds of soliciting reviews, so the process can drag on, especially at lower quality journals. Although patience is a virtue, authors are not being unreasonable to expect that journals complete the review process within a productive timeframe. So if you have not heard from a journal within two weeks of submission, feel free to contact the Managing Editor and ask if the manuscript has been sent out for peer review. And if you have not received a decision letter within two months after submission, feel free to ask the Managing Editor what is causing the delay [1, 21]. Regrettably, you often do need to remain politely vigilant that the process moves ahead in a timely manner, especially at lower level journals.

At any good journal, the majority of manuscripts will be rejected in the first decision letter from the Editor, most without external peer review [2, 6, 18]. With very rare exceptions, the rest will receive a decision letter somewhere in that gray zone calling for revision and resubmission [7, 10, 11, 14–17]. If you never resubmit your manuscript to that journal, then there is zero chance that that journal will publish it [7, 9]. If you resubmit your manuscript without seriously doing the revisions, your chances of publication at that journal are only infinitesimally better. If you do the recommended revisions (as explained in subsequent chapters) and resubmit your manuscript, the journal review process will resume again, usually with the same peer reviewers and Editor. The evaluation cycle continues repeating until either you give up or the Editor-in-Chief reaches a black-or-white decision to either reject or accept the manuscript.

References

1. Groves T. Why submit your research to the BMJ. BMJ. 2007; 334: 4-5.
2. Groves T, Abbasi K. Screening research papers by reading abstracts. BMJ. 2004; 329: 470-471.
3. Ketcham CM, Hardy RW, Rubin B, Siegal GP. What editors want in an abstract. Lab Invest. 2010; 90: 4-5.
4. Cals JWL, Kotz D. Effective writing and publishing scientific papers, part II: title and abstract. J Clin Epidemiol. 2013; 66: 585.
5. Langdon-Neuner E. Hangings at the *bmj*: What editors discuss when deciding to accept or reject research papers. The Write Stuff. 2008; 17: 84-85.
6. Making the most of peer review. Nat Neurosci. 2000; 3: 629.
7. Pierson DJ. The Top 10 Reasons Why Manuscripts Are Not Accepted for Publication. Respir Care. 2004; 49: 1246-1252.
8. Coates R, Sturgeon B, Bohannan J, Pasini E. Language and publication in *Cardiovascular Research* articles. Cardiovasc Res. 2002; 53: 279-285.
9. Woolley KL, Barron JP. Handling Manuscript Rejection: Insights From Evidence and Experience. Chest. 2009; 135: 573-577.
10. Williams HC. How to reply to referees' comments when submitting manuscripts for publication. J Am Acad Dermatol. 2004; 51: 79-83.
11. DeMaria A. Manuscript Revision. J Am Coll Cardiol. 2011; 57: 2540-2541.
12. Graf C, Deakin L, Docking M, Jones J, Joshua S, McKerahan T, Ottmar M, Stevens A, Wates E, Wyatt D. Best practice guidelines on publishing ethics: a publisher's perspective, 2nd edition. Int J Clin Pract. 2014; 68: 1410-1428.
13. Bourne PE. Ten Simple Rules for Getting Published. PLoS Comput Biol. 2005; 1: e57.
14. Cummings P, Rivara FP. Responding to Reviewers' Comments on Submitted Articles. Arch Pediatr Adolec Med. 2002; 156: 105-107.

15. MacDonald NE, Ford-Jones L, Friedman JN, Hall J. Preparing a manuscript for publication: A user-friendly guide. Paediatr Child Health. 2006; 11: 339-342.
16. Morgan PP. The joys of revising a manuscript. CMAJ. 1986; 134: 1328.
17. Langdorf MI, Hayden SR. Turning Your Abstract into a Paper: Academic Writing Made Simpler. West J Emerg Med. 2009; 10: 120-123.
18. Kravitz RL, Franks P, Feldman MD, Gerrity M, Byrne C, Tierney WM. Editorial Peer Reviewers' Recommendations at a General Medical Journal: Are They Reliable and Do Editors Care? PLoS One. 2010; 5: e10072.
19. Lock S. Peer review weighed in the balance. BMJ. 1982; 285: 1224-126.
20. International Committee of Medical Journal Editors. Recommendations for the Conduct, Reporting, Editing, and Publication of Scholarly Work in Medical Journals. Philadelphia: American College of Physicians; 1978, 2017. Accessed on 12 January 2018 at: www.icmje.org/icmje-recommendations.pdf
21. Saper CB. Academic Publishing, Part III: How to Write a Research Paper (So That It Will Be Accepted) in a High-Quality Journal. Ann Neurol. 2015; 77: 8-12.

Chapter 54
Peer Review

Peer review is the process of verifying that statements are true or reasonable, to the best of current human knowledge, before putting them into general circulation. Science is not scientific because researchers follow a formal methodology, or gather data, or perform statistical analysis, or report their findings in a special format. Many other kinds of non-scientific writings also contain those elements. Furthermore, anyone can write, print, and claim whatever they want, and there is plenty of junk science and pseudo-science out there. Epistemologically, peer review is what makes science scientific. Peer review is a process of intersubjective verification, whereby other qualified scientists independently review the study conclusions (and all other assertions) and decide whether they appear to be valid knowledge, rather than mere personal opinion or mistaken "knowledge" not corresponding to external reality. This independent intersubjective expert verification is what raises a report up to the level of scientific knowledge, …at least in theory.

In practice, peer review today is usually only a measure of quality improvement, and it is almost always shoddy and incomplete [1–3]. The fundamental problem is that peer reviewers are never paid for the time they devote to reviewing manuscripts, nor rewarded in any other meaningful way. The consequence is that they often do not spend as much time on the process as they know they could and should, understandably so, since they are volunteering their precious time to do a thankless task. If you are fortunate, your manuscript will be reviewed by kind colleagues, with a genuine interest in your topic, who therefore provide a fair and professional assessment of your manuscript, along with an itemized list of constructive feedback for further improvement. If you are unfortunate, your manuscript will be reviewed by someone with more ego than competence, who begrudgingly accepts the task, skims your manuscript several weeks later, misconstrues it entirely, and then quickly fires off his or her "expert" review with half a dozen misspelled reasons why the journal should stop sending him or her such terrible manuscripts [3–6]. (And if you are completely cursed, he or she will then steal your manuscript's ideas and publish them as his or her own or use them in a grant application [7–11].)

© Springer Nature Switzerland AG 2019
M. Hanna, *How to Write Better Medical Papers*,
https://doi.org/10.1007/978-3-030-02955-5_54

For researchers who have not already seen peer review feedback on dozens of manuscripts, reading such peer review is often disorienting and difficult to interpret correctly. The feedback from a peer reviewer should normally contain three parts. First, professional reviewers will start their comments by providing a neutrally phrased capsule summary of the paper, to make it clear to the Editor and the authors what the study did and what the paper is about. If you receive peer review that does not start with such a summary (and often they do not), your paper was reviewed by an amateur. Truly competent reviewers will also explicitly state that they have no relevant conflicts-of-interests (or will disclose them if they do). Next, the peer reviewer normally provides an overall global assessment of the worth of the paper. Those remarks are usually brief but essentially amount to the reviewer's opinion to the Editor about which of the four levels of decision the journal should issue, although it is never explicitly phrased in those terms. Finally, the reviewer will use the rest of the review to provide detailed feedback on specific points of the manuscript, in the form of recommendations for improvement, questions, and criticism. In this final part, reviewers almost never waste time praising anything they find good, because that is not their assignment [1]. The review focuses entirely on what needs further improvement. So try to not become discouraged – the review is usually not nearly as bad as it first seems. Some reviewers hit all the big issues first and then provide a list of points on minor details. Other reviewers simply list all their comments together in the order they occur in the manuscript. Peer review can sometimes run up to a page of feedback per reviewer. If instead the feedback from a reviewer is brief (a single short paragraph or less), this usually indicates that the journal turned to someone without much experience or interest in providing peer review or that the reviewer did not want to spend much time on your manuscript. If you manuscript receives feedback from fewer than three reviewers, that is often a sign that either the Editor was not really interested in publishing your paper (and therefore did not want to consume the time of his or her pool of volunteer peer reviewers) or that several peer reviewers looked at it and declined the Editors' request to provide peer review – thereby signaling what they felt the Editor should do too.

In any case, there are two important points to keep in mind. One, as explained in the previous chapter, the decision about publication is made by the Editor, not by the peer reviewers [12–15]. So regardless of how positive or negative the reviewer comments are, the bottom line about how you should proceed is contained in the decision letter from the Editor, which may or may not be consistent with the viewpoints of the reviewers. Two, the intended purpose of peer review is to improve the quality of your manuscript [16], (and to weed out papers that cannot be considered sufficiently scientific, due to unfixable major flaws). Unless a study is indeed irremediably unscientific, revising the manuscript in light of feedback from other experts can only make it better, regardless of how unpleasant the process might sometimes seem. So if you received peer review feedback, the next step is to get to work on improving your manuscript in light of that expert feedback, either for resubmission to the same journal or, if clearly rejected, to submit to a new journal.

References

1. Kassirer JP, Campion EW. Peer Review: Crude and Understudied, but Indispensable. JAMA. 1994; 272: 96-97.
2. Moher D, Altman DG. Four Proposals to Help Improve the Medical Research Literature. PLoS Med. 2015; 12: e1001864.
3. Bacchetti P. Peer review of statistics in medical research: the other problem. BMJ. 2002; 324: 1271-1273.
4. Ernst E. A beginner's guide to criticism: A brief taxonomy of reviewers, and how to deal with them. MJA. 2007; 187: 649.
5. Kelly BD. Dear Editor – a note from any imaginary author in response to any referee. Med Hypotheses. 2009; 72: 359.
6. Shashok K. Content and communication: How can peer review provide helpful feedback about the writing. BMC Med Res Methodol. 2008; 8: 3.
7. Resnik DB. A Troubled Tradition. In: Baker JF, ed. For the Record: *American Scientist* Essays on Scientific Publication. Research Triangle Park, NC, USA: Sigma Xi; 2011, pp. 7-14.
8. Ready T. Plagiarize or perish? Nat Med. 2006; 12: 494.
9. Maddox J. Plagiarism is worse than mere theft. Nature. 1995; 376: 721.
10. Sigma Xi. Honor in Science. Research Triangle Park, NC, USA: Sigma Xi; 2000.
11. Dansinger M. Dear Plagiarist: A Letter to a Peer Reviewer Who Stole and Published Our Manuscript as His Own. Ann Intern Med. 2017; 166: 143.
12. Groves T. Why submit your research to the BMJ. BMJ. 2007; 334: 4-5.
13. Kravitz RL, Franks P, Feldman MD, Gerrity M, Byrne C, Tierney WM. Editorial Peer Reviewers' Recommendations at a General Medical Journal: Are They Reliable and Do Editors Care? PLoS One. 2010; 5: e10072.
14. Lock S. Peer review weighed in the balance. BMJ. 1982; 285: 1224-126.
15. International Committee of Medical Journal Editors. Recommendations for the Conduct, Reporting, Editing, and Publication of Scholarly Work in Medical Journals. Philadelphia: American College of Physicians; 1978, 2017. Accessed on 12 January 2018 at: www.icmje.org/icmje-recommendations.pdf
16. Berk RN. Preparation of Manuscripts for Radiology Journals: Advice to First-Time Authors. AJR. 1992; 158: 203-208.

Chapter 55
Doing the Revisions

Many inexperienced researchers get discouraged and/or lazy when their paper is sent back with a long list of criticisms and an ambiguous decision letter from the Editor. Sometimes, they give up and simply submit the same (unchanged) manuscript to another journal. That is usually a bad decision, because an opportunity to improve and publish the paper (with the previous journal) is thereby lost and the new journal is unlikely to offer a more positive assessment. A paper is not "done" until some journal actually publishes it, and part of the work for *every* paper is making revisions after peer review. Virtually no manuscript ever gets accepted as is on the first submission [1–8]. So no matter how good your paper is, the reviewers will find at least a few details that should be improved. More likely, they will find a long list of substantial deficiencies in your manuscript. But if you are lucky, they will be insightful, specific, and constructive about how the paper should be improved. Revision often requires a substantial amount of time and effort [3]; (especially when insufficient time and effort was invested before submission). But the process of review and revision should increase the quality.

So when you are writing a paper, always plan ahead for the further work to improve the paper after review. Do not become demoralized by reviewer comments; stay focused on the scientific contents in their comments and the ways your manuscript can be improved. And no matter how negative the reviewers were, do not let that deter you from resubmitting your manuscript to that same journal, if the Editor has permitted it. The final decision about publication rests only with the Editor, who would have already rejected your paper if there was little chance of publication after revision. Never submit the manuscript to another journal merely to avoid the work of revisions; that new journal would be equally demanding or might even just reject your manuscript [3]. So if the Editor allows you to resubmit the manuscript after revision, revise and resubmit to that same journal. Ideally, you should immediately stop everything else you are doing, so you can complete the revisions and resubmission promptly, while your manuscript is still fresh in the

© Springer Nature Switzerland AG 2019
M. Hanna, *How to Write Better Medical Papers*,
https://doi.org/10.1007/978-3-030-02955-5_55

memory of the Editors and peer reviewers [5–7]. But you should never rush the revision and resubmission [9], in the sense of sending in the manuscript without carefully doing every last bit of revision recommended.

In theory, journals distinguish between expecting "minor" revisions or "major" revisions, though the division line can seem blurry. "Minor" revisions usually mean just editing the manuscript in a variety of ways. "Major" revisions by contrast usually involve doing new statistical analyses, replacing figures and tables, rewriting entire parts of the paper to include new content, or even reporting on additional data. When reviewers call for minor revisions, it is usually easier and faster to just comply and do it than to resist and debate it, even if you are not entirely convinced that the reviewer is more right than you are. When reviewers call for major revisions, you must either do them or offer a solid scientific defense why not. If you do not do those revisions (and do not provide convincing explanations why not), then you supply the Editor with an easy justification for rejecting your paper. At all legitimate journals, the number of manuscripts permitted to revise and resubmit substantially exceeds the number that the journal will eventually agree to publish [10, 11].

So if the reviewers' recommendations are constructive attempts to help you make your report better, then you should follow their advice. You can even incorporate reviewer comments directly into your manuscript; reviewers will never complain about that, especially if you also thank them in the Acknowledgments for that contribution. If a reviewer asks you to cite a specific paper, it is often because he or she is a co-author of that paper. Read that paper and if it is applicable to your topic, then try to work it in somewhere sensible if possible. (If it is really not relevant, do not cite it simply to please the reviewer [12–15].) If the Editor asks you to reduce your manuscript length, reread chapter 41, "Cut It Down", and reduce the length of your manuscript [7]. Editors are virtually never wrong about that judgment. The only exception is when they offer to publish your manuscript if it is resubmitted as a mere letter. That is your choice – you can either reduce the manuscript down to a letter or you can resubmit the full manuscript elsewhere [3]. If your sample size is less than 20 or your topic is obscure, you should probably pursue the offer to publish as a letter.

If you really disagree with some point by one of the peer reviewers, you should solicit the viewpoint of your co-authors and other senior colleagues. There is no obligation to make every change the reviewers recommend, especially if you have a good scientific explanation why not. After all, it is your research and your paper, not theirs. Furthermore, reviewers do sometimes call for changes that would make the paper worse or would be wrong methodologically, and in those cases, their recommendations should be politely declined with explanations. But mere laziness or stubbornness is never a legitimate reason to not do the revisions, and Editors are not fooled by resubmitting the same manuscript with mere cosmetic changes [4, 16 (p. 210)]. If you decide to not do some major revision they recommended, you will need to provide good scientific reasons why not [7]. Furthermore, if more than one reviewer raises the same question or criticism, that is a clear indication that there is indeed a real problem in your manuscript, not merely an idiosyncratic opinion of a quirky reviewer. In those cases, you really should try to correct the problem; it is not sensible to try to dispel such points in the reply-to-review without changing the manuscript [11]. Editors themselves rarely suggest changes to a manuscript. So when they do, the most prudent course of action is to follow their advice completely and gratefully [17].

There is one exception about doing revisions: if a peer reviewer called for you to collect additional new data, he or she is probably going too far. If you truly agree with him or her that more data needs to be collected, and you have the willingness and resources to collect that additional data, feel free to pursue that course. Otherwise, just write back in the reply-to-review letter that the reviewer's suggestion is a very good one but regrettably is not possible due to insufficient availability of research funding to do that additional work. The current viewpoint of most Editors is that calling for additional data collection is an unproductive position in peer review [5, 18]. It is always possible to think of further research that could be done, but additional research is usually neither feasible nor essential. If the journal believes that the current version of the manuscript is really not publishable without additional data collection, then they should just reject it [18, 19].

You can of course make additional revisions to your manuscript that the peer reviewers did not propose. But if those revisions are more than just minor editing of the writing, then you should point them out in the reply-to-review letter somewhere, so the Editor and peer reviewers are aware of those additional substantial revisions that you made. If possible, try to relate your additional changes somehow or other to the remarks of the reviewers.

If the journal Editor rejected your paper after peer review, then you should still revise the manuscript in light of any reviewer feedback [7, 17, 20–22]. Doing so will make your manuscript better. But no matter how supportive the reviewers were, do not waste the journal's time resubmitting the manuscript to that journal, if the Editor has already turned it down [5, 7, 11, 15, 22, 23]. You will never convince the Editor to change his or her mind. And a review of studies on the subject shows that the majority of rejected manuscripts are subsequently published in another journal, (albeit more than a year later on average) [22]. So just chose another journal and move along. There are many good journals and all of them are available on the internet and indexed in all major databases. So there is never any reason to fixate on any one specific journal. The goal is to just get your paper published so people can read it.

References

1. MacDonald NE, Ford-Jones L, Friedman JN, Hall J. Preparing a manuscript for publication: A user-friendly guide. Paediatr Child Health. 2006; 11: 339-342.
2. Pierson DJ. The Top 10 Reasons Why Manuscripts Are Not Accepted for Publication. Respir Care. 2004; 49: 1246-1252.
3. Williams HC. How to reply to referees' comments when submitting manuscripts for publication. J Am Acad Dermatol. 2004; 51: 79-83.
4. Morgan PP. The joys of revising a manuscript. CMAJ. 1986; 134: 1328.
5. DeMaria A. Manuscript Revision. J Am Coll Cardiol. 2011; 57: 2540-2541.

6. Langdorf MI, Hayden SR. Turning Your Abstract into a Paper: Academic Writing Made Simpler. West J Emerg Med. 2009; 10: 120-123.

7. Cummings P, Rivara FP. Responding to Reviewers' Comments on Submitted Articles. Arch Pediatr Adolec Med. 2002; 156: 105-107.

8. Kravitz RL, Franks P, Feldman MD, Gerrity M, Byrne C, Tierney WM. Editorial Peer Reviewers' Recommendations at a General Medical Journal: Are They Reliable and Do Editors Care? PLoS One. 2010; 5: e10072.

9. Bauchner H. The Rush to Publication: An Editorial and Scientific Mistake. JAMA. 2017; 318: 1109-1110.

10. Lock S. How editors survive. BMJ. 1976; 2 (6044): 1118-1119.

11. Making the most of peer review. Nat Neurosci. 2000; 3: 629.

12. International Committee of Medical Journal Editors. Recommendations for the Conduct, Reporting, Editing, and Publication of Scholarly Work in Medical Journals. Philadelphia: American College of Physicians; 1978, 2017. Accessed on 12 January 2018 at: www.icmje. org/icmje-recommendations.pdf

13. Council of Science Editors. CSE's White Paper on Promoting Integrity in Scientific Journal Publications, 2012 Update, 3rd Revised Edition. Wheat Ridge, CO: Council of Scientific Editors; 2012.

14. ALLEA – All European Academies. The European Code of Conduct for Research Integrity, Revised Edition. Berlin: ALLEA; 2017. Accessed on 5 November 2017 at: www.allea.org/wp-content/uploads/2017/04/ALLEA-European-Code-of-Conduct-for-Research-Integrity-2017.pdf

15. Graf C, Deakin L, Docking M, Jones J, Joshua S, McKerahan T, Ottmar M, Stevens A, Wates E, Wyatt D. Best practice guidelines on publishing ethics: a publisher's perspective, 2nd edition. Int J Clin Pract. 2014; 68: 1410-1428.

16. Booth WC, Colomb GC, Williams JM. The Craft of Research, 3rd ed. Chicago: University of Chicago Press; 1995, 2008.

17. Elefteriades JA. Twelve Tips on Writing a Good Scientific Paper. Inter J Angiol. 2002; 11: 53-55.

18. Rockman HA. Waste not, want not. J Clin Invest. 2014; 124: 463.

19. Ploegh H. End the wasteful tyranny of reviewer experiments. Nature. 2011; 472: 391.

20. Roberts WC. Revising Manuscripts After Studying Reviewers' Comments. Am J Cardiol. 2006; 98: 989.

21. Berk RN. Preparation of Manuscripts for Radiology Journals: Advice to First-Time Authors. AJR. 1992; 158: 203-208.

22. Woolley KL, Barron JP. Handling Manuscript Rejection: Insights From Evidence and Experience. Chest. 2009; 135: 573-577.

23. Bourne PE. Ten Simple Rules for Getting Published. PLoS Comput Biol. 2005; 1: e57.

Chapter 56
The Reply-to-Review Letter

When journals express a willingness to see your manuscript again after revision, they always ask you to send in a "point-by-point" reply to the reviewer comments. At this stage, your manuscript is close to publication, but final acceptance is dependent upon making your manuscript better, so it will meet the high standards of the peer reviewers and Editors. Acceptance of your manuscript depends primarily upon improving the quality of your manuscript. Yet the reply-to-review letter plays an essential supporting role, because it should show the peer reviewers and Editors that you took their feedback seriously and did everything possible to improve your manuscript. There is a certain art and style to the reply-to-review letter, which will help ensure that your manuscript is actually accepted for publication, rather than sent back to you again for more revisions, or worse.

Start by copying all the reviewer comments into a neat new document, and set them in bold font. You should then intersperse your replies, typed in normal font, to each little suggestion or comment the reviewers made. Do not skip a reviewer remark simply because you did not like it [1–3]. That will not work; they will notice, especially if they numbered their comments to you. If you made a change to your manuscript, you should usually quote the new version in the reply-to-review letter. If you are quoting the new revised version of your manuscript, put that quote in italics or red, so it can be quickly identified as such.

If you look closely at the kinds of comments made by any one reviewer, it is usually possible to determine if he or she is primarily a clinician, a scientist, or a methodologist (statisticians, epidemiologists, psychologists, and so on). That insight can be useful in thinking about how to respond to his or her feedback. In rare instances, one of the journal Editors might also add some brief remarks to the peer review. If so, those remarks should be taken very seriously.

Nearly all reviewer comments can be categorized into five kinds of comments: compliments, suggestions for improvement, collegial questions, off-topic opinions, or criticism. Each of these types of comments has its own corresponding way of responding in the reply-to-review letter.

© Springer Nature Switzerland AG 2019
M. Hanna, *How to Write Better Medical Papers*,
https://doi.org/10.1007/978-3-030-02955-5_56

Whenever reviewers compliment your paper, thank them politely and humbly [1]. This shows diplomacy, builds positive rapport, and draws attention to the quality of your paper.

When reviewers make constructive suggestions for improvement, you should do the revision (if at all possible) and thank the reviewer for his or her ("insightful", "helpful", "expert", "beneficial") recommendation. If the reviewer's suggestion was necessary due to commonplace negligence on your part (e.g. misspelling, math errors in a table), then you should also humbly apologize for your negligence and thank the reviewer for pointing it out. If the reviewer asks you to address something that is already addressed in your manuscript, just politely point it out [1]. Reviewers are busy; they cannot always read every manuscript as if it were a newly discovered lost essay from Socrates.

Sometimes reviewers simply ask collegial questions. This usually occurs when the reviewer is not sure what other feedback to give. Always make a warm, collegial response. Do not skip the question or hurry past it with a too brief reply. And do not be pedantic or condescending (regardless of how ridiculous the question might seem). The reviewer spent precious time reading your paper, and now he or she is trying to discuss your work with you collegially, so your manuscript will seem attractive to the Editor. Be grateful that the reviewer is showing an interest in your work, and respond collegially.

Similarly, sometimes you paper makes a reviewer start thinking about something else, and he or she writes some opinions and comments about something that is not really part of your paper. It is important to read such remarks again closely ("between the lines"), because sometimes they do contain implicit calls for improvement or criticisms buried somewhere in the reviewer's "thinking aloud to myself" remarks [4]. In that case, you probably should try to revise your paper accordingly. But if the reviewer really is talking about something else unrelated to your paper, just express your agreement and move on.

In contrast to "suggestions for improvement" (above), "criticism" simply asserts that what you did is invalid or low quality, without making any recommendations for correction. When reviewers make criticisms, you can either find ways to revise your paper or you can defend it. You and your co-authors must decide for yourselves whether you find the reviewer's criticism justified. If it is justified, then you should revise your paper and reply as you would to a suggestion for improvement. If instead you disagree with the criticism, then you should just defend your manuscript in the reply-to-review letter [1, 3, 5–7]. But you must do this in a scientific and collegial way [1, 3, 7]. This is not the occasion to argue unprofessionally with the reviewer. You should acknowledge the reviewer's point as best you can. Then you should explain why you did your research the way that you did. Respond with evidence [1]. Cite the published scientific literature that supports your approach and perspective. If you cannot find any such literature to cite, you should probably reconsider your opinion that the reviewer is wrong. If needed, you should present further data and statistical analysis that was not presented in your paper. Oftentimes, a reviewer's criticism is simply due to insufficient information about your research and thinking, and he or she simply needs to hear more about what you did and why. Other times, reviewers will still disagree with you, but they – or the Editor – will accept your defense as a scientifically legitimate difference of opinion. If you present your defense in an unprofessional way though, the reviewer may be provoked to fire back further criticism. That does not bring you closer to your goal of a published paper, especially if the reviewer is a personal friend of the Editor.

The entire reply-to-review is an exercise in diplomacy. Every reply you make should take a positive, appreciative, collegial tone. If you are going to tell the reviewers that you disagree with them, start by first telling them that they are right and you agree with them, and then explain why nonetheless your view diverges just a little bit from theirs [1]. You should repeatedly thank the reviewers for their helpful expert guidance. The reviewers do not get rewarded for their service. They have volunteered their precious time to help you make your paper better. So you should always be genuinely grateful to them, even if you disagree with them [3]. Moreover, your goal is to get your paper accepted for publication. If your reply letter is unprofessional or argumentative, you will only make your own life more difficult. But if you write your reply-to-review letter in a collegial and diplomatic way, you will maximize your chances of getting your paper accepted without further revision.

Finally, remain aware that some reviewers are, regrettably, arrogant jerks (or simply having a bad day) [1, 8, 9]. Emboldened by the anonymity of peer review, they do sometimes make obnoxious comments or unnecessarily harsh criticism. Avoid taking such remarks to heart. Furthermore, the reply-to-review is not the place to pick a fight. If a reviewer writes something that seems clearly rude, unprofessional, too personally critical, or otherwise inappropriate, double-check your interpretation with your co-authors or other colleagues. If they agree with your interpretation, just politely contact the journal Editor-in-Chief directly to take note of the reviewer's unacceptable conduct, and ask the Editor to not send your manuscript to that reviewer again. There is no place in modern research for any such unprofessional personal hostility [10, 11].

One final suggestion. Before you send your reply-to-review letter to the journal, consider the fact that you might never get another chance to revise your manuscript again for that journal. No matter how great your research is, the reviewers and Editor can live just fine without it ever being published. You get one chance to do your best revision and write your best reply-to-review. Even if you do all the revision the peer reviewers recommend, the Editor might still reject your manuscript [3]. If you only do 80% of the revisions, haggle pointlessly about 10%, and simply ignore another 10%, the journal decision will be swift and painful. So do it completely the first time [1, 2, 12]. And use the reply-to-review to show them that you are serious about meeting the high standards of the journal.

References

1. Williams HC. How to reply to referees' comments when submitting manuscripts for publication. J Am Acad Dermatol. 2004; 51: 79-83.
2. Bourne PE. Ten Simple Rules for Getting Published. PLoS Comput Biol. 2005; 1: e57.
3. Cummings P, Rivara FP. Responding to Reviewers' Comments on Submitted Articles. Arch Pediatr Adolec Med. 2002; 156: 105-107.
4. Roberts WC. Revising Manuscripts After Studying Reviewers' Comments. Am J Cardiol. 2006; 98: 989.
5. Woolley KL, Barron JP. Handling Manuscript Rejection: Insights From Evidence and Experience. Chest. 2009; 135: 573-577.
6. Morgan PP. The joys of revising a manuscript. CMAJ. 1986; 134: 1328.
7. DeMaria A. Manuscript Revision. J Am Coll Cardiol. 2011; 57: 2540-2541.
8. Resnik DB. A Troubled Tradition. In: Baker JF, ed. For the Record: *American Scientist* Essays on Scientific Publication. Research Triangle Park, NC, USA: Sigma Xi; 2011, pp. 7-14.
9. Ernst E. A beginner's guide to criticism: A brief taxonomy of reviewers, and how to deal with them. MJA. 2007; 187: 649.
10. Council of Science Editors. CSE's White Paper on Promoting Integrity in Scientific Journal Publications, 2012 Update, 3rd Revised Edition. Wheat Ridge, CO: Council of Scientific Editors; 2012.
11. Graf C, Deakin L, Docking M, Jones J, Joshua S, McKerahan T, Ottmar M, Stevens A, Wates E, Wyatt D. Best practice guidelines on publishing ethics: a publisher's perspective, 2nd edition. Int J Clin Pract. 2014; 68: 1410-1428.
12. Making the most of peer review. Nat Neurosci. 2000; 3: 629.

Chapter 57
Correcting the Printer's Proofs

After the journal finally accepts your paper, they will send you printer's proofs to double-check and approve. You should read those carefully, because small errors can often still be found in a manuscript even at this late stage. In particular, you should double-check that every statement and number in the Abstract still matches the main paper. Many papers undergo substantial revision for peer review. If you made changes to the main paper but did not change the Abstract accordingly, then the final Abstract will not accurately reflect the final paper. That lack of consistency occurs frequently [1–7], surely because authors do not bother to check the printer's proofs.

Furthermore, many journals have copy-editors, and they often make numerous small changes to a manuscript. Oftentimes that is helpful, especially if English grammar is not your forte, because the copy-editors generally have a strong command of grammar and an attentive eye for details. Unfortunately, most of them have no training in medicine or science, and their edits can often change the sense of what your paper says – sometimes quite substantially. (In particular, major biomedical publishers based in the Netherlands have a reputation for copy-editing over aggressively – a point worth considering prior to submitting your manuscript.) Do not hesitate to correct their corrections – copy-editors do not have the scientific competence or legal right to make meaningful changes without your approval. Above all, you should also verify that the typeset version of your figures and tables are still readable and correctly formed, because the published versions often appear quite different than the manuscript versions [8].

But you should not make any new changes beyond correcting objective errors, (or reversing undesired changes made by the journal). Correcting the printer's proofs is not an opportunity to make new revisions, however tempting. If something substantial truly must be revised at this stage, you need to ask the Editor's permission and explain why.

Meticulously checking the printer's proofs and making tiny corrections can often feel tedious, but it is your last chance to do so in a way that eliminates the error from sight. After your paper is published, any further corrections will only be published

© Springer Nature Switzerland AG 2019
M. Hanna, *How to Write Better Medical Papers*,
https://doi.org/10.1007/978-3-030-02955-5_57

as an additional Correction or *Erratum* in some other issue of the journal, while leaving the original error intact [9–12] – a "solution" that is virtually useless. So find the time to check the printer's proofs carefully.

References

1. Fontelo P, Gavino A, Sarmiento RF. Comparing data accuracy between structured abstracts and full-text journal articles: implications in their use for informing clinical decisions. Evid Based Med. 2013; 18: 207-211.
2. Estrada CA, Bloch RM, Antonacci D, Basnight LL, Patel SR, Patel SC, Wiese W. Reporting and Concordance of Methodologic Criteria Between Abstracts and Articles in Diagnostic Test Studies. J Gen Intern Med. 2000; 15: 183-187.
3. Pitkin RM, Branagan MA, Burmeister LF. Accuracy of Data in Abstracts of Published Research Articles. JAMA. 1999; 281: 1110-1111.
4. Pitkin RM, Branagan MA. Can the accuracy of abstracts be improved by providing specific instructions? A randomized controlled trial. JAMA. 1998; 280: 267-269.
5. Ward LG, Kendrach MG, Price SO. Accuracy of abstracts for original research articles in pharmacy journals. Ann Pharmacother. 2004; 38: 1173-1177.
6. Harris AHS, Standard S, Brunning JL, Casey SL, Goldberg JH, Oliver L, Ito K, Marshall JM. The Accuracy of Abstracts in Psychology Journals. J Psychol. 2002; 136: 141-148.
7. Altwairgi AK, Booth CM, Hopman WM, Baetz TD. Discordance Between Conclusions Stated in the Abstract and Conclusions in the Article: Analysis of Published Randomized Controlled Trials of Systemic Therapy in Lung Cancer. J Clin Oncol. 2012; 30: 3552-3557.
8. Bullimore MA. Love the Data, Hate the Figures. Optom Vis Sci. 2004; 81: 642-643.
9. Christiansen S, Flanagin A. Correcting the Medical Literature: "To Err is Human, to Correct Divine". JAMA. 2017; 318: 804-805.
10. Scarlat MM. Erratum, corrigenda et emendatio or "mistake, correction and amendment". Int Orthop. 2017; 41: 1071-1072.
11. Pulverer B. When things go wrong: correcting the scientific record. EMBO J. 2015; 34: 2483-2485.
12. The *PLoS Medicine* Editors. Getting Closer to a Fully Correctable and Connected Research Literature. PLoS Med. 2013; 10: e1001408.

Chapter 58
Rereading the Published Paper

Generally, your paper will become available on the internet as an "in press" pre-print within about a month after you confirm the final printer's proofs. Depending on how unmodern and unprofessional the publisher is, it can be up to several months before the final print version of your paper becomes available. But when it does, you should read it again. At this point, it is too late to make any further corrections to the printed version, and most publishers will therefore also not alter the electronic version (except in cases of serious ethical, safety, or legal concerns). But journals can and will print a *Corrigendum* (your fault) or an *Erratum* (their fault), even for tiny details, especially if an error has meaningful implications [1–4]. So it is worth the effort to check the quality of your final paper, because that is the only version anyone else is ever going to read. Moreover, reading the final printed version (months later) may give you a different impression and/or a feel of satisfaction for your work.

References

1. Christiansen S, Flanagin A. Correcting the Medical Literature: "To Err is Human, to Correct Divine". JAMA. 2017; 318: 804-805.
2. Scarlat MM. Erratum, corrigenda et emendatio or "mistake, correction and amendment". Int Orthop. 2017; 41: 1071-1072.
3. Pulverer B. When things go wrong: correcting the scientific record. EMBO J. 2015; 34: 2483-2485.
4. The *PLoS Medicine* Editors. Getting Closer to a Fully Correctable and Connected Research Literature. PLoS Med. 2013; 10: e1001408.

© Springer Nature Switzerland AG 2019
M. Hanna, *How to Write Better Medical Papers*,
https://doi.org/10.1007/978-3-030-02955-5_58

Chapter 59
Dissemination

So now your paper has been published in the latest issue of the journal. At this point, you must be done writing your paper, right? Your paper is already published. What else could there possibly be to do now? There is one more thing to do: disseminate your paper to the scientific community and possibly the general public too. After all, you did not go through all that work only to have your paper remain rarely read and never cited.

Start first by posting the capsule summary of your paper and links to the full publication on your website, your institute's webpage, and/or any online profiles you use. If permitted by your agreements with the journal publisher, post the full paper to those sites and any repositories you use. Second, you should compile a list of all your colleagues who would have an interest in the paper, and you should send them a link to the paper with a brief personal note. Third, if your paper would be of interest to a particular non-scientific audience (e.g. a particular patient population), send links to the organizations that work with them. Similarly, if you believe your paper might be of interest to the general public, work together with your institute's communication officer to prepare a press release for journalists.

Disseminating your published paper enables you to strengthen your professional networks and to better ensure that your papers are widely read.

© Springer Nature Switzerland AG 2019
M. Hanna, *How to Write Better Medical Papers*,
https://doi.org/10.1007/978-3-030-02955-5_59

Chapter 60
Conclusion

The Introduction of this book stated that the published journal literature of medicine, including the related life and health sciences, is plagued with substantial errors, nonsensical statements, lethal omissions, illogical reasoning, false discoveries, and misleading conclusions [1–11]. Furthermore, over half the research studies that are completed are never published in a scientific journal at all [12–15]. The Introduction of this book then asserted that there were two closely related reasons for the low quality of the medical scientific literature, and explained that one of those two reasons is that the university system does not provide medical researchers with sufficient education and training in the specific subjects and skills needed to report medical research. No one single book can substitute for years of education and training, but hopefully this book has provided you with enough practical knowledge to fully justify the time you have spent reading it.

The catchphrase, "Publish or perish", is often heard in the world of academic medical research [16–19]. The idea expressed by this phrase is that job appointments in medical schools (and related settings) and research funding are both strongly dependent on the candidates' track record of scientific publications, and therefore, anyone who does not publish enough papers will be out of work with no chance of returning. In the world of medical research, there seems to be no doubt that this phrase accurately reflects the current occupational atmosphere. And medical researchers often quote this phrase with a note of sadomasochistic glee in their voices.

In the medical literature, the "publish or perish" atmosphere in medical research is often viewed as the root cause of the low quality of the published medical literature [5–7, 9, 20–23], as well as transgressions of research ethics [24–33]. (The explanation is that everyone is under pressure to publish as many papers as possible, regardless of their quality. So the proposed solution is to encourage hiring/promotion committees and grant-awarding agencies to limit the number of publications considered and focus on their importance instead.) But the "publish or perish" orientation does not and cannot explain the low quality of the medical literature if we simply take "publish or perish" at face value, as those past commentaries have done.

© Springer Nature Switzerland AG 2019
M. Hanna, *How to Write Better Medical Papers*,
https://doi.org/10.1007/978-3-030-02955-5_60

We need to critically dissect the notion of "publish or perish" before it is able to shed any light on the real cause for the low quality of the medical literature.

The phrase, "publish or perish" has caught on as a popular catchphrase in medical academia, because almost everyone who starts exploring a career in medical research (including the life and health sciences) soon realizes that there is a sparsity of funding and positions, despite all the major opportunities to improve the population's health through medical research. Aside from research reports in high-impact journals, most published papers declare "None" as their "Source of Funding", even though they do usually contain useful new knowledge. Most medical doctors are not provided with sufficient protected time to do research [34, 35]. Even when a resident or junior faculty member is expected to do some research as part of their appointment at a university hospital, they often will receive only one day per week of protected time for academic development [35–37]. That amounts to about 400 hours per year – perhaps enough to write and publish 2–4 papers – if all the data was already collected and ready to analyze and all the protected time could be directed to that research work. For most medical doctors there is neither protected time nor funding to write up scientific journal articles, so there is very little incentive to do it [38]. Thus the "publish or perish" phrase expresses the occupational situation resulting from the woefully inadequate levels of funding that society provides for the medical research it craves.

In the Introduction of this book it was asserted that there are two closely related reasons for the low quality of the medical research literature. One of those reasons is that society does not provide adequate education and training specifically on medical research to most of the people actually involved in doing that work, as discussed already in the Introduction. The other reason for the poor quality of the medical literature is simply what is being discussed here – that most research has inadequate funding to be performed and reported well. Or more precisely: society fails to provide even a fraction of the funding needed to ensure that all this medical research is performed and reported at an appropriate level of quality. The vastly insufficient funding to do the research leads to projects being abandoned, or performed and reported hastily with low quality, or handed over to other people (students, research assistants, etc.) with insufficient education and training to do it properly.

The inadequate funding of medical research creates the "publish or perish" atmosphere. The consequence is that many people who gain some initial training and experience in medical research do indeed exit from the world of medical research. But it is nonsensical to imagine that they "perish". Anyone who is working in medical research must already have a substantial amount of education and skills, compared to most other people of their same age. So when they start to notice the "publish or perish" climate in medical research, they often just start looking into other career pathways that will make more rewarding use of their many talents and abilities. And even if they never publish anything at all, they will normally find many other good opportunities to use their education and skills in other well-paid careers – in patient care, government, business, and so on.

The people who "perish" (or suffer for years) are instead the patients who have medical problems for which there is no cure or inadequate prevention, therapy, or care-provision. If there was more funding for medical research, better quality research could be performed and reported, and more progress could be made on improving the population's medical care and health. So the medical community ought to be telling society, "If you want better progress in medical treatment, society needs to provide the funding to do the research – and to better train and retain more specialists to do it well."

But instead, the "publish or perish" catchphrase mindlessly accepts society's failure to direct its resources toward the vital medical research that will improve their health. Compared to past centuries, the developed world is not poor these days. But society wastes a lot of its money on other things and activities, such as entertainment, wars, gadgets, advertising, and bureaucracy. Expenditures in these areas do not improve anyone's lives, nor the future of human life on earth.

If societies want better medical care and better health, they need to invest into it. That includes paying to train all medical researchers better in methodology, ethics, statistics, logic, and communication. Medical researchers need to improve the quality of their scientific writings. But we also need to communicate better with the general lay public about the role that medical research plays in improving their healthcare – and therefore their lives.

References

1. Collins FS, Tabak LA. NIH plans to enhance reproducibility. Nature. 2014; 505: 612-613.
2. Berwanger O, Ribeiro RA, Finkelsztejn A, Watanabe M, Suzumura EA, Duncan BB, Devereaux PJ, Cook D. The quality of reporting of trial abstracts is suboptimal: survey of major general medical journals. J Clin Epidemiol. 2009; 62: 387-392.
3. Golder S, Loke YK, Wright K, Norman G. Reporting of Adverse Events in Published and Unpublished Studies of Health Care: A Systematic Review. PLoS Med. 2016; 13: e1002127.
4. Jonville-Béra AP, Giraudeau B, Autret-Leca E. Reporting of Drug Tolerance in Randomized Clinical Trials: When Data Conflict with Authors' Conclusions. Ann Intern Med. 2006; 144: 306-307.
5. Altman DG. The scandal of poor medical research. BMJ. 1994; 308: 283-284.
6. Bailar JC III. Science, Statistics, and Deception. Ann Intern Med. 1986; 104: 259-260.
7. Marušić M, Marušić A. Good Editorial Practice: Editors as Educators. Croat Med J. 2001; 42: 113-120.
8. The *PLoS Medicine* Editors. An Unbiased Scientific Record Should Be Everyone's Agenda. PLoS Med. 2009; 6: 0119-0121.
9. O'Donnell M. Evidence-based illiteracy: time to rescue "the literature". Lancet. 2000; 355: 489-491.
10. Knight J. Clear as mud. Nature. 2003; 423: 376-378.
11. Chalmers I, Glasziou P. Avoidable waste in the production and reporting of research evidence. Lancet. 2009; 374: 86-89.
12. von Elm E, Costanza MC, Walder B, Tramèr MR. More insight into the fate of biomedical meeting abstracts: a systematic review. BMC Med Res Methodol. 2003; 3: 12.
13. Weber EJ, Callaham ML, Wears RL, Barton C, Young G. Unpublished Research from a Medical Specialty Meeting: Why Investigators Fail to Publish. JAMA. 1998; 280: 257-259.

14. Sprague S, Bhandari M, Devereaux PJ, Swiontkowski MF, Tornetta P III, Cook DJ, Dirschl D, Schemitsch EH, Guyatt GH. Barriers to Full-Text Publication Following Presentation of Abstracts at Annual Orthopaedic Meetings. J Bone Joint Surg Am. 2003; 85-A: 158-163.
15. Smith MA, Barry HC, Williamson J, Keefe CW, Anderson WA. Factors Related to Publication Success Among Faculty Development Fellowship Graduates. Fam Med. 2009; 41: 120-125.
16. Brandon AN. "Publish or Perish". Bull Med Libr Assoc. 1963; 51: 109-110.
17. Munro CL, Savel RH. Publish (High-Quality Evidence For Clinical Practice) or (Patients May) Perish. Am J Crit Care. 2013; 22: 182-184.
18. Schachman HK. From "Publish or Perish" to "Patent and Prosper". J Biol Chem. 2006; 281: 6889-6903.
19. Morales P, Bosch F. ¿Editar o perecer? Desafíos en la edición biomédica. Gac Sanit. 2005; 19: 258-261.
20. Angell M. Publish or Perish: A Proposal. Ann Intern Med. 1986; 104: 261-262.
21. Tallis RC. Researchers forced to do boring research... BMJ. 1994; 308: 591.
22. Matheson NA. ...while poor leadership fuels mediocrity. BMJ. 1994; 308: 591.
23. Halperin EC. Publish or Perish—and Bankrupt the Medical Library While We're at It. Acad Med. 1999; 74: 470-472.
24. Neill US. Publish or perish, but at what cost? J Clin Invest. 2008; 118: 2368.
25. Qiu J. Publish or perish in China. Nature. 2010; 463: 142-143.
26. Jafarey A. Deceit and fraud in medical research – Publish or perish culture is to blame. Int J Surg. 2006; 4: 132.
27. Currie C. Author saw fraud, misconduct, and unfairness to more junior staff. BMJ. 1997; 315: 747-748.
28. Koshland DE Jr. Fraud in Science. Science. 1987; 235: 141.
29. The insider's guide to plagiarism. Nat Med. 2009; 15: 707.
30. Beautification and fraud. Nat Cell Biol. 2006; 8: 101-102.
31. Accurately reporting research. Nat Cell Biol. 2009; 11: 1045.
32. Baethge C. Gemeinsam veröffentlichen oder untergehen. Dtsch Arztebl. 2008; 105: 380-383.
33. Dansinger M. Dear Plagiarist: A Letter to a Peer Reviewer Who Stole and Published Our Manuscript as His Own. Ann Intern Med. 2017; 166: 143.
34. North American Primary Care Research Group Committee on Building Research Capacity, The Academic Family Medicine Organizations Research Subcommittee. What Does It Mean to Build Research Capacity? Fam Med. 2002; 34: 678-684.
35. Young RA, DeHaven MJ, Passmore C, Baumer JG. Research Participation, Protected Time, and Research Output by Family Physicians in Family Medicine Residencies. Fam Med. 2006; 38: 341-348.
36. Smythe WR. Protected time. Surgery. 2004; 135: 232-234.
37. Flood CG, Faught JW, Schulz JA. Reflection on Academic Protected Time: An Opportunity to Integrate Educational Programs. J Obstet Gynaecol Can. 2006; 28: 295-298.
38. Asher R. Six Honest Serving Men for Medical Writers. JAMA. 1969; 208: 83-87.

Acknowledgments

I would like to thank the following people for their contributions to this project (in the chronological order of the timepoint of their contributions):

Harry Sinnamon, PhD, (Emeritus Professor and Co-Chair of Neuroscience & Behavior at Wesleyan University; Middletown, CT, USA), for providing background guidance long ago on substantial parts of the approach described in the chapter on the elevator speech;

Fernando Pérez, ScD, (Biólogo; Cologne, Germany), for discussion and support of the production of an earlier version of this book;

the many academic departments and professional conferences that have hosted my talks on this subject and thereby provided many opportunities to refine the material and receive audience feedback, especially the Office of the Research Dean at the University Hospital of Cologne, Germany;

the many readers who provided feedback on various aspects of an earlier version of this book, in particular Laurel Dezieck (Wesleyan University; Middletown, CT, USA) and also the Fall 2009 Research Fellows of the Division of Spine Surgery at New York University;

Jasna Blažičko-Milčić, MA, (Zagreb, Croatia), for providing proof-reading feedback on an earlier version of this book;

Margaret Moore, BA, (Springer; New York, NY, USA), the Acquisitions Editor for this book, for facilitating the publication of this book with Springer, providing intensive support for the project during the printing preparation phase, and ensuring that I compiled an index for the book.

© Springer Nature Switzerland AG 2019
M. Hanna, *How to Write Better Medical Papers*,
https://doi.org/10.1007/978-3-030-02955-5

About the Author

Michael Hanna, PhD, is an independent Medical Writer and Research Consultant from New York City. He has over a decade of experience designing studies, conducting literature reviews, performing statistical analysis, and writing and editing scientific papers across the spectrum of medical specialties. He has lectured widely in Europe and North America on medical writing and has mentored many researchers and medical residents on scientific writing.

Michael Hanna earned a doctoral degree in Clinical Psychology from the University of Cologne, Germany, and completed a post-doctoral fellowship at Cornell University's medical school in New York City. Previously, he earned a Master's degree in Psychology from the University of Paris VIII and a Bachelor's degree in Neuroscience and in French Studies from Wesleyan University in Middletown, CT, USA.

Prior to becoming a professional Medical Writer and Research Consultant, Michael Hanna taught at the University Hospital of Aachen, Germany. He also acquired clinical and scientific experience at the University of Cologne, Germany; the Raymond Poincaré Hospital in Paris, France; and other specialized clinics in America and Europe. He is fluent in German, French, and Spanish.

Dr. Hanna can be contacted at: michael.hanna@mercury-mrw.com

Disclosures of Potential Conflicts of Interest

The author discloses the following potential conflicts of interest related to the subject matter of this book:

1. receipt of royalties from the publisher (Springer) on sales of this book;
2. receipt of fees from numerous university researchers, for-profit medical product companies, and some other non-profit institutions and organizations for providing medical writing, scientific editing, statistical analysis, data visualization, study design, publication consulting, and other related services for the development of scientific medical publications;
3. receipt of fees from numerous universities and professional societies for lecturing and mentoring about medical scientific writing.

© Springer Nature Switzerland AG 2019
M. Hanna, *How to Write Better Medical Papers*,
https://doi.org/10.1007/978-3-030-02955-5

Bibliography

This bibliography contains all works either that are cited in this book or that I have read and believe would be of interest to medical researchers wishing to improve their medical scientific journal papers. Further works I read in the process of preparing this book are not listed in the bibliography if they were considered to be too specialized, too flawed, or too outdated to be of any interest to medical researchers just trying to improve their own scientific writing. (Nonetheless, this bibliography cannot in any sense be considered a thorough or balanced guide to this vast literature. Surely there are hundreds of articles and books with direct relevance to this topic that I have never even seen, while many items in this bibliography clearly reflect the idiosyncrasies of my own personal reading habits.)

The bibliography contains 590 items. To assist readers in identifying the literature that will be of most use to them, two asterisks (**) are placed in front of entries that I consider among the top 2% (n=12) in this bibliography, while one asterisk (*) is placed in front of all other entries (n=47) that I consider among the top 10% in this list. These asterisks refer to the literature considered to be most helpful for medical researchers to write better journal papers, not merely which bibliographic entries are the best overall or most important to read in general.

A picture worth a thousand words (of explanation). Nat Methods. 2006; 3: 237. [A brief editorial about the need for researchers to be more conscientious and restrained in their editing of data images.]

Abdulla R. Conveying Science: Original Studies Versus Case Reports. Pediatr Cardiol. 2013; 34: 1761. [An editorial with a brief historical view of the role of case reports in medical science and a very short statement of why this journal decided to stop publishing them.]

Abraham P. Duplicate and salami publications. J Postgrad Med. 2000; 46: 67-69. [A good introductory editorial about duplicate and "salami" publication.]

Accurately reporting research. Nat Cell Biol. 2009; 11: 1045. [An editorial about inappropriate image manipulation, long-term preservation of raw data, plagiarism, and proper citation.]

Ad Hoc Working Group for Critical Appraisal of the Medical Literature. A Proposal for More Informative Abstracts of Clinical Articles. Ann Intern Med. 1987; 106: 598-604. [The original proposal that led journals to adopt a structured format for abstracts; the advice here has since been superseded, but the sample abstract revision and the glossary of terms are still useful.]

© Springer Nature Switzerland AG 2019
M. Hanna, *How to Write Better Medical Papers*,
https://doi.org/10.1007/978-3-030-02955-5

Afifi M. Plagiarism is not fair play. Lancet. 2007; 369: 1428. [An honorable letter, by a non-native speaker of English, arguing against leniency for plagiarism by non-native speakers of English.]

Alasbali T, Smith M, Geffen N, Trope GE, Flanagan JG, Jin Y, Buys YM. Discrepancy between Results and Abstract Conclusions in Industry- vs Nonindustry-Funded Studies Comparing Topical Prostaglandins. Am J Ophthalmol. 2009; 147: 33-38. [This small study of some ophthalmology literature documents industry spin by showing that papers with industry funding frequently had abstract conclusions that were not consistent with the main results, while papers without industry funding had similar main results yet no discrepancy in the study conclusion.]

Albert T, Wager E. How to handle authorship disputes: a guide for new researchers. In: Committee on Publication Ethics. The COPE Report 2003. Norfolk, England: Committee on Publication Ethics; 2003, pp. 32-34. [This set of suggestions about authorship disputes from two very well-known medical writers/trainers without doctoral-level qualifications is interesting and mostly helpful, but it suffers fatally from ethical spinelessness, perhaps due to lack of scientific/scholarly authoritativeness.]

Alberti C, Boulkedid R. Describing ICU data with tables. Intensive Care Med. 2014; 40: 667-673. [This basic tutorial paper about the construction of tables (for any medical field) is neither original nor inspiring, but it is consistently correct and usable.]

ALLEA – All European Academies. The European Code of Conduct for Research Integrity, Revised Edition. Berlin: ALLEA; 2017. Accessed on 5 November 2017 at: www.allea.org/wp-content/uploads/2017/04/ALLEA-European-Code-of-Conduct-for-Research-Integrity-2017.pdf [A brief but solid and authoritative code of research ethics.]

* Altman DG. Practical Statistics for Medical Research. Boca Raton, FL, USA: CRC Press; 1991, 1999. [Although this introductory-level textbook is written very clearly and sensibly by one of the leading medical statisticians, it is not really addressed to researchers on the middle of the bell curve; highly recommended for people dedicated to a career in medical research, but for everyone else, some other textbook of medical statistics would probably be a more suitable starting point.]

* Altman DG. The scandal of poor medical research. BMJ. 1994; 308: 283-284. [This brief editorial about the unacceptably low quality of most medical research is somewhat scattershot in its attempt to identify the causes of this problem but is on-target about its diagnosis and sense of the gravity of the problem; worth reading and seriously reflecting on.]

* Altman DG, Bland JM. Absence of evidence is not evidence of absence. BMJ. 1995; 311: 485. [An important editorial explaining how negative findings in clinical or epidemiological studies are often due to lack of statistical power and should not be interpreted as evidence of lack of effects.]

Altman D, Bland JM. Confidence intervals illuminate absence of evidence. BMJ. 2004; 328: 1016-1017. [This letter illuminates how confidence intervals provide information about the possible range of the results in the population from which the study sample was drawn.]

Altman DG, Bland JM. Missing data. BMJ. 2007; 334: 424. [This basic introduction to the problem of missing data is perhaps useful for initial familiarity but is too cursory to rely upon for statistical analysis or reporting.]

Altman DG, Bland JM. Presentation of numerical data. BMJ. 1996; 312: 572. [A good brief tutorial article, mostly about how to present numerical results but also with some remarks about figures and tables.]

Altman DG, Bland JM. The normal distribution. BMJ. 1995; 310: 298. [A useful brief introduction to the Normal distribution of data – a presupposition of many statistical tests.]

Altman DG, Deeks JJ, Sackett DL. Odds ratios should be avoided when events are common. BMJ. 1998; 317: 1318. [A letter about appropriate and inappropriate use and reporting of odds ratios.]

Altman DG, Gardner MJ. More Informative Abstracts. Ann Intern Med. 1987; 107: 790-791. [An informative letter criticizing the paper cited above by the Ad Hoc Working Group for Critical Appraisal of the Medical Literature, especially their example of revising an abstract to be structured.]

Altman DG, Goodman SN, Schroter S. How Statistical Expertise Is Used in Medical Research. JAMA. 2002; 287: 2817-2820. [A large survey study about the involvement of statistical experts in research, including issues of recognizing their contributions.]

* Altman DG, Royston P. The cost of dichotomizing continuous variables. BMJ. 2006; 332: 1080. [This brief essay explains why continuous variables should never be transformed into categories – a dreadfully commonplace error with no excuse.]

Altman DG, Schulz KF, Moher D, Egger M, Davidoff F, Elbourne D, Gøtzsche PC, Lang T; for CONSORT Group. The Revised CONSORT Statement for Reporting Randomized Trials: Explanation and Elaboration. Ann Intern Med. 2001; 134: 663-694. [A detailed explanation for an earlier version of the CONSORT guidelines; useful but not the most current version.]

Altwairgi AK, Booth CM, Hopman WM, Baetz TD. Discordance Between Conclusions Stated in the Abstract and Conclusions in the Article: Analysis of Published Randomized Controlled Trials of Systemic Therapy in Lung Cancer. J Clin Oncol. 2012; 30: 3552-3557. [This study of oncology literature documents that the conclusion of randomized controlled trials sometimes differs substantially in the abstract versus the main body of the paper.]

American Academy of Dermatology. Position Statement on Photographic Enhancement. 1997, 2007. Accessed on 11 May 2018 at: http://www.aad.org/Forms/Policies/Uploads/PS/ PS-Photographic%20Enhancement.pdf [This brief document provides the position of this professional society on what is or is not acceptable alteration of medical photographs in scientific communications.]

American Psychological Association. Guidelines for Ethical Conduct in the Care and Use of Nonhuman Animals in Research. 2012. Accessed on 8 January 2018 at: https://www.apa.org/ science/leadership/care/care-animal-guidelines.pdf [These ethical guidelines on the use of animals in research are more useful for the behavioral sciences than the basic life sciences; medical researchers collecting outcome data from animals that is behavioral (rather than biological) will also find them useful.]

Amos KA. The ethics of scholarly publishing: exploring differences in plagiarism and duplicate publication across nations. J Med Lib Assoc. 2014; 102: 87-91. [A somewhat shoddy study reporting the proportion of retractions in 20 countries due to plagiarism or duplicate publication – mispresented as the "rate of retraction".]

Angell M. Publish or Perish: A Proposal. Ann Intern Med. 1986; 104: 261-262. [An editorial criticizing the academic culture that induces quick but trivial research, salami publication, inflated co-author lists, and duplicate publication.]

Annesley TM. The Abstract and the Elevator Talk: A Tale of Two Summaries. Clin Chem. 2010; 56: 521-524. [An excellent tutorial paper, mostly about writing good abstracts, but also briefly describing elevator speeches.]

Appelbaum PS, Roth LH, Lidz C. The Therapeutic Misconception: Informed Consent in Psychiatric Research. Int J Law Psychiatry. 1982; 5: 319-329. [A small but interesting study illustrating the therapeutic misconception in two samples of psychiatric patients.]

Appelbaum PS, Roth LH, Lidz CW, Benson P, Winslade W. False Hopes and Best Data: Consent to Research and the Therapeutic Misconception. Hastings Cent Rep. 1987; 17: 20-24. [This early narrative review of the problem of the therapeutic misconception in research provides useful practical suggestions on how to attenuate it.]

Aristotole. Nicomachean Ethics. [Translated from the Ancient Greek by Irwin T.] Indianapolis, IN, USA: Hackett Publishing; (ca. 350 BCE), 1985. [The foundational book of ethics, by the grandfather of all science; important reading for anyone seeking knowledge.]

Aristotle. Posterior Analytics. [Translated from the Ancient Greek by Barnes J.] Oxford: Oxford University Press; (ca. 350 BCE), 1975, 2002. [The foundational book of scientific reasoning; regrettably, much of the material will seem antiquated and opaque to contemporary researchers, yet the rest of it remains fundamentally relevant.]

Aristotle. On Rhetoric. [Translated from the Ancient Greek by Kennedy GA.] Oxford: Oxford University Press; (ca. 355 BCE), 2007. [A foundational book on ethics, persuasion, argumentation, and communicative style; surely of interest to scholars of these subjects and perhaps of some practical use to advanced scientific writers.]

Asher R. Six Honest Serving Men for Medical Writers. JAMA. 1969; 208: 83-87. [A classic tutorial article on how to approach the writing of a paper; most useful for beginners but enjoyable reading for anyone.]

* Asher R. Straight and crooked thinking in medicine. BMJ. 1954; 2 (4885): 460-462. [This lucid edito-
    rial on logical and illogical thinking in clinical medicine and research is one of the rare pieces of
    writing to directly address this vast and crucial dimension of medical science; highly recommended.]
Asher R. Why are medical journals so dull? BMJ. 1958; 2 (5094): 502-503. [This classic article,
    which criticizes various aspects of the journals themselves and the incomprehensible papers
    they publish, is mostly just as relevant today as it was then, unfortunately.]
Asher SL, Iserson KV, Merck LH, for the Society for Academic Emergency Medicine Ethics
    Committee. Society for Academic Emergency Medicine Statement on Plagiarism. Acad Emerg
    Med. 2017; 24: 1290-1292. [A statement from a professional medical society, mostly about
    what constitutes redundant publication.]
Assmann SF, Pocock SJ, Enos LE, Kasten LE. Subgroup analysis and other (mis)uses of baseline
    data in clinical trials. Lancet. 2000; 355: 1064-1069. [A small study of the literature document-
    ing the poor reporting and misuse of patient baseline data in statistical analysis.]
* Aurelius M. Meditations. [Translated from the Latin by Hard R.] Oxford: Oxford University
    Press; (ca. 170-180), 2011. [An excellent ethical and philosophical treatise to get you through
    any moral quagmires you might encounter in medical research.]
Authorship without authorization. Nat Mater. 2004; 3: 743. [An editorial against guest authorship,
    published without any specific author names.]
Aydıngöz Ü. Figures, tables, and references: integral but sometimes neglected components of sci-
    entific articles. Diagn Interv Radiol. 2005; 11: 67-68. [An editorial about the preparation of
    figures, tables, and references; mostly unoriginal and focused on small detail aspects.]
Ayer AJ. Language, Truth and Logic. London: Penguin Books; 1936, 1990. [This book of phi-
    losophy serves as useful background reading for a deeper understanding of scientific writing.]
Bacchetti P. Peer review of statistics in medical research: the other problem. BMJ. 2002; 324:
    1271-1273. [An accurate and useful essay about peer reviewers making unfounded criticisms
    of statistical aspects of manuscripts and research proposals.]
Baerlocher MO, O'Brien J, Newton M, Gautam T, Noble J. Data integrity, reliability and fraud in
    medical research. Eur J Intern Med. 2010; 21: 40-45. [This survey study about data reliability
    and fraud contains many interesting empirical insights and reflections on these topics; worth
    further reflection.]
Baethge C. Gemeinsam veröffentlichen oder untergehen. Dtsch Arztebl. 2008; 105: 380-383. [A
    critical essay, by the Editor of this journal, about the inflation of author lists.]
Bagley SC, White, H, Golomb BA. Logistic regression in the medical literature: Standards for use
    and reporting, with particular attention on one medical domain. J Clin Epidemiol. 2001; 54:
    979-985. [A useful literature review on one particular medical topic to illustrate how logistic
    regressions are often inadequately reported and/or performed; essential reading for anyone
    reporting a logistic regression analysis.]
Bahrami H. The Value of p-Value. Am J Gastroenterol. 2005; 100: 1427-1428. [A useful but
    unoriginal letter about p-values and confidence intervals.]
* Bailar JC III. Science, Statistics, and Deception. Ann Intern Med. 1986; 104: 259-260. [An astute
    essay asserting that various inappropriate approaches to statistical analysis, although common-
    place, are deceptive and therefore unethical and unscientific.]
Baille J. On Writing: Write the Abstract, and a Manuscript Will Emerge From It! Endoscopy. 2004;
    36: 648-650. [This tutorial paper on the writing of conference abstracts is full of bad advice and
    riddled with errors; not recommended.]
Baker JF, ed. For the Record: *American Scientist* Essays on Scientific Publication. Research
    Triangle Park, NC, USA: Sigma Xi; 2011. [A collection of ethics essays, all reprinted from
    American Scientist and accordingly breezy in style, about honesty, peer review, co-authorship
    falsification problems in international collaborations, development of codes of research ethics
    by professional societies, the transformation of scientific publication by computerization, and
    teaching publication ethics.]
Balon R. Guest Authorship, Mortality Reporting, and Integrity in Rofecoxib Studies. JAMA. 2008;
    300: 902. [A letter about the unfair direct and indirect financial gains of guest authors.]

Balshem H, Helfand M, Schünemann HJ, Oxman AD, Kunz R, Brozek J, Vist GE, Falck-Ytter Y, Meerpohl J, Norris S, Guyatt GH. GRADE guidelines: 3. Rating the quality of evidence. J Clin Epidemiol. 2011; 64: 401-406. [This article from the GRADE system about rating the quality of evidence in a systematic review is also useful for anyone reporting original clinical research.]

Barnard JA. Protected Time: A Vital Ingredient for Research Career Development. J Pediatr Gastroenterol Nutr. 2015; 60: 292-293. [This brief essay provides a clear picture of the funding and protected time needed by early career-phase doctors during the residency and fellowship years to become independent investigators.]

Baron JH. Plagiarism. BMJ. 1999; 319: 1494. [A brief surrealist narrative account of the experience of being plagiarized.]

Barratt A, Wyer PC, Hatala R, McGinn T, Dans AL, Keitz S, Moyer V, Guyatt G; for Evidence-Based Medicine Teaching Tips Working Group. Tips for learners of evidence-based medicine: 1. Relative risk reduction, absolute risk reduction, and number needed to treat. CMAJ. 2004; 171: 353-358. [A well-written tutorial paper explaining the calculations of "relative risk reduction", "absolute risk reduction", and "number needed to treat".]

Barry HC, Ebell MH, Shaughnessy AF, Slawson DC, Nietzke F. Family Physicians' Use of Medical Abstracts to Guide Decision Making: Style or Substance? J Am Board Fam Pract. 2001; 14: 437-442. [An empirical study suggesting that the format of abstracts does not affect the rates at which the abstract contents change physicians' approach to treatment of the illness discussed in the abstract.]

Bartholomew RE. Science for sale: the rise of predatory journals. J R Soc Med. 2014; 107: 384-385. [A good editorial about the problem of predatory journals.]

* Bates AW. "Author pays" publishing model: Not all authors will gain. BMJ. 2003; 327: 53. [A letter rightly arguing against the notion that authors should bear the costs of publication.]

Battisti WP, Wager E, Baltzer L, Bridges D, Cairns A, Carswell CI, Citrome L, Gurr JA, Mooney LaVA, Moore J, Peña T, Sanes-Miller CH, Veitch K, Woolley KL, Yarker YE. Good Publication Practice for Communicating Company-Sponsored Medical Research: GPP3. Ann Intern Med. 2015; 163: 461-464. [Guidelines for reporting research supported by for-profit entities.]

Bauchner H. The Rush to Publication: An Editorial and Scientific Mistake. JAMA. 2017; 318: 1109-1110. [A convincing editorial explaining how the rush to publish quickly compromises scientific quality with no offsetting gains for public health.]

Baxt WG, Waeckerle JF, Berlin JA, Callaham ML. Who Reviews the Reviewers? Feasibility of Using a Fictitious Manuscript to Evaluate Peer Reviewer Performance. Ann Emerg Med. 1998; 32: 310-317. [A study showing that peer reviewers frequently fail to identify even major errors in a manuscript.]

Beall J. Ban predators from the scientific record. Nature. 2016; 534: 326. [A letter proposing mechanisms to repel predatory publishers from the scientific literature.]

Beall J. Medical Publishing Triage – Chronicling Predatory Open Access Publishers. Ann Med Surg. 2013; 2: 47-49. [An essay describing predatory publishers and their ruses; despite being published in a very new journal, this essay is an accurate and reliable set of warnings about predatory publishers.]

Beall J. Predatory publishers are corrupting open access. Nature. 2012; 489: 179. [A generally good editorial about predatory publishing, marred by a couple remarks with the author's ideological biases against open-access publishing.]

Beautification and fraud. Nat Cell Biol. 2006; 8: 101-102. [An editorial mostly about an infamous case of scientific fraud involving image manipulation.]

Begley CG, Ellis LM. Raise standards for preclinical cancer research. Nature. 2012; 483: 531-533. [This commentary paper reports that Amgen was rarely able to reproduce "landmark" preclinical studies on cancer and discusses the many improvements that are needed to make preclinical research more reproducible.]

** Benjamin W. Poliklinik. In: Einbahnstrasse. Frankfurt: Suhrkamp Verlag; 1928, 2009, p. 59. [A brilliant little literary portrayal of editing as performing surgery on a text.]

Benjamini Y, Hochberg Y. Controlling the False Discovery Rate: a Practical and Powerful Approach to Multiple Testing. J R Statist Soc B. 1995; 57: 289-300. [An advanced-level paper for statisticians demonstrating that controlling the false discovery rate is a more powerful (less conservative) solution to the problem of multiple hypothesis testing than Bonferroni correction.]

Bennie MJ, Lim CW. Salami publication. BMJ. 1992; 304: 1314. [This letter provides a convincing defense of legitimate reasons to publish more than one paper from a single study.]

Berger M, Cirasella J. Beyond Beall's List: Better understanding predatory publishers. College & Research Libraries News. 2015; 76: 132-135. [This reliable and informative essay accurately identifies the ideological biases of Beall and provides a more comprehensive and balanced approach to evaluating whether a journal is predatory – a point which has gained importance since Beall removed his blacklists from the internet.]

Bergmeier L. Animal welfare is not just another bureaucratic hoop. Nature. 2007; 448: 251. [A thoughtful letter about animal research and reporting its ethical aspects in journal papers.]

Berk RN. Preparation of Manuscripts for Radiology Journals: Advice to First-Time Authors. AJR. 1992; 158: 203-208. [This editorial is full of good advice about the preparation and submission/publishing phases of writing papers in any medical field, (but its advice about the contents of papers is too scant and dated).]

Bernal-Delgado E, Fisher ES. Abstracts in high profile journals often fail to report harm. BMC Med Res Methodol. 2008; 8: 14. [A study documenting that the abstracts of clinical trials often fail to report harm.]

Berwanger O, Ribeiro RA, Finkelsztejn A, Watanabe M, Suzumura EA, Duncan BB, Devereaux PJ, Cook D. The quality of reporting of trial abstracts is suboptimal: survey of major general medical journals. J Clin Epidemiol. 2009; 62: 387-392. [This study of the literature showed that the abstracts of randomized controlled trials published in the the leading medical journals very frequently fail to report important information about the methods and results.]

Bhandari M, Einhorn TA, Swiontkowski MF, Heckman JD. Who Did What? (Mis)Perceptions About Authors' Contributions to Scientific Articles Based on Order of Authorship. J Bone Joint Surg Am. 2003; 85-A: 1605-1609. [A small but interesting survey of how this journal's editorial board interprets the probable contributions of co-authors of a manuscript in the absence of any explicit statement about their contributions.]

Bhopal RS, Rankin JM, McColl E, Stacy R, Pearson PH, Kaner EFS, Thomas LH, Vernon BG, Rodgers H. Team approach to assigning authorship order is recommended. BMJ. 1997; 314: 1046. [This letter proposes an interesting mechanism to improve the fairness of the order of authorship, but it has the pitfall of promoting unfounded inflation of the authorship list, as evidenced also by the fact that this letter with only about 360 words lists 9 co-authors.]

Bhopal R, Rankin J, McColl E, Thomas L, Kaner E, Stacy R, Pearson P, Vernon B, Rodgers H. The vexed question of authorship: views of researchers in a British medical faculty. BMJ. 1997; 314: 1009-1012. [A small single-site survey of British university medical faculty that documented almost complete ignorance of the criteria for authorship of research papers.]

Billings JS. An Address on Our Medical Literature. BMJ. 1881; 2: 262-268. [This historical essay (and bibliographic study) about the state of medical publications and the conduct of research is of very little practical use to contemporary medical authors, but it provides a fascinating perspective on "the medical literature".]

Bland M. An Introduction to Medical Statistics, 4th ed. Oxford: Oxford University Press; 2015. [Written by one of the leading medical statisticians, this is a good introductory textbook – for students of statistics or health sciences; for clinicians and other practicing professionals, this book might be useful to deepen a preexisting knowledge of statistics but otherwise is not a good first starting point, because this book puts more emphasis on the underlying mathematics than on the practical applications.]

* Bland JM, Altman DG. Statistics Notes: Bootstrap resampling methods. BMJ. 2015; 350: h2622. [A very brief and very useful introduction to the important statistical method of bootstrapping.]

Bland CJ, Schmitz CC. Characteristics of the Successful Researcher and Implications for Faculty Development. J Med Educ. 1986; 61: 22-31. [An interesting narrative literature review about the characteristics of productive researchers; essential reading for anyone wanting to pursue a career as a researcher.]

Boerma T. New authorship practices are needed in developing countries. BMJ. 1997; 315: 745-746. [A letter about the problems of authorship credit in developing countries, with a small informal survey from Tanzania as supporting evidence.]

Bogdonoff MD. The Need for Faculty Protected Time. Arch Intern Med. 1972; 129: 363-365. [An editorial asserting that teachers of medical students need protected time for research and reflection; historical but surely still as relevant as ever.]

Bohannon J. Who's Afraid of Peer Review? Science. 2013; 342: 60-65. [A delightfully well-written special report about how predatory publishers will publish anything.]

Boiselle PM. A Fond Farewell to *JTI* Case Reports. J Thorac Imaging. 2012; 27: 337-338. [A quick and informative editorial about why this journal, like so many others, stopped publishing case reports.]

Bono CM. Reporting and statistically comparing averages of a patient cohort: the glass may really be half empty. Spine J. 2010; 10: 811-812. [A critical commentary on a clinical study, illustrating why titles should not contain conclusions, and many other commonplace deficiencies in statistical analysis and reporting.]

Booth WC, Colomb GC, Williams JM. The Craft of Research, 3rd ed. Chicago: University of Chicago Press; 1995, 2008. [Written by three professors of English language and literature, this introductory-level book about conducting and reporting research in the humanities and social sciences explains how to conduct bibliographic research, how to make logical arguments, and how to write a research report; although this book only sporadically mentions medicine or life sciences, it is probably as good or better than most such books written explicitly for those fields.]

Boquiren F, Creed F, Shapiro C. Plagiarism: Digging to the root of the problem. J Psychosom Res. 2006; 61: 431. [An editorial advising authors against submitting manuscripts with plagiarized material.]

Bosch X, Hernández C, Pericas JM, Doti P, Marušić A. Misconduct Policies in High-Impact Biomedical Journals. PLoS One. 2012; 7: e51928. [An empirical study of journal policies on research misconduct.]

Bourne PE. Ten Simple Rules for Getting Published. PLoS Comput Biol. 2005; 1: e57. [This editorial has mostly good advice on how to write and publish papers, but it is all underdeveloped, and some of the advice is dubious; worth reading nonetheless.]

Boyce M. Observational study of 353 applications to London multicentre research ethics committee 1997-2000. BMJ. 2002; 325: 1081. [A brief empirical report of the decisions of a research ethics committee on research proposals.]

Braitman LE. Confidence Intervals Assess Both Clinical Significance and Statistical Significance. Ann Intern Med. 1991; 114: 515-517. [A very good tutorial paper about confidence intervals, using several examples.]

Bramstedt KA. A guide to informed consent for clinician-investigators. Cleve Clin J Med. 2004; 71: 907-910. [A cursory, magazine-style introduction to the dual-role conflict of clinician investigators and the contents and style of informed consent forms, with a 3/11 self-citation rate.]

Brandon AN. "Publish or Perish". Bull Med Libr Assoc. 1963; 51: 109-110. [Although addressed to medical librarians, this brief and well-written exhortation to write and publish may help inspire any procrastinating novice.]

Branson RD. Anatomy of a Research Paper. Respir Care. 2004; 49: 1222-1228. [This tutorial paper discusses what should be included in each main section of a paper, as well as other relevant aspects of the manuscript; much of the advice here is quite good, but some of it is outdated or misleading.]

Brice J, Bligh J. 'Dear Editor…': advice on writing a covering letter. Med Educ. 2005; 39: 876. [A helpful editorial with numerous tips on what to write in the cover letter accompanying a manuscript submitted to a journal.]

Briscoe MH. Preparing Scientific Illustrations, 2nd ed. New York: Springer; 1996. [Substantial portions of this basic book are outdated and some of it is simply erroneous, but overall it remains a handy little guide on making all kinds of figures for reports and presentations; weakest on topics of data graphing, while better for other kinds of figures and general formatting issues.]

Buffel du Vaure C, Boutron I, Perrodeau E, Ravaud P. Reporting funding source or conflict of interest in abstracts of randomized controlled trials, no evidence of a large impact on general practitioners' confidence in conclusions, a three-arm randomized controlled trial. BMC Med. 2014; 12: 69. [This study acknowledges that disclosures should be made in the abstract but concludes that they have no influence on readers; the authors then relegate their own disclosures to another part of the manuscript.]

Bullimore MA. Love the Data, Hate the Figures. Optom Vis Sci. 2004; 81: 642-643. [A useful brief editorial about quality deficiencies in graphs.]

Burke JF, Sussman JB, Kent DM, Hayward RA. Three simple rules to ensure reasonably credible subgroup analyses. BMJ. 2015; 351: h5651. [A Bayesean argument against most subgroups analyses.]

Byrne DW. Common Reasons for Rejecting Manuscripts at Medical Journals: A Survey of Editors and Peer Reviewers. Sci Ed. 2000; 23 (2): 39-44. [This small survey of journal Editors and peer reviewers about the reasons for manuscript rejection is unreliable and outdated as research, but it remains nonetheless useful for authors by pointing to problems that usually do lead to manuscript rejection.]

Callaham ML. A New Feature for Readers: Capsule Summaries. Ann Emerg Med. 2003; 42: 609-610. [Although addressed to readers rather than authors, this brief editorial is an excellent explanation of what a capsule summary should contain and why they are needed.]

Callaham ML. Whole Bowel Irrigation and the Capsule Summary. Ann Emerg Med. 2004; 44: 667. [This Editor's reply to a letter explains the composition and limitation of capsule summaries written by editorial teams.]

Cals JWL, Kotz D. Effective writing and publishing scientific papers, part II: title and abstract. J Clin Epidemiol. 2013; 66: 585. [A brief tutorial paper with mostly good advice about writing the title and abstract.]

Cals JWL, Kotz D. Effective writing and publishing scientific papers, part IX: authorship. J Clin Epidemiol. 2013; 66: 1319. [A useful tutorial essay on managing the practical aspects of co-authorship.]

Cals JWL, Kotz D. Literature review in biomedical research: useful search engines beyond PubMed. J Clin Epidemiol. 2016; 71: 115-116. [An informative letter about background literature reviews, search engines, and predatory journals.]

Cameron C, Deming SP, Notzon B, Cantor SB, Broglio KR, Pagel W. Scientific Writing Training for Academic Physicians of Diverse Language Backgrounds. Acad Med. 2009; 84: 505-510. [This narrative article describes the development of a scientific writing training program primarily for non-native speakers of English and their responses to it; useful for anyone charged with developing a scientific writing course.]

Caramelli B. Abstract – the trailer of scientific communication. Rev Assoc Med Bras. 2011; 57: 593. [A brief editorial with acceptable advice about abstracts, despite the regrettable title.]

Carlisle JB. Data fabrication and other reasons for non-random sampling in 5087 randomised, controlled trials in anaesthetic and general medical journals. Anaesthesia. 2017; 72: 944-952. [A vast exploratory study on improbable results for baseline patient characteristics.]

Carroll L. Alice's Adventures in Wonderland. New York: Signet; 1865, 2000. [A fabulous introduction to logical thinking and communicational clarity, written by a world-renowned mathematician and literary genius.]

Carroll L. Symbolic Logic; The Game of Logic. Mineola, NY, USA: Dover Publications; 1897, 1958. [Two books, republished together here, that may help train readers to see the reasoning underlying sets of propositions.]

Castillo M. Vanity Press and Other Scams That Make You Feel Cool. AJNR Am J Neuroradiol. 2011; 32: 423-429. [An editorial making the case against using vanity presses.]

Chakravarty K. Excluding authors may be impossible. BMJ. 1997; 315: 748. [A letter, based on the author's personal experiences, warning of the possible problems if authorship agreements are not made from the outset of the research.]

* Chalmers I, Glasziou P. Avoidable waste in the production and reporting of research evidence. Lancet. 2009; 374: 86-89. [An excellent essay about choosing clinically important research topics, designing studies well, and publishing them completely in a timely and unbiased way.]

Chalmers TC, Frank CS, Reitman D. Minimizing the Three Stages of Publication Bias. JAMA. 1990; 263: 1392-1395. [A wide-ranging essay about various factors – before, during, and after the publication of research – that can bias selection of the medical scientific knowledge that becomes available to read.]

Champ R. Plain English. Brit J Gen Pract. 2008; 58: 436. [A brief letter with good advice for crafting the "take-home message", elevator speech, or capsule summary of a paper, not actually about plain English.]

Chapman S. "Author pays" publishing model: Model is concerned with vanity and profit. BMJ. 2003; 327: 54. [A letter, from a journal Editor, against charging fees to authors.]

Charon R. Narrative and Medicine. NEJM. 2004; 350: 862-864. [An essay providing a brief overview of narrative competencies and their benefits for clinical practice; a useful framework for writing some case reports and any narrative articles about medical practice.]

Charon R. Narrative Medicine: A Model for Empathy, Reflection, Profession, and Trust. JAMA. 2001; 286: 1897-1902. [An essay providing explanations of how narrative competencies improve a physician's relations to various other types of people; potentially useful for the writing of case reports and any narrative articles about medical practice.]

Chaudhry S, Schroter S, Smith R, Morris J. Does declaration of competing interests affect readers' perceptions? A randomised trial. BMJ. 2002; 325: 1391-1392. [A study showing that declaring conflicts of interest does have a moderate and statistically significant negative effect on readers' perception of the study.]

Chen JJ, Roberson PK, Schell MJ. The False Discovery Rate: A Key Concept in Large-Scale Genetic Studies. Cancer Control. 2010; 17: 58-62. [An introductory-level tutorial paper about the false discover rate technique; useful for anyone making multiple tests for statistical significance in the same study.]

Chiu K, Grundy Q, Bero L. 'Spin' in published biomedical literature: A methodological systematic review. PLoS Biol. 2017; 15: e2002173. [A systematic review of mostly review papers showing that "spin" is commonplace in the medical literature, especially when results are non-significant; curiously, this paper itself contains spin: the main hypothesis that industry funding was associated with spin is clearly refuted in the main text but presented as "inconclusive" in the abstract.]

Christiansen S, Flanagin A. Correcting the Medical Literature: "To Err is Human, to Correct Divine". JAMA. 2017; 318: 804-805. [An informative introduction to the various types of correction notices and retractions that journals use to correct various kinds of errors in the published literature.]

Citrome L. Compelling or irrelevant? Using number needed to treat can help decide. Acta Psychiatr Scand. 2008; 117: 412-419. [An extensive but mostly mediocre presentation of NNT, perhaps of interest to psychiatrists.]

Clamp down on copycats. Nature. 2005; 438: 2. [A brief editorial urging more intervention against plagiarism.]

Clarke M, Chalmers I. Discussion Sections in Reports of Controlled Trials Published in General Medical Journals: Islands in Search of Continents? JAMA. 1998; 280: 280-282. [A small literature study providing some evidence that many reports of clinical trials do not relate their results to previous reviews of the literature.]

* Cleveland WS. The Elements of Graphing Data. Murray Hill, NJ, USA: AT&T Bell Laboratories; 1994. [A fundamental and authoritative book about the graphing of data; strongly recommended for anyone making graphs from numerical data.]

Coates R, Sturgeon B, Bohannan J, Pasini E. Language and publication in *Cardiovascular Research* articles. Cardiovasc Res. 2002; 53: 279-285. [An empirical study on the rates of various language errors in manuscripts submitted to this journal by native speakers of English versus non-native speakers and the relation of those errors to manuscript acceptance rates; this article also serves as a useful overview of the kinds of commonplace language errors that derail manuscripts.]

* Cohen J. The Earth Is Round ($p < .05$). Am Psychol. 1994; 49: 997-1003. [This informal article, by a leading authority of statistics in Psychology, discusses the major problems with null hypothesis testing and the binary threshold of significance of p<0.05; it is not recommended

for beginners (too complex and muddled), but it may be quite interesting for researchers with training in statistics who are unfamiliar with these problems.]

Cole TJ. Too many digits: the presentation of numerical data. Arch Dis Child. 2015; 100: 608-609. [A very useful article about the precise issue of how many numerical digits to report in research papers.]

Collier L. Be clear, concise, and correct. BMJ. 1997; 314: 753-754. [A letter asserting that scientific papers should be written in a clear and concise style.]

Collins FS, Tabak LA. NIH plans to enhance reproducibility. Nature. 2014; 505: 612-613. [An essay, from the Director and Principal Deputy Director of the US NIH, about the widespread problem of the irreproducibility of preclinical research and the measures the NIH planned to take to reduce that problem.]

Collins G, Davis J, Swift O. Publishing a medical book: Authorship from a medical student perspective. Med Teach. 2015; 37: 100. [A brief letter about the authors' personal experience writing a book as medical students; perhaps interesting for medical students who enjoy writing and want to learn more about it.]

Colt HG, Mulnard RA. Writing an Application for a Human Subjects Institutional Review Board. Chest. 2006; 130: 1605-1607. [A brief, general introduction to writing a proposal for a Research Ethics Committee.]

* Committee on Publication Ethics (COPE). Guidelines on good publication practice. In: White C, ed. The COPE Report 2003. London: BMJ Books; 2004, pp. 69-73. [A very well written set of recommended best practices on a range of ethical issues in biomedical publishing, authored by a well-established British committee formed to advise journal Editors about ethical issues; well-worth the small amount of time needed to read it.]

Cooper ID. How to write an original research paper (and get it published). J Med Lib Assoc. 2015; 103: 67-68. [A brief tutorial paper, addressed to medical librarians.]

Cooper L. Better writing and more space needed online. Nature. 2008; 455: 26. [A letter arguing that journals should eliminate length limits of articles in online journals, based on the mostly mistaken premise that this would improve the quality of scientific communication.]

Copi IM. Introduction to Logic. New York: Macmillan; 1982. [A solid textbook on logical reasoning, which plays a crucial but neglected role in scientific writing.]

Council for International Organizations of Medical Sciences, International Council for Laboratory Animal Science. International Guiding Principles for Biomedical Research Involving Animals, December 2012. Accessed on 7 January 2018 at: iclas.org/wp-content/uploads/2013/03/CIOMS-ICLAS-Principles-Final.pdf [This set of 10 ethical principles provides fundamental guidance for research involving animals; essential reading for anyone conducting research on animals.]

Council of Science Editors. CSE's White Paper on Promoting Integrity in Scientific Journal Publications, 2012 Update, 3rd Revised Edition. Wheat Ridge, CO: Council of Scientific Editors; 2012. [A long, broad, somewhat dated, and mostly unoriginal overview of ethical aspects of scientific publishing.]

Cressey D. Informed consent on trial. Nature. 2012; 482: 16. [A news story about how informed consent forms for research have become too long and incomprehensible.]

Cromey DW. Avoiding Twisted Pixels: Ethical Guidelines for the Appropriate Use and Manipulation of Scientific Digital Images. Sci Eng Ethics. 2010; 16: 639-667. [This article presents an in-depth technical and scholarly discussion of what is and is not scientifically acceptable digital processing of images; recommended reading for anyone working with photographs or images as figures.]

Cummings P, Rivara FP. Reporting Statistical Information in Medical Journal Articles. Arch Pediatr Adolec Med. 2003; 157: 321-324. [A substantial editorial with many good recommendations about how to report statistical information in papers; worthwhile reading.]

Cummings P, Rivara FP. Responding to Reviewers' Comments on Submitted Articles. Arch Pediatr Adolec Med. 2002; 156: 105-107. [A substantial editorial with many good recommendations about how to respond to peer review; worthwhile reading.]

Currie C. Author saw fraud, misconduct, and unfairness to more junior staff. BMJ. 1997; 315: 747-748. [An informative letter providing a critical overview of the types of misconduct observed by this research officer of a medical school.]

Dansinger M. Dear Plagiarist: A Letter to a Peer Reviewer Who Stole and Published Our Manuscript as His Own. Ann Intern Med. 2017; 166: 143. [An open letter to a peer reviewer who published under his name a manuscript he had reviewed by the author of this letter.]

Davis AJ. Readers don't have to come from overseas to benefit from plain English. BMJ. 1997; 314: 753. [A letter asserting that writing in plain English will make a text more easily understood by patients and English native speaking doctors too.]

DeAngelis CD. The Roman Article: Read It Again – in the Same Journal. JAMA. 2009; 301: 1382-1383. [A brief editorial against redundant publication.]

DeAngelis C, Drazen JM, Frizelle FA, Haug C, Hoey J, Horton R, Kotzin S, Laine C, Marušić A, Overbeke AJPM, Schroeder TV, Sox HC, Van Der Weyden MB. Clinical Trial Registration: A Statement from the International Committee of Medical Journal Editors. NEJM. 2004; 351: 1250-1251. [An editorial explaining why registration of clinical trials became a requirement for publication in ICMJE member journals.]

del Carmen MG, Joffe S. Informed Consent for Medical Treatment and Research: A Review. Oncologist. 2005; 10: 636-641. [A basic introduction to informed consent, in the American context, with particular focus on patient populations with reduced competence to provide it.]

DeMaria A. Manuscript Revision. J Am Coll Cardiol. 2011; 57: 2540-2541. [A useful editorial about this journal's decision-making process, manuscript revision, and the reply-to-review letter.]

DeMaria AN. Of Abstracts and Manuscripts. J Am Coll Cardiol. 2006; 47: 1224-1225. [An interesting editorial about how even the best of conference abstracts are low quality when judged by the standards of journal peer review.]

Derish P, Eastwood S. A Clarity Clinic for Surgical Writing. J Surg Res. 2008; 147: 50-58. [A very useful collection of recommendations on how to revise manuscripts for language issues, with abundant examples.]

de Sa P. Bhopal and colleagues' suggested method of ordering authors wouldn't work. BMJ. 1997; 315: 745. [A well-reasoned, scholarly letter demonstrating that voting methods are not reliable for determining the order of authorship.]

Detsky AS, Sackett DL. When Was a 'Negative Clinical Trial Big Enough? How Many Patients You Needed Depends on What You Found. Arch Intern Med. 1985; 145: 709-712. [An excellent article, from leading authorities of evidence-based medicine, about negative trial results, type II errors, and post hoc power calculations; recommendable.]

Dindo D, Demartines N, Clavien P-A. Classification of Surgical Complications: A New Proposal With Evaluation in a Cohort of 6336 Patients and Results of a Survey. Ann Surg. 2004; 240: 205-213. [A sensible schema for grading the severity of postoperative complications; useful for reporting harms.]

Doctors and medical statistics. Lancet. 2007; 370: 910. [A brief, simple editorial asserting that most clinicians have inadequate understanding of statistics to correctly understand the research literature.]

Dowek G. La logique. Paris: Éditions Le Pommier; 1995, 2015. [A very short and accessible book about reasoning, which is an essential component of scientific research.]

Doyle DJ. Search engines for scholarly research: a brief update for clinicians. Can J Anesth. 2007; 54: 336-341. [A mostly outdated but otherwise well-written bilingual narrative overview of PubMed, Google Scholar, and other (now mostly defunct) search engines.]

Drazen JM. Authorship Limits. NEJM. 2002; 347: 1118. [The Editor's reply to a letter from readers, clarifying the journal's position about who should decide the authorship of manuscripts.]

Drazen JM. Believe the Data. NEJM. 2012; 367: 1152-1153. [An editorial commentary asserting that the credibility of clinical studies should be based on their methodological quality, not on their funding source.]

Drazen JM, de Leeuw PW, Laine C, Mulrow C, DeAngelis CD, Frizelle FA, Godlee F, Haug C, Hébert PC, James A, Kotzin S, Marušić A, Reyes H, Rosenberg J, Sahni P, Van Der Weyden M, Zhaori G. Toward More Uniform Conflict Disclosures — The Updated ICMJE Conflict of Interest Reporting Form. NEJM. 2010; 363: 188-189. [An editorial presenting the current revised version of the ICMJE form for disclosures of conflicts of interest.]

Drotar D. Thoughts on Improving the Quality of Manuscripts Submitted to the Journal of Pediatric Psychology: Writing a Convincing Introduction. J Pediatr Psychol. 2009; 34: 1-3. [This editorial about how to write more compelling introductions is addressed to readers of that particular journal but is easily transferable to other specialty journals; recommendable for anyone trying to improve their Introduction sections.]

Drug targets slip-sliding away. Nature. 2011; 17: 1155. [A balanced editorial about the high rate of irreproducibility of published preclinical research on possible drug-targets.]

Dubé CE, Lapane KL. Lay Abstracts and Summaries: Writing Advice for Scientists. J Cancer Educ. 2014; 29: 577-579. [A very brief tutorial paper about how to write a summary of a study for a lay audience.]

Durbin CG Jr. Effective Use of Tables and Figures in Abstracts, Presentations, and Papers. Respir Care. 2004; 49: 1233-1237. [A useful tutorial paper about the visual design of graphs and tables for journal papers and conference presentations.]

* Eco U, et al. Interpretation and Overinterpretation. Cambridge, UK: Cambridge University Press; 1992. [Written by world-renowned literary theorists, this engaging book about the interpretation of literary texts surely serves as deeper training for scientists trying to *interpret* what research results (their own or other people's) really mean, or do not mean.]

Efron B, Tibshirani R. Statistical Data Analysis in the Computer Age. Science. 1991; 253: 390-395. [An interesting article about how the computing power of our era now enables us to perform more sophisticated forms of statistical analysis, such as bootstrapping and advanced forms of regression analysis; recommendable reading for anyone who already has a solid foundation in statistical analysis.]

Ehara S. Assessing the scientific and educational value of case reports: an editor's view. Jpn J Radiol. 2011; 29: 1-2. [A brief editorial about which types of case reports might be worth publishing versus which are not.]

Eisenach JC. Case Reports Are Leaving Anesthesiology, but Not the Specialty. Anesthesiology. 2013; 118: 479-480. [An editorial with an ultrabrief historical view of the role of case reports in medical science and an explanation of why this journal decided to relegate them to a spin-off journal.]

Elefteriades JA. Twelve Tips on Writing a Good Scientific Paper. Inter J Angiol. 2002; 11: 53-55. [An essay with tips on how to write a good journal paper, at least 11 of which are quite good; well recommended for beginner and intermediate level authors.]

Emanuel EJ. Institutional Review Board Reform. NEJM. 2002; 347: 1285-1286. [A letter making a good case against continued use of the term "Institutional Review Board".]

Enfield KB, Truwit JD. The Purpose, Composition, and Function of an Institutional Review Board: Balancing Priorities. Respir Care. 2008; 53: 1330-1336. [A good introductory overview of Research Ethics Committees in the context of the USA.]

Ernst E. A beginner's guide to criticism: A brief taxonomy of reviewers, and how to deal with them. MJA. 2007; 187: 649. [A satirical yet useful description of types of negative peer reviewers and tips on how to respond to them.]

Erren TC. The Long and Thorny Road to Publication in Quality Journals. PLoS Comput Bio. 2007; 3: e251. [A substantial letter asserting, correctly, that it is difficult for anyone without experience publishing scientific papers to get published in high impact journals.]

Estrada CA, Bloch RM, Antonacci D, Basnight LL, Patel SR, Patel SC, Wiese W. Reporting and Concordance of Methodologic Criteria Between Abstracts and Articles in Diagnostic Test Studies. J Gen Intern Med. 2000; 15: 183-187. [A small study of the literature that documents inconsistency of information in the abstract and main text, among other reporting deficiencies.]

Evans JG, Beck P. Informed consent in medical research. Clin Med. 2002; 2: 267-272. [An illuminating medical history article on when the ethical theories of informed consent finally became standard practice for medical research.]

Ezsias A. Authorship is influenced by power and departmental politics. BMJ. 1997; 315: 746. [A letter describing the problems of dilution and loss of authorship credit of junior researchers to senior clinicians or institutes that claim ownership of the raw data.]

Falagas ME, Pitsouni EI, Malietzis GA, Pappas G. Comparison of PubMed, Scopus, Web of Science, and Google Scholar: strengths and weaknesses. FASEB J. 2008; 22: 338-342. [A comparison of these four literature search engines.]

Fanelli D. How Many Scientists Fabricate and Falsify Research? A Systematic Review and Meta-Analysis of Survey Data. PLoS One. 2009; 4: e5738. [A solid systematic review and metaanalysis of surveys of scientists about the rates of fabricated and falsified research data and results.]

Flaherty A. A brief proposal, 150 words. Nature. 2007; 450: 1156. [This letter, by a Neurologist at Harvard, about a way that journals could (supposedly) pressure authors to use shorter words serves as good anecdotal evidence that affiliation at a world-class university facilitates the publication of unfounded and trivial remarks at top-tier journals.]

Flanagin A, Carey LA, Fontanaros PB, Phillips SG, Pace BP, Lundberg GD, Rennie D. Prevalence of Articles With Honorary Authors and Ghost Authors in Peer-Reviewed Medical Journals. JAMA. 1998; 280: 222-224. [An empirical study on the prevalence of guest authors and ghost authors in a large sample of articles from six American medical journals.]

Flood CG, Faught JW, Schulz JA. Reflection on Academic Protected Time: An Opportunity to Integrate Educational Programs. J Obstet Gynaecol Can. 2006; 28: 295-298. [A small survey about the contents of academic protected time curricula for residents in Canadian OB/GYN programs.]

Fontelo P, Gavino A, Sarmiento RF. Comparing data accuracy between structured abstracts and full-text journal articles: implications in their use for informing clinical decisions. Evid Based Med. 2013; 18: 207-211. [A small study of the literature assessing the prevalence and severity of inaccuracies in abstracts.]

Foote MA. The Proof of the Pudding: How to Report Results and Write a Good Discussion. Chest. 2009; 135: 866-868. [This tutorial paper on how to write the Results and Discussion sections of a paper has some good tips, but the advice is generally insufficient and the fictive examples are weak; not recommendable in the current era.]

Frank E. Publish or perish: the moral imperative of journals. CMAJ. 2016: 188: 675. [This brief editorial simultaneously calls for increased rates of publication and increased rigor of peer review, without noticing the inconsistency between these two laudable goals.]

* Frankfurt HG. On Bullshit. Princeton, NJ, USA: Princeton University Press; 2005. [Despite the seemingly facetious title, this is an earnest philosophical reflection on general trends in contemporary communication, which have clear relevance to serious and frequent issues of scientific misconduct such as "spin", bias, and data fudging.]

Frazier ALB, Toth L. AALAS Publications: Write for All Readers. J Am Assoc Lab Anim Sci. 2017; 56: 710. [A brief editorial with useful tips and general remarks about copyediting for clear English.]

Frege G. Über die wissenschaftliche Berechtigung einer Begriffsschrift. In: Frege G. Funktion, Begriff, Bedeutung: Fünf logische Studien. Göttingen, Germany: Vandenhoeck & Ruprecht; (1892), 1962, 2008, pp. 70-76. [A short philosophical essay about why the sciences need to use unambiguous terminology.]

Frege G. Über Sinn und Bedeutung. In: Frege G. Funktion, Begriff, Bedeutung: Fünf logische Studien. Göttingen, Germany: Vandenhoeck & Ruprecht; (1892), 1962, 2008, pp. 23-46. [A philosophical essay about the meaning versus sense of language.]

Friedman JN. The case for ... writing case reports. Paediatr Child Health. 2006; 11: 343-344. [A brief and helpful tutorial paper on how to write and publish a case report, along with an unconvincing set of reasons why one should.]

Fuess BS Jr., ed. How to Use the Power of the Printed Word. New York: Anchor Books; 1985. [An anthology of brief essays, by famous Americans, with some useful advice for aspiring writers.]

Fye WB. Medical Authorship: Traditions, Trends, and Tribulations. Ann Intern Med. 1990; 113: 317-325. [A scholarly essay, mostly providing an American medical history perspective on various issues and problems with authorship and medical scientific publishing.]

Galal S. How Arabic became the international language of science. The UNESCO Courier. 1977; 30 (11): 46-52. [A short and interesting humanities essay about Arabic as the main language of the medical sciences from about the 8th to the 13th century.]

Garcia-Doval I, Ingram JR, Naldi L, Anstey A. Case reports in dermatology: loved by clinicians, loathed by editors, and occasionally important. Br J Dermatol. 2016; 175: 449-451. [An editorial describing various types of case reports that might contain valuable knowledge.]

* Gardner MJ, Altman DG. Confidence intervals rather than P values: estimation rather than hypothesis testing. BMJ. 1986; 292: 746-750. [An article, by two leading medical statisticians, explaining why more emphasis should be given to calculating and reporting confidence intervals rather than p-values; recommended reading for anyone who is not already well-informed about this point.]

Garfield E. Journal impact factor: a brief review. CMAJ. 1999; 161: 979-980. [This essay about journal impact factors, written by their co-creator, is neither current nor balanced.]

Garfield E. The Ethics of Scientific Publication: Authorship Attribution and Citation Amnesia. In: Essays of an information scientist, volume 5. Philadelphia: ISI Press; 1982, pp. 622-626. [A dated but useful ethics essay about authorship attribution and plagiarism, authored by the inventor of the impact factor, with a 9/25 self-citation rate.]

Gasparyan AY, Ayvazyan L, Kitas GD. Authorship problems in scholarly journals: considerations for authors, peer reviewers and editors. Rheumatol Int. 2013; 33: 277-284. [A mostly correct but somewhat poorly written narrative review of various ethical issues about authorship.]

** Gawande A. Better. New York: Metropolitan Books; 2007. [This collection of commented narrative stories illustrates what it means to do better quality work in healthcare; besides being enjoyable reading for anyone in medicine or research, this book should provide readers with invaluable character formation.]

GBD 2015 LRI Collaborators. Estimates of the global, regional, and national morbidity, mortality, and aetiologies of lower respiratory tract infections in 195 countries: a systematic analysis for the Global Burden of Disease Study 2015. Lancet Infect Dis. 2017; 17: 1133-1161. [An epidemiological study cited here as part of an example in the chapter, "Searching the Literature"; not otherwise germane to the topics of this book.]

GBD 2016 Causes of Death Collaborators. Global, regional, and national age-sex specific mortality for 264 causes of death, 1980-2016: a systematic analysis for the Global Burden of Disease Study 2016. Lancet. 2017; 390: 1151-1210. [An epidemiological study cited here as part of an example in the chapter, "Searching the Literature"; not otherwise germane to the topics of this book.]

Giglia E. Beyond PubMed: Other free-access biomedical databases. Eura Medicophys. 2007; 43: 563-569. [A guide article to many free biomedical databases (not literature search engines); perhaps still useful, but presumably quite dated.]

Gillan DJ, Wickens CD, Hollands JG, Carswell CM. Guidelines for Presenting Quantitative Data in HFES Publications. Hum Factors. 1998; 40: 28-41. [These guidelines provide detailed advice on the design of basic data graphs; although the illustrations are simplistic and a bit dated, the general principles and much of the advice remains entirely valid and useful.]

* Gillman MA. Checking for plagiarism, duplicate publication, and text recycling. Lancet. 2011; 377: 1403. [A letter asserting, quite correctly, that academic institutions will cover up research misconduct to protect their reputations.]

Giustini D, Barsky E. A look at Google Scholar, PubMed, and Scirus: comparisons and recommendations. JCHLA / JABSC. 2005; 26: 85-89. [An informal review of the advantages and limitations of Google Scholar and some main alternative search engines.]

Glass RM. Guest authors: no place in any journal. Nature. 2010; 468; 765. [A brief letter against guest authorship.]

Glatstein E. Restrictions of a Statistical Mind: Clinical Relevance versus *P* Values or When Less is More. Int J Radiation Oncology Biol Phys. 2007; 68: 322-323. [A short and simple essay on the difference between statistical significance and clinical relevance.]

Godlee F. Publishing study protocols: making them visible will improve registration, reporting and recruitment. BMC News and Views. 2001; 2: 4. [An editorial explaining why researchers should publish their study protocols.]

Golder S, Loke YK, Wright K, Norman G. Reporting of Adverse Events in Published and Unpublished Studies of Health Care: A Systematic Review. PLoS Med. 2016; 13: e1002127. [This systematic review of studies comparing the rates of adverse events reported in published versus unpublished sources provides strong evidence that harms often remain unreported in the medical literature.]

Goodman NW. Survey of fulfillment of criteria for authorship in published medical research. BMJ. 1994; 309: 1482. [A brief report of a survey of first-authors documenting that co-authors often do not fulfill the criteria of authorship.]

Goodman NW, Edwards MB. Medical Writing: A Prescription for Clarity, 3rd ed. Cambridge: Cambridge University Press; 1991, 2006. [This book provides good guidance on editing medical texts for better word choices and sentence composition.]

Goodman SN. Toward Evidence-Based Medical Statistics. 1: The *P* Value Fallacy. Ann Intern Med. 1999; 130: 995-1004. [A long essay, written clearly by a staunch Bayesian, criticizing the standard approaches to statistics in medicine and all other sciences; perhaps of some historical interest to statisticians and methodologists.]

Goodman SN, Berlin J, Fletcher SW, Fletcher RH. Manuscript Quality before and after Peer Review and Editing at *Annals of Internal Medicine*. Ann Intern Med. 1994; 121: 11-21. [An empirical assessment of manuscripts showing that peer review improves the quality of manuscripts that are ultimately accepted for publication.]

Goodman SN, Royall R. Evidence and Scientific Research. Am J Public Health. 1988; 78: 1568-1574. [An essay with some interesting reflections on what constitutes scientific evidence, frequently muddled by the authors' agenda of converting people to their Bayesian approaches; not recommended.]

Gøtzsche PC, Hróbjartsson A, Johansen HK, Haahr MT, Altman DG, Chan A-W. Ghost Authorship in Industry-Initiated Randomised Trials. PLoS Med. 2007; 4: 0047-0051. [A small publication study showing that statisticians of industry-supported trials are almost never given the credit they deserve for their contributions.]

Gøtzsche PC, Kassirer JP, Woolley KL, Wager E, Jacobs A, Gertel A, Hamilton C. What Should Be Done To Tackle Ghostwriting in the Medical Literature? PLoS Med. 2009; 6: 0122-0125. [Three separate viewpoint editorials about how to eliminate ghostwriting from the medical literature.]

** GRADE Working Group. Grading quality of evidence and strength of recommendations. BMJ. 2004; 328: 1490. Note: Beware the five-page abridged print version that can also be found online; the full eight-page version was accessible on 7 April 2018 at: www.bmj.com/content/bmj/328/7454/1490.full.pdf [This introductory summary of the GRADE system for evaluating the quality of evidence and strength of recommendations is highly useful for understanding the methodological quality of one's own research and any other studies one might cite; recommended reading for all researchers.]

Graf C, Deakin L, Docking M, Jones J, Joshua S, McKerahan T, Ottmar M, Stevens A, Wates E, Wyatt D. Best practice guidelines on publishing ethics: a publisher's perspective, 2nd edition. Int J Clin Pract. 2014; 68: 1410-1428. [A comprehensive (but relatively unoriginal) overview of all the ethical issues of scientific publishing, written by a publisher for the editorial staff of its journals.]

Greenbaum S, Nelson G. An Introduction to English Grammar, 3rd ed. Harlow, England: Pearson; 1999, 2009. [A concise and authoritative textbook of English grammar and usage.]

* Greenland P, Fontanarosa PB. Ending Honorary Authorship. Science. 2012; 337: 1019. [An excellent editorial – written by two leading journal Editors and published in one of the absolute foremost scientific journals – about the ethical imperative of ending guest authorship; essential reading for anyone working in research.]

Gregory AT. Peer review: where science meets the arts of war, politics and ancient history. MJA. 2007; 187: 684. [A light-hearted article quoting some flowery remarks from peer reviewers; not particularly interesting.]

Gregory AT. Supernovas of style. MJA. 2006; 185: 651. [A light-hearted article quoting some flowery remarks from peer reviewers; somewhat amusing and occasionally instructive; worth a look.]

Grierson HJC. Rhetoric and English Composition. Edinburgh: Oliver & Boyd; 1945. [A short and useful book on English writing style.]

Griscom NT. Your research: How to get it on paper and in print. Pediatr Radiol. 1999; 29: 81-86. [This tutorial paper provides almost entirely useless guidance on what to write in a paper, sandwiched between much good advice on the *process* of writing a paper; in other words, this paper is useless if you need to help deciding *what* to write, but is useful if you need help figuring out *how* to go about doing the writing.]

Gross RA. Style, spin, and science. Neurology. 2015; 85: 10-11. [A brief but very useful editorial, mainly about word choices, "spin", and proper reporting of statistical significance.]

Gross RA, Johnston KC. Levels of evidence. Neurology. 2009; 72: 8-10. [This editorial presents a brief overview of the levels of evidence system and an explanation of why this journal started tagging all research articles with their level of evidence.]

Groves T. Why submit your research to the BMJ. BMJ. 2007; 334: 4-5. [An editorial providing many useful insights on the brutal efficiency of manuscript review at high-quality journals that take their job seriously.]

Groves T, Abbasi K. Screening research papers by reading abstracts. BMJ. 2004; 329: 470-471. [An illuminating editorial explaining how Editors often triage submitted manuscripts based on reading only the abstracts.]

Grube K. Author ship. Nat Mater. 2004; 3: 743. [An amusing and illuminating satirical illustration.]

Guidelines for the treatment of animals in behavioral research and teaching. Animal Behavior. 2012; 83: 301-309. [Semi-anonymously written and revised several times on behalf of the Association for the Study of Animal Behavior and the Animal Behavior Society, this thoughtful guidelines article on the ethical treatment of animals is addressed primarily to scientists of behavior or ecology but is easily applicable to biomedical research, and it includes a useful list of further resources.]

Guimarães CA. Structured Abstracts: Narrative Review. Acta Cir Bras. 2006; 21: 263-268. [Mostly a set of insert boxes with examples of various structured abstracts, as well as a narrative review of some of the literature about structured abstracts; this weak article adds very little to the literature.]

Gunzburg R, Szpalski M, Aebi M. The impact factor: publish, be cited or perish... Eur Spine J. 2002; 11: S1. [A brief editorial, vaguely critical of impact factors, and lacking any clear rationale or message.]

Gustavii B. How to Write and Illustrate a Scientific Paper. Cambridge, UK: Cambridge University Press; 2003. [A good short book, primarily for life scientists, with special emphasis on figures.]

Guyatt G, Jaeschke R, Heddle N, Cook D, Shannon H, Walter S. Basic statistics for clinicians: 1. Hypothesis testing. CMAJ. 1995; 152: 27-32. [A very basic yet very solid explanation of hypothesis testing, p-values, and possible errors with such statistical tests.]

Guyatt G, Jaeschke R, Heddle N, Cook D, Shannon H, Walter S. Basic statistics for clinicians: 2. Interpreting study results: confidence intervals. CMAJ. 1995; 152: 169-173. [A well-written basic explanation of confidence intervals, in particular how they help to interpret how definitive a study was; highly recommended reading for anyone who does not already have a strong understanding of confidence intervals.]

Guyatt G, Oxman AD, Akl EA, Kunz R, Vist G, Brozek J, Norris S, Falck-Ytter Y, Glasziou P, deBeer H, Jaeschke R, Rind D, Meerpohl J, Dahm P, Schünemann HJ. GRADE guidelines: 1. Introduction—GRADE evidence profiles and summary of findings tables. J Clin Epidemiol. 2011; 64: 383-394. [An introduction to the important GRADE system, which is used to evaluate evidence in systematic reviews and guidelines.]

Guyatt GH, Oxman AD, Kunz R, Atkins D, Brozek J, Vist G, Alderson P, Glasziou P, Falck-Ytter Y, Schünemann HJ. GRADE guidelines: 2. Framing the question and deciding on important outcomes. J Clin Epidemiol. 2011; 64: 395-400. [Although written for authors of systematic reviews and guidelines, this article from the GRADE system may also be useful to researchers designing new studies or writing original clinical reports.]

Guyatt GH, Oxman AD, Kunz R, Brozek J, Alonso-Coello P, Rind D, Devereaux PJ, Montori VM, Freyschuss B, Vist G, Jaeschke R, Williams JW Jr., Murad MH, Sinclair D, Falck-Ytter Y, Meerpohl J, Whittington C, Thorlund K, Andrews J, Schünemann HJ. GRADE guidelines 6. Rating the quality of evidence—imprecision. J Clin Epidemiol. 2011; 64: 1283-1293. [Although written for authors of systematic reviews and guidelines, this article from the GRADE system is broadly useful for understanding how to interpret the meaning and implications of confidence intervals (which represent the precision of study results).]

Guyatt GH, Oxman AD, Kunz R, Woodcock J, Brozek J, Helfand M, Alonso-Coello P, Glasziou P, Jaeschke R, Akl EA, Norris S, Vist G, Dahm P, Shukla VK, Higgins J, Falck-Ytter Y, Schünemann HJ; GRADE Working Group. GRADE guidelines: 7. Rating the quality of evidence—inconsistency. J Clin Epidemiol. 2011; 64: 1294-1302. [An article from the GRADE system, for systematic reviewers and guideline developers, about inconsistency between studies.]

Guyatt GH, Oxman AD, Kunz R, Woodcock J, Brozek J, Helfand M, Alonso-Coello P, Falck-Ytter Y, Jaeschke R, Vist G, Akl EA, Post PN, Norris S, Meerpohl J, Shukla VK, Nasser M, Schünemann HJ; GRADE Working Group. GRADE guidelines: 8. Rating the quality of evidence—indirectness. J Clin Epidemiol. 2011; 64: 1303-1310. [Although written for authors of systematic reviews and guidelines, this article from the GRADE system is broadly useful for designing studies and reporting the methodological details about the patient population, intervention, and outcome measures.]

Guyatt GH, Oxman AD, Montori V, Vist G, Kunz R, Brozek J, Alonso-Coello P, Djulbegovic B, Atkins D, Falck-Ytter Y, Williams JW Jr., Meerpohl J, Norris SL, Akl EA, Schünemann HJ. GRADE guidelines: 5. Rating the quality of evidence—publication bias. J Clin Epidemiol. 2011; 64: 1277-1282. [This article from the GRADE system covers the generally intriguing topic of publication bias and how systematic reviews should examine it.]

Guyatt GH, Oxman AD, Schünemann HJ. GRADE guidelines—an introduction to the 10th–13th articles in the series. J Clin Epidemiol. 2013; 66: 121-123. [The second half of this brief article contains an interesting illustration of how expert medical researchers reflect about their word choices for terminology.]

Guyatt GH, Oxman AD, Sultan S, Glasziou P, Akl EA, Alonso-Coello P, Atkins D, Kunz R, Brozek J, Montori V, Jaeschke R, Rind D, Dahm P, Meerpohl J, Vist G, Berliner E, Norris S, Falck-Ytter Y, Murad MH, Schünemann HJ; GRADE Working Group. GRADE guidelines: 9. Rating up the quality of evidence. J Clin Epidemiol. 2011; 64: 1311-1316. [A useful article from the GRADE system about three features of study results that increase the quality of evidence from those studies.]

Guyatt GH, Oxman AD, Vist G, Kunz R, Brozek J, Alonso-Coello P, Montori V, Akl EA, Djulbegovic B, Falck-Ytter Y, Norris SL, Williams JW Jr., Atkins D, Meerpohl J, Schünemann HJ. GRADE guidelines: 4. Rating the quality of evidence—study limitations (risk of bias). J Clin Epidemiol. 2011; 64: 407-415. [This article from the GRADE system about evaluating study limitations within a systematic review may also be useful for anyone reporting original clinical research.]

Guyatt G, Walter S, Shannon H, Cook D, Jaeschke R, Heddle N. Basic statistics for clinicians: 4. Correlation and regression. CMAJ. 1995; 152: 497-504. [A good basic introduction to correlation coefficients and regression analysis.]

Haidich A-B, Birtsou C, Dardavessis T, Tirodimos I, Arvanitidou M. The quality of safety reporting in trials is still suboptimal: Survey of major general medical journals. J Clin Epidemiol. 2011; 64: 124-135. [This study of the literature shows that randomized controlled trials on medications published in leading medical journals usually fall short of the reporting standards set by the CONSORT extension for the reporting of harms.]

Hakoum MB, Jouni N, Abou-Jaoude EA, Hasbani DJ, Abou-Jaoude EA, Lopes LC, Khaldieh M, Hammoud MZ, Al-Gibbawi M, Anouti S, Guyatt G, Akl EA. Characteristics of funding clinical trials: cross-sectional survey and proposed guidance. BMJ Open. 2017; 7: e015997. [A study of the way funding sources are reported in the literature, along with a proposal for how they should be.]

Hall T. Without a putative contributor, would the integrity of the work change? BMJ. 1997; 315: 746-747. [A lengthy letter making a good brief point about deciding who should be named in the acknowledgments section of a paper.]

Halperin EC. Publish or Perish — and Bankrupt the Medical Library While We're at It. Acad Med. 1999; 74: 470-472. [A viewpoint article mainly arguing that academic medicine's "publish or perish" culture leads to a costly proliferation of journal publications with little or no relevance.]

Hamilton CW. On the Table. Chest. 2009; 135: 1087-1089. [A useful tutorial article on creating good tables.]

Hanna M. Matching Taxpayer Funding to Population Health Needs. Circ Res. 2015; 116: 1296-1300. [A data-based essay about the politics of medical research funding.]

Hanna M. More About the Teaching of Scientific Writing. Acad Med. 2010; 85: 4. [This letter asserts that good scientific writing is not quick and easy to learn, so most researchers should work together with someone who already has that specialized skill.]

Hanna M. Solo scientists are not all hippies. Intelligent Life. 2008 (Winter); 2 (2): 14. [A letter about research and productivity inside versus outside of academia.]

Hare D. Giving credit where credit is due — Authorship versus acknowledgment. Can Vet J. 2001; 42: 249-250. [A brief, basic, bilingual editorial about properly deciding whose contributions merit authorship.]

Harris AHS, Standard S, Brunning JL, Casey SL, Goldberg JH, Oliver L, Ito K, Marshall JM. The Accuracy of Abstracts in Psychology Journals. J Psychol. 2002; 136: 141-148. [This study of the literature from several American psychology journals documented that information or claims in the abstracts of research articles are sometimes inconsistent with or missing from the main body of the article.]

Hartley J. Current findings from research about structured abstracts. J Med Libr Assoc. 2004; 92: 368-371. [A narrative literature review of research on structured versus unstructured abstracts; perhaps of historical interest to specialists.]

Hartley J. Current findings from research on structured abstracts: an update. J Med Libr Assoc. 2014; 102: 146-148. [A brief and informal narrative review providing an update to the previous citation; perhaps of interest to specialists.]

Hayes SN, Redberg RF. Dispelling the Myths: Calling for Sex-Specific Reporting of Trial Results. Mayo Clin Proc. 2008; 83: 523-525. [This editorial / commentary makes the case for reporting trial results stratified by sex.]

Haynes RB. More informative abstracts: current status and evaluation. J Clin Epidemiol. 1993; 46: 595-599. [A brief narrative review of the early response to and evaluation of structured abstracts.]

** Haynes RB, Mulrow CD, Huth EJ, Altman DG, Gardner MJ. More Informative Abstracts Revisited. Ann Intern Med. 1990; 113: 69-76. [This essay provides the last proposal for the use of structured abstracts, along with appendices providing detailed instructions for the contents of abstracts; although this classic article is no longer entirely current in all details, it remains highly worthwhile reading on the most important part of papers.]

Henderson AR. Testing experimental data for univariate normality. Clin Chim Acta. 2006; 366: 112-129. [A solid, advanced-level review and assessment of the various methods for testing if data is Normally distributed.]

Heneghan MBJ. Plain English and minimal Latin may explain readability of 1950s paper... BMJ. 2004; 329: 352. [A little letter encouraging and illustrating the use of plain English.]

Hess DR. How to Write an Effective Discussion. Respir Care. 2004; 49: 1238-1241. [A brief and clear explanation of the usual template approach to the Discussion section, along with some good advice about pitfalls to avoid; perhaps useful for novice researchers or those with difficulty composing a coherent essay.]

Hesselmann F, Graf V, Schmidt M, Reinhart M. The visibility of scientific misconduct: A review of the literature on retracted journal articles. Curr Sociol. 2017; 65: 814-845. [A review paper of studies about retractions, sandwiched between an attempt to interpret retractions in terms of sociological theory of visibility of deviance; potentially of some use to other scholars of the topic.]

Hidalgo B, Goodman M. Multivariate or Multivariable Regression? Am J Pub Health. 2013; 103: 39-40. [A short but long-winded paper explaining the difference between the terms "multivariable" and "multivariate".]

Hochberg Y, Benjamini Y. More Powerful Procedures for Multiple Significance Testing. Stat Med. 1990; 9: 811-818. [An advanced-level discussion of statistical approaches to controlling for multiple comparisons that are superior to Bonferroni correction.]

Hoen WP, Walvoort HC, Overbeke AJPM. What Are the Factors Determining Authorship and the Order of the Authors' Names? A Study Among Authors of the *Nederlands Tijdschrift voor Geneeeskunde* (Dutch Journal of Medicine). JAMA. 1998; 280: 217-218. [A large Dutch survey documenting widespread ignorance of the criteria of authorship and failure to fulfill them.]

Hollands JG, Spence I. Judgments of Change and Proportion in Graphical Perception. Hum Factors. 1992; 34: 313-334. [An experimental study comparing viewers' ability to perceive proportions and change in line graphs, pie charts, and various bar graphs.]

Hooijmans C, de Vries R, Leenaars M, Ritskes-Hoitinga M. The Gold Standard Publication Checklist (GSPC) for improved design, reporting and scientific quality of animal studies: GSPC versus ARRIVE guidelines. Lab Anim. 2011; 45: 61. [A brief essay providing a good introduction to two important guidelines for the reporting of animal studies.]

Hooijmans CR, Leenaars M, Ritskes-Hoitinga M. A Gold Standard Publication Checklist to Improve the Quality of Animal Studies, to Fully Integrate the Three Rs, and to Make Systematic Reviews More Feasible. Altern Lab Anim. 2010; 38: 167-182. [Guidelines for the reporting of studies on animals; essential reading for anyone reporting such studies.]

* Hopewell S, Clarke M, Moher D, Wagner E, Middleton P, Altman DG, Schulz KF; and CONSORT Group. CONSORT for Reporting Randomized Controlled Trials in Journal and Conference Abstracts: Explanation and Elaboration. PLoS Med. 2008; 5: e20. [Authoritative guidelines for what to write in the abstract of a randomized controlled trial, including point-by-point examples and explanations; also more broadly useful for the reporting of any clinical trial.]

Hopewell S, Collins GS, Boutron I, Yu L-M, Cook J, Shanyinde M, Wharton R, Shamseer L, Altman DG. Impact of peer review on reports of randomised trials published in open peer review journals: retrospective before and after study. BMJ. 2014; 349: g4145. [A study of the literature showing that peer review has only a modest beneficial effect on the reporting of trials and often fails to catch important shortcomings.]

* Horton R. The rhetoric of research. BMJ. 1995; 310: 985-988. [Setting aside this eminent Editor's own rhetorical goals here, this essay provides a very useful introduction to sophisticated issues of how to write compelling research papers, especially Discussion sections; highly recommended for experienced authors.]

Hosking JRM. L-moments: Analysis and Estimation of Distributions using Linear Combinations of Order Statistics. J R Statist Soc B. 1990; 52: 105-124. [An advanced-level paper for statisticians about this approach to assessing the distribution of data.]

* How experts communicate. Nat Neurosci. 2000; 3: 97. [This editorial explains why science requires a clear writing style and illustrates how to achieve such a style; illuminating and enjoyable to read.]

Howick J, Chalmers I, Glasziou P, Greenhalgh T, Henghan C, Liberati A, Moschetti I, Phillips B, Thornton H. The 2011 Oxford CEBM Levels of Evidence: Introductory Document. Accessed on 18 February 2018 at: https://www.cebm.net/wp-content/uploads/2014/06/CEBM-Levels-of-Evidence-Introduction-2.1.pdf [A poorly written, self-published introduction to the important and widely used schema of levels of evidence.]

Howie JW. How I read. BMJ. 1976; 2 (6044): 1113-1114. [An account of how this author reads journal papers, including some useful tips for writers and much advice that is either outdated or dubious.]

Huth EJ. Irresponsible Authorship and Wasteful Publication. Ann Intern Med. 1986; 104: 257-259. [A classic editorial against false authorship lists, salami publication, and repetitive publication.]

Ibrahim JG, Chu H, Chen M-H. Missing Data in Clinical Studies: Issues and Methods. J Clin Oncol. 2012; 30: 3297-3303. [A well-written intermediate-level article on ways to deal with missing data, including examples.]

In pursuit of comprehension. Nature. 1996; 384: 497. [This editorial, about *Nature*'s efforts to make its papers easier to read, is itself written in a convoluted style that would surely make the current Editors of *Nature* smirk and wince.]

International Association of Veterinary Editors. Consensus Author Guidelines on Animal Ethics and Welfare for Veterinary Journals. Accessed on 13 January 2018 at: https://static1.squarespace. com/static/53e16b74e4b0528c244ec998/t/543acda6e4b094d04bcacacd/1413139878532/ IAVE-AuthorGuidelines.pdf [A rather brief and general set of ethics criteria for journals to reject or consider reviewing manuscripts reporting research on animals.]

** International Committee of Medical Journal Editors. Recommendations for the Conduct, Reporting, Editing, and Publication of Scholarly Work in Medical Journals. Philadelphia: American College of Physicians; 1978, 2017. Accessed on 12 January 2018 at: www.icmje. org/icmje-recommendations.pdf [This very important guidelines document from the ICMJE about the preparation of manuscripts for scientific medical journals is essential reading for all medical researchers; in recent years, updated annually in December.]

Ioannidis JPA. The Proposal to Lower *P* Value Thresholds to .005. JAMA. 2018; 314: 1429-1430. [A rather unconvincing opinion piece about how to solve the problems arising from the current overreliance on dividing all results as "significant" versus "non-significant" based on a threshold of p<0.05.]

** Ioannidis JPA, Evans SJW, Gøtzsche PC, O'Neill RT, Altman DG, Schulz K, Moher D; for CONSORT Group. Better Reporting of Harms in Randomized Trials: An Extension of the CONSORT Statement. Ann Intern Med. 2004; 141: 781-788. [Although written for randomized trials, these guidelines on the reporting of harms are broadly applicable to all clinical trials and quite useful.]

Ioannidis JPA, Mulrow CD, Goodman SN. Adverse Events: The More You Search, the More Your Find. Ann Intern Med. 2006; 144: 298-300. [A good editorial explaining how the rates of harms depend on how they are measured.]

* Iverson C, Christianse S, Flanagin A, Fontanarosa PB, Glass RM, Gregoline B, Lurie SJ, Meyer HS, Winker MA, Young RK, eds. AMA Manual of Style: A Guide for Authors and Editors, 10th ed. Oxford: Oxford University Press; 2007. [A large and comprehensive style guide from the American Medical Association about all aspects of the style and formatting of medical publications; an invaluable reference manual, especially for editors and copy-editors.]

Jafarey A. Deceit and fraud in medical research – Publish or perish culture is to blame. Int J Surg. 2006; 4: 132. [A letter asserting that research misconduct in the developing world is due to financial incentives to publish and insufficient teaching of ethics.]

Jain SH. Negotiating Authorship. J Gen Intern Med. 2011; 26: 1513-1514. [An interesting narrative account of the author's experience reclaiming authorship from a senior supervisor who tried to steal it away from him.]

Japiassú AM. How to prepare and submit abstracts for scientific meetings. Rev Bras Ter Intensiva. 2013; 25: 77-80. [This tutorial article provides advice on what to write in an abstract for conferences; the quality of advice here is not great, but overall it is probably more helpful than not for anyone preparing a conference abstract.]

Jia J-D. Fierce disputes about order of authors sometimes occur in China. BMJ. 1997; 315: 746. [A brief letter about disputes about first authorship in China.]

Johnson ES, Stratton IM. Recommendations for designing tables that report randomized trials. Diabet Med. 2007; 24: 1309-1312. [This brief tutorial article on the design of tables for trial reports adds nothing useful beyond what can be found (in much better form) in the CONSORT guidelines and the books by Tufte (both listed in this bibliography) and occasionally has some poor advice.]

* Jones R, Scouller J, Grainger F, Lachlan M, Evans S, Torrance N. The scandal of poor medical research: sloppy use of literature often to blame. BMJ. 1994; 308: 591. [This brief letter describes three common deficiencies in publications' use of past literature; it serves to make authors aware of a widespread but generally neglected major problem in scientific reporting.]

* Jonville-Béra AP, Giraudeau B, Autret-Leca E. Reporting of Drug Tolerance in Randomized Clinical Trials: When Data Conflict with Authors' Conclusions. Ann Intern Med. 2006; 144:

306-307. [This substantial letter, reanalyzing the reporting of adverse events from two randomized controlled trials, illustrates why it is often dangerously erroneous to make conclusions about the safety of treatments; very worthwhile cautionary reading.]

Junker CA. Adherence to Published Standards of Reporting: A Comparison of Placebo-Controlled Trials Published in English or German. JAMA. 1998; 280: 247-249. [This study compares the quality of reporting of trials in German vs. English and shows that, although there is little difference between them, there is substantial room for improvement for almost all published papers; especially worthwhile to see which deficiencies are most frequent.]

Kallet RH. How to Write the Methods Section of a Research Paper. Respir Care. 2004; 49: 1229-1232. [This tutorial paper about what to write in the methods section of an experimental study (not clinical or observational studies) provides solid, introductory-level advice for clinician-researchers or bioengineers reporting on experimental studies, and perhaps to a lesser-degree also for basic scientists reporting in medical journals.]

Kant I. Grundlegung zur Metaphysik der Sitten. Leipzig: Verlag von Felix Meiner; 1785, 1792, 1947. [This foundational treatise of moral philosophy serves as one possible basis for many of the ethical issues discussed in the present book.]

Kapoor VK. Polyauthoritis giftosa. Lancet. 1994; 346: 1039. [A substantial letter criticizing the inflation of author lists and proposing excellent remedies.]

Kassirer JP, Angell M. Redundant Publication: A Reminder. NEJM. 1995; 333: 449-450. [An editorial mostly about salami publication, with helpful examples.]

Kassirer JP, Campion EW. Peer Review: Crude and Understudied, but Indispensable. JAMA. 1994; 272: 96-97. [An old and preliminary, but nonetheless interesting, attempt, by two Editors from the NEJM, to elucidate peer review as a cognitive process of assessing the validity of a manuscript.]

Katchburian E. Publish or perish: a provocation. Sao Paulo Med J. 2008; 126: 202-203. [An interesting editorial criticizing the approach of assessing the value of publications according to how often they are cited.]

Kelly BD. Dear editor – a note from any imaginary author in response to any referee. Med Hypotheses. 2009; 72: 359. [A satirical reply-to-review letter that is vaguely amusing but juvenile, excessively bitter, and lacking subtlety.]

Kennedy D. Multiple Authors, Multiple Problems. Science. 2003; 301: 733. [An editorial about the problems with long lists of authors.]

Kesselheim AS, Robertson CT, Myers JA, Rose SL, Gillet V, Ross KM, Glynn RJ, Joffe S, Avorn J. A Randomized Study of How Physicians Interpret Research Funding Disclosures. NEJM. 2012; 367: 1119-1127. [A well-designed study on how the declared source of funding of a study influences physicians' interpretation of the study.]

Ketcham CM, Hardy RW, Rubin B, Siegal GP. What editors want in an abstract. Lab Invest. 2010; 90: 4-5. [This editorial provides valuable insights about the pivotal role of the abstract in journals' evaluation of submitted manuscripts, along with some advice of mixed quality about what to write in an abstract.]

Kicinski M, Springate DA, Kontopantelis E. Publication bias in meta-analysis from the Cochrane Database of Systematic Reviews. Stat Med. 2015; 34: 2781-2795. [This statistical modeling study of a large sample of metaanalyses from the Cochrane library provides strong evidence that there is publication bias in favor of studies that report superior efficacy of experimental treatment vs. placebo or that report no statistically significant difference of safety outcomes.]

Kick the bar chart habit. Nat Methods. 2014; 11: 113. [This recommendable editorial urges scientists to replace dynamite-plunger graphs with box-and-whisker plots; it suffers from a complete lack of example figures, but the text addresses an important topic incisively.]

Kilkenny C, Browne WJ, Cuthill IC, Emerson M, Altman DG. Improving Bioscience Research Reporting: The ARRIVE Guidelines for Reporting Animal Research. PLoS Biol. 2010; 8: e1000412. [Very useful guidelines with a checklist of the items to include in reports on animal research; essential reading for any report of animal research.]

Kingori P, Gerrets R. Morals, morale and motivations in data fabrication: Medical research fieldworkers views and practices in two Sub-Saharan African contexts. Soc Sci Med. 2016; 166:

150-159. [A strong and illuminating social science study about why medical research field-workers fabricate data.]

* Kirkman J. Confine yourself to forms of English that are easily understood. BMJ. 1996; 313: 1321-1322. [A convincing invited editorial, with examples, urging writers to avoid words and phrases that are colloquial, specific to a single culture, or otherwise difficult for non-native speakers to comprehend.]

Kittisupamongkol W. Guest authorship in the literature. J Am Acad Dermatol. 2009; 60: 876-877. [A mostly unoriginal but correct letter about guest authorship.]

* Knight J. Clear as mud. Nature. 2003; 423: 376-378. [A news article about why scientific papers are so difficult to read and remedies for that problem.]

Knol MJ, Groenwold RHH, Grobbee DE. *P*-values in baseline tables of randomised controlled trials are inappropriate but still common in high impact journals. Eur J Prev Cardiol. 2012; 19: 231-232. [A very brief literature study documenting that the mistake of calculating p-values for comparisons of baseline variables of study groups is still commonplace.]

Knottnerus JA, Tugwell P. Better data presentation in graphs and tables is possible and needed. J Clin Epidemiol. 2010; 63: 585-586. [Mostly an editorial overview of the articles in that issue of that journal, only some of which dealt with data presentation; limited usefulness beyond the all-too-true point of the title.]

Kohli P, Cannon CP. The Importance of Matching Language to Type of Evidence: Avoiding Pitfalls of Reporting Outcomes Data. Clin Cardiol. 2012; 35: 714-717. [An editorial explaining which types of terms are appropriate for reporting results, depending on the study design.]

Kohli P, Chandrashekhar Y, Narula J. *Vini, Vidi, Vici...* Restructured Format for Condensed Abstracts. JACC Cardiovasc Imaging. 2013; 6: 1220-1221. [An editorial, essentially about capsule summaries; comparatively thin on content.]

Koshland DE Jr. Fraud in Science. Science. 1987; 235: 141. [This editorial condemning fraud in science is outdated and unscientific in its sense of the scope of the problem but quite accurate in its analysis of the causes.]

Kotz D, Cals JWL. Effective writing and publishing scientific papers, part VII: tables and figures. J Clin Epidemiol. 2013; 66: 1197. [A short tutorial paper with mostly good advice about tables and figures, but some small flaws too.]

Kravitz RL, Franks P, Feldman MD, Gerrity M, Byrne C, Tierney WM. Editorial Peer Reviewers' Recommendations at a General Medical Journal: Are They Reliable and Do Editors Care? PLoS One. 2010; 5: e10072. [A large study showing that peer reviewers agree with each other barely more often than by chance and Editors sometimes ignore their unanimous recommendations anyway.]

Krzywinski M, Altman N. Visualizing samples with box plots. Nat Methods. 2014; 11: 119-120. [A tutorial article on box-and-whisker plots with mostly dubious or bad advice; not recommendable.]

* Kuhn TS. The Structure of Scientific Revolutions. Chicago: University of Chicago Press; 1962, 1970. [A landmark book of theory on how scientific knowledge advances; useful as background reading for thinking about how to approach research.]

Kwok LS. The White Bull effect: abusive coauthorship and publication parasitism. J Med Ethics. 2005; 31: 554-556. [A mostly successful scholarly attempt to characterize the fraudulent behavior and underlying psychopathology of senior researchers claiming unearned authorship credit, as well as the surrounding institutional defects that facilitate it.]

Lachenbruch PA. Proper metrics for clinical trials: transformations and other procedures to remove non-normality effects. Stat Med. 2003; 22: 3823-3842. [An advanced-level study comparing statistical approaches to analyzing data with various non-Normal distributions.]

Laine C, Horton R, DeAngelis CD, Drazen JM, Frizelle FA, Godlee F, Haug C, Hébert PC, Kotzin S, Marušić A, Sahni P, Schroeder TV, Sox HC, Van Der Weyden MB, Verheugt FWA. Clinical Trial Registration — Looking Back and Moving Ahead. NEJM. 2007; 356: 2734-2736. [This editorial, which provides an update on clinical trial registration two years after it became a requirement for publication in ICMJE member journals, is of limited interest today.]

Landewé RBM. How Publication Bias May Harm Treatment Guidelines. Arthritis Rheumatol. 2014; 66: 2661-2663. [A good editorial / study commentary about publication bias.]

Landis SC, Amara SG, Asadullah K, Austin CP, Blumenstein R, Bradley EW, Crystal RG, Darnell RB, Ferrante RJ, Fillit H, Finkelstein R, Fisher M, Gendelman HE, Golub RM, Goudreau JL, Gross RA, Gubitz AK, Hesterlee SE, Howells DW, Huguenard J, Kelner K, Koroshetz W, Krainc D, Lazic SE, Levine MS, Macleod MR, McGall JM, Moxlex RT III, Narasimhan K, Noble LJ, Perrin S, Porter JD, Steward O, Unger E, Utz U, Silberberg SD. A call for transparent reporting to optimize the predictive value of preclinical research. Nature. 2012; 490: 187-191. [Guidelines, developed in a major stakeholder meeting, for the reporting of methods of preclinical research; essential reading for anyone reporting on animal studies.]

Lane DM, Sándor A. Designing Better Graphs by Including Distributional Information and Integrating Words, Numbers, and Images. Psychol Methods. 2009; 14: 239-257. [A substantial article with illustrated advice about how to improve the quality of some commonly used data graphs; this intermediate-level article requires some previous familiarity with statistics and graphing but otherwise should be quite accessible and applicable for most medical researchers.]

Lang JM, Rothman KJ, Cann CI. That Confounded P-Value. Epidemiology. 1998; 9: 7-8. [This useful article explains why this journal prefers that authors report an effect size and confidence interval instead of a p-value.]

Lang TA, Secic M. How to Report Statistics in Medicine, 2nd ed. Philadelphia: American College of Physicians; 2006. [A thorough book explaining the proper way to report statistical results.]

Langdon-Neuner E. Hangings at the *bmj*: What editors discuss when deciding to accept or reject research papers. The Write Stuff. 2008; 17: 84-85. [This informal magazine article describes how the Editors of BMJ discuss manuscripts at their weekly meeting, and thus it provides some interesting insights into the (generally opaque) process of manuscript selection by journals.]

Langdorf MI, Hayden SR. Turning Your Abstract into a Paper: Academic Writing Made Simpler. West J Emerg Med. 2009; 10: 120-123. [This tutorial paper, from two Editors-in-Chief, about what to write in a journal paper and how to write it, contains mostly good advice, (despite the regrettable title), especially about matters of English writing style.]

Larson MG. Descriptive Statistics and Graphical Displays. Circulation. 2006; 114: 76-81. [Despite a couple errors and an impoverished reference list, this tutorial paper provides a good basic introduction to descriptive statistics and a few commonly usable graphs.]

LaValley MP. Logistic Regression. Circulation. 2008; 117: 2395-2399. [A reasonably good tutorial paper about how to perform logistic regression analyses.]

Lawrence PA. Rank injustice. Nature. 2002; 415: 835-836. [A critical essay mainly about senior authors taking credit for work done by junior authors.]

Lazarus C, Haneef R, Ravaud P, Boutron I. Classification and prevalence of spin in abstracts of non-randomized studies evaluating an intervention. BMC Med Res Methodol. 2015; 15: 85. [An empirical study on the frequency of spin in abstracts.]

Lemaire F. Do All Types of Human Research Need Ethics Committee Approval? Am J Respir Crit Care Med. 2006; 174: 363-364. [An editorial affirming and illustrating that research will not be published in scientific journals if it did not obtain approval of an ethics committee but should have according to universal ethical guidelines, even if the researchers' local laws and/or culture did not require approval by an ethics committee.]

Lengauer T, Nussinov R. How to Write a Presubmission Inquiry. PLoS Comput Biol 2015; 11: e1004098. [This tutorial paper provides useful advice on how to write a presubmission inquiry – a practice that is rarely advisable.]

Lentz J, Kennett M, Perlutter J, Forrest A. Paving the way to a more effective informed consent process: Recommendations from the Clinical Trials Transformation Initiative. Contemp Clin Trials. 2016; 49: 65-69. [A project report, based mostly on the level-5 evidence of expert opinion, on ways to improve the informed consent process for research, with many suggestions worthy of further consideration and study.]

Leopold SS. Case Closed—Discontinuing Case Reports in *Clinical Orthopaedics and Related Research*. Clin Orthop Relat Res. 2015; 473: 3074-3075. [A brief editorial explaining why this journal stopped publishing case reports.]

Li T, Hutfless S, Scharfstein DO, Daniels MJ, Hogan JW, Little RJA, Roy JA, Law AH, Dickersin K. Standards should be applied in the prevention and handling of missing data for patient-centered outcomes research: a systematic review and expert consensus. J Clin Epidemiol. 2014; 67: 15-32. [This article contains a very useful overview of 39 recommendations for dealing with missing data based on a systematic review of the literature, as well as a sometimes mis-guided reduction of that list down to 10 recommendations based on the authors' opinions.]

Lidz CW, Appelbaum PS. The Therapeutic Misconception: Problems and Solutions. Med Care. 2002; 40: V55-V63. [A good introductory overview to the problem of therapeutic misconception when obtaining informed consent for participation in research.]

Lilleyman J, Lowe D. Editorial: Structured abstracts. J Clin Pathol. 1992; 45: 8. [A brief editorial about why this journal introduced a structured format for abstracts.]

Link AM. US and Non-US Submissions: An Analysis of Review Bias. JAMA. 1998; 280: 246-247. [A brief report on two years of manuscript reviews at a specialty journal providing some evidence that there is essentially no discriminatory bias by reviewers from the US or by reviewers from all other countries when considering how each of those two groups assesses manuscripts from the US versus from all other countries.]

Lippert S, Callaham ML, Lo B. Perceptions of Conflict of Interest Disclosures among Peer Reviewers. PLoS One. 2011; 6: e26900. [A survey of peer reviewers on how authors' declared conflicts of interest influence the peer reviewers' assessment of the manuscript.]

** Little RJ, D'Agostino R, Cohen ML, Dickersin K, Emerson SS, Farrar JT, Frangakis C, Hogan JW, Molenberghs G, Murphy SA, Neaton JD, Rotnitzky A, Scharfstein D, Shih WJ, Siegel JP, Stern H. The Prevention and Treatment of Missing Data in Clinical Trials. NEJM. 2012; 367: 1355-1360. [A summary of a major report on the important problem of missing data, including recommendations for how to prevent, account for, and adjust for missing data.]

Loader SM. I don't know. BMJ. 2004; 328: 1016. [A clever little metacognitive letter about scientific ignorance.]

Lock S. Authors of the world, unite... BMJ. 1982; 284: 1726-1727. [A brief editorial about why journal Editors agreed to unify the formatting requirements for references in the Vancouver style.]

Lock S. Failure of communication. BMJ. 1985; 291: 761. [A brief editorial criticizing the tedious writing style of a major committee report calling on scientists to communicate more clearly with the general public.]

Lock S. How editors survive. BMJ. 1976; 2 (6044): 1118-1119. [A somewhat dated editorial about peer review, good English, and the difference between conference presentations and journal papers.]

Lock S, ed. Peer review at work. BMJ. 1985; 290: 1555-1561. [In order to provide some behind-the-scenes insight into how peer review works, this article published a study report that the BMJ had rejected three times after peer review, along with the peer reviewer comments and correspondence between the Editors, authors, peer reviewers, and statisticians; interesting reading, but historical, in particular because no journal today would tolerate so much dispute from an author about their decision.]

Lock S. Peer review weighed in the balance. BMJ. 1982; 285: 1224-126. [An editorial with reflections on the shortcomings and possible improvements of peer review and journal decision making.]

Lock S. Repetitive publication: a waste that must stop. BMJ. 1984; 288: 661-662. [An editorial criticizing the various forms of repetitive publication.]

Lock S. Structured abstracts: Now required for all papers reporting clinical trials. BMJ. 1988; 297: 156. [A brief editorial about why the BMJ adopted a structured format for abstracts.]

* Loftus GR. A picture is worth a thousand *p* values: On the irrelevance of hypothesis testing in the microcomputer age. Behav Res Methods. 1993; 25: 250-256. [This tutorial article explains why

making graphs is a superior to generating p-values as an approach to data analysis; although the case illustrations are from Psychology and some material is rather dated, the fundamental point of this article is important and explained well.]

Lundberg GD, Paul MC, Fritz H. A Comparison of the Opinions of Experts and Readers as to What Topics a General Medical Journal (JAMA) Should Address. JAMA. 1998; 280: 288-290. [A study comparing the topics that JAMA's editorial board members versus readers felt were most important.]

Lunt M. Introduction to statistical modelling: linear regression. Rheumatology. 2015; 54: 1137-1140. [A basic but mathy introduction to linear regression that confusingly switches its discussion of its figure 1c and 1d.]

MacCallum CJ. Reporting Animal Studies: Good Science and a Duty of Care. PLoS Biol. 2010; 8: e1000413. [An editorial from the Senior Editor of this journal about the widespread deficiencies in the reporting of animal research and emerging remedies for that.]

MacDonald NE, Ford-Jones L, Friedman JN, Hall J. Preparing a manuscript for publication: A user-friendly guide. Paediatr Child Health. 2006; 11: 339-342. [This guide to writing journal papers contains useful advice for students and novices about the psychological and social aspects of how to get the writing work done and how to cope with the responses from journals, but the other tips it provides are somewhat spotty and it lacks any guidance on the actual substance of journal papers; best suited for trainees who need to do some writing but have no intentions of remaining in research.]

Machin D, Campbell MJ, Walters SJ. Medical Statistics: A Textbook for the Health Sciences. West Sussex, England: John Wiley & Sons; 2007. [A useful introductory-level textbook about statistical analysis in medicine, and also about study design.]

Maddox J. Plagiarism is worse than mere theft. Nature. 1995; 376: 721. [This mixed news-story / editorial fails to make the case that plagiarism is *worse* than theft, but it does clearly show that plagiarism *is* theft of other people's intellectual work and the monetary rewards for that work.]

Mahajan RP, Hunter JM. Case reports: should they be confined to the dustbin? Br J Anaesth. 2008; 100: 744-746. [An editorial about which types of case reports may be valuable and why this journal had to become more selective about their publication.]

Maisonneuve H. Guest Authorship, Mortality Reporting, and Integrity in Rofecoxib Studies. JAMA. 2008; 300: 902. [A research letter reporting on lack of awareness in France of the criteria for authorship, based on Pignatelli et al. cited below]

* Making the most of peer review. Nat Neurosci. 2000; 3: 629. [A brief editorial packed with very valuable advice about how to get through peer review and maximize the chances of publication.]

Maltenfort MG. Understanding a Normal Distribution of Data. J Spinal Disord Tech. 2015; 28: 377-378. [A brief basic introduction to this topic, which is correct but entirely lacking both originality and references to the literature.]

Maltenfort MG. Understanding a Normal Distribution of Data (Part 2). Clin Spine Surg. 2016; 29: 30. [A very good brief overview of advanced methods for analyzing data that is not Normally distributed.]

Marcelo A, Gavino A, Isip-Tan IT, Apostol-Nicodemus L, Mesa-Gaerlan FJ, Firaza PN, Faustorilla JF Jr, Callaghan FM, Fontelo P. A comparison of the accuracy of clinical decisions based on full-text articles and on journal abstracts alone: a study among residents in a tertiary care hospital. Evid Based Med. 2013; 18: 48-53. [An empirical study showing that reading journal abstracts or full articles substantially improves the ability of medical residents to correctly answer questions on case-based clinical tests.]

Marco CA, Schmidt TA. Who Wrote This Paper? Basics of Authorship and Ethical Issues. Acad Emerg Med. 2004; 11: 76-77. [A good editorial clarifying the basic ethical issues of authorship.]

Marcus E. A New Year and a new Era for *Cell*. Cell. 2004; 116: 1-2. [An editorial, mostly about the journal *Cell* itself, but also containing some interesting remarks on what makes a paper scientifically important.]

* Marcus E. Credibility and Reproducibility. Cell. 2014; 159: 965-966. [An editorial, from the Editor-in-Chief of *Cell*, about the widespread problem of irreproducibility of basic research

and the threat it poses to the credibility of science; highly recommended for all laboratory scientists.]

Marcus E. June is the Cruelest Month. Cell. 2013; 154: 9-10. [An editorial reminding everyone why impact factors and other citations metrics are not so important.]

Marcus E. Taming Supplemental Material. Cell. 2009; 139: 10-11. [An editorial providing useful guidance for how to think about what is or is not appropriate to present as supplemental files.]

Marincola FM. In support of descriptive studies; relevance to translational research. J Transl Med. 2007; 5: 1. [An editorial calling for more descriptive research before hypotheses-testing research.]

Marušić A, Marušić M. Teaching Students How to Read and Write Science: A Mandatory Course on Scientific Research and Communication in Medicine. Acad Med. 2003; 78: 1235-1239. [A narrative paper describing the development and implementation of a scientific writing course into the medical schools of Croatia.]

* Marušić M, Marušić A. Good Editorial Practice: Editors as Educators. Croat Med J. 2001; 42: 113-120. [This substantial editorial discusses how scientific journals in developing countries could serve a positive role in improving the quality of local science but usually have the opposite effect of reinforcing local low quality; in addition to providing useful reflections about scientific journals in the developing world, this article is now also more generally thought-provoking about why scientific quality is so important in an era of exploding opportunities for quick-and-easy publication in junk journals, preprint servers, and other dubious formats.]

* Masterson GR, Ashcroft GS. Better libraries and more journal clubs would help. BMJ. 1994; 308: 592-593. [A letter about the inadequate facilities, training, and funding that leads to poor quality medical research publications, with a small informal survey as supporting evidence.]

Matheson NA. ...While poor leadership fuels mediocrity. BMJ. 1994; 308: 591. [A somewhat foggy letter, the main point of which seems to be that academic doctors' clinical capabilities suffer because career advancement is based mainly on the length of their publication lists.]

Mathieu S, Giraudeau B, Soubrier M, Ravaud P. Misleading abstract conclusions in randomized controlled trials in rheumatology: comparison of the abstract conclusions and the results section. Joint Bone Spine. 2012; 79: 262-267. [A study of the literature showing that abstract conclusions are often misleading because they are not supported by the primary outcome.]

Matthews JNS, Altman DG, Campell MJ, Royston P. Analysis of serial measurements in medical research. BMJ. 1990; 300: 230-235. [A tutorial paper describing one approach to statistical analysis in studies that make repeated measures on the subjects; worthwhile reading for any such study design.]

McCloskey M. Scheme with little funding and no protected time will be forced on GPs. BMJ. 1998; 317: 1454. [A letter from a GP criticizing some plan for required CME without funding for participation.]

McDonald JC. Charts, Graphs and Tables – Reporting the Data. Radiat Prot Dosimetry. 2001; 95: 291-293. [This editorial about various types of graphs and graphic aspects of figures has some good advice toward the end, but the lack of illustrations renders the rest of it unsuitable for beginners.]

McGough JJ, Faraone SV. Estimating the Size of Treatment Effects: Moving Beyond *P* Values. Psychiatry. 2009; 6 (10): 21-29. [A very clear and useful review of five measures of effects sizes, including Cohen's d, relative risk, and number needed to treat.]

McKneally M. Put my name on that paper: Reflections on the ethics of authorship. J Thorac Cardiovasc Surg. 2006; 131: 517-519. [An editorial providing guidance about accurate and truthful authorship claims.]

McNamee R. Regression Modelling and Other Methods to Control Confounding. Occup Environ Med. 2005; 62: 500-506. [A good intermediate-level paper on the exact topic of its title.]

McQuay HJ, Moore RA. Work done by junior researchers gives rise to problems. BMJ. 1997; 315: 745. [This thoughtful letter about acknowledging the contributions of research assistants is most valuable for its suggestion that the final manuscript be read aloud and discussed by everyone involved just prior to submission – a rare best practice that should be universally adopted.]

Meier GF. Versuch einer allgemeinen Auslegungskunst. Hamburg: Felix Meiner Verlag; 1757, 1996. [A book of fundamental theory about meaning and interpretation; as background reading for advanced scholar-scientists, this work provides a deeper understanding of the process of the interpretation of data and also communication with readers.]

Meyer J, Shamo MK, Gopher D. Information Structure and the Relative Efficacy of Tables and Graphs. Hum Factors. 1999; 41: 570-587. [This experimental study suggests that graphs are better than tables if there are patterns in the data, while tables are better than graphs for transmitting specific information.]

Miedzinski LJ, Davis P, Al-Shurafa H, Morrison JC. A Canadian faculty of medicine and dentistry's survey of career development needs. Med Educ. 2001; 35: 890-900. [This survey of full-time faculty at a Canadian medical school reported that their top three perceived career development needs were effective writing of grant and publications, time management, and effective oral and written communication.]

Mireles-Cabodevila E, Stoller JK. Research During Fellowship. Chest. 2009; 135: 1395-1399. [A well-written article with 10 pieces of advice about the practical difficulties of carrying out research; highly recommended reading for anyone who wants to lead a research study.]

Mišak A, Marušić M, Marušić A. Manuscript editing as a way of teaching academic writing: Experience from a small scientific journal. J Second Lang Writ. 2005; 14: 122-131. [A narrative article, by the Editors of the Croatian Medical Journal, about how English language editors can contribute much more to the improvement of scientific communication than mere language editing.]

Moher D, Altman DG. Four Proposals to Help Improve the Medical Research Literature. PLoS Med. 2015; 12: e1001864. [Although this article's four proposals to improve the quality of medical research literature are interesting and worthwhile ideas, mostly they could only be implemented by people in positions of leadership at journals or universities; limited practical use for researchers just trying to write better papers.]

Moher D, Hopewell S, Schulz KF, Montori V, Gøtzsche PC, Devereaux PJ, Elbourne D, Egger M, Altman DG. CONSORT 2010 Explanation and Elaboration: updated guidelines for reporting parallel group randomised trials. BMJ. 2010; 340: c869. [Extended explanation of authoritative guidelines for the reporting of randomized trials; essential reading for anyone writing up a randomized trial, and broadly useful for reporting other prospective clinical studies too.]

Moher D, Liberati A, Tetzlaff J, Altman DG; and PRISMA Group. Preferred Reporting Items for Systematic Reviews and Meta-Analyses: The PRISMA Statement. PLoS Med. 2009; 6: e1000097. [Reporting guidelines for systematic reviews and metaanalyses; important for anyone writing such articles, and useful for readers of such articles too.]

Morales P, Bosch F. ¿Editar o perecer? Desafíos en la edición biomédica. Gac Sanit. 2005; 19: 258-261. [This article summarizes a small meeting of various professionals to discuss the state of biomedical publishing in Spain; it is somewhat cursory but raises interesting issues, considering how many medical researchers around the world read and write Spanish better than English.]

Morgan PP. The joys of revising a manuscript. CMAJ. 1986; 134: 1328. [An editorial about revising manuscripts for journal review and writing a reply-to-review letter; outdated in some details but otherwise still relevant.]

Morgan PP. Why case reports? CMAJ. 1985; 133: 353. [An outdated editorial about what case reports should contain to be publishable.]

Morris JA. Theory must drive experiment. BMJ. 1994; 308: 592. [A somewhat arcanely formulated letter making the good underlying point that research studies without good questions yield trivial data.]

Mullee MA, Lampe FC, Pickering RM, Julious SA. Statisticians should be coauthors. BMJ. 1995; 310: 869. [A letter explaining why statisticians should be involved and credited as coauthors on research papers.]

Munro CL, Savel RH. Publish (High-Quality Evidence For Clinical Practice) or (Patients May) Perish. Am J Crit Care. 2013; 22: 182-184. [An editorial explaining that the primary purpose of publishing medical research is to improve patient care, while advancing one's own career is only secondary.]

Nakayama T, Hirai N, Yamazaki S, Naito M. Adoption of structured abstracts by general medical journals and format for a structured abstract. J Med Lib Assoc. 2005; 93: 237-242. [A study of the literature in regards to the frequency and form of structured abstracts in journals of general medicine; perhaps of some interest to specialists.]

National Institute of Health. Principles and Guidelines for Reporting Preclinical Research. Accessed on 13 January 2018 at: https://www.nih.gov/research-training/rigor-reproducibility/principles-guidelines-reporting-preclinical-research [An important but somewhat cursory set of principles for the policies journals should adopt about the reporting of preclinical research.]

Neff MJ. Informed Consent: What Is It? Who Can Give It? How Do We Improve It? Respir Care. 2008; 53: 1337-1341. [A good, basic introduction to informed consent for research in the American context.]

Neill US. Publish or perish, but at what cost? J Clin Invest. 2008; 118: 2368. [An editorial discussing the ethical problems of redundant publication and text recycling and how this journal's editorial board responds to such conduct.]

Neill US. Stop misbehaving! J Clin Invest. 2006; 116: 1740-1741. [This editorial calls on researchers to desist from inappropriate image manipulation and a variety of commonplace forms of research misconduct related to the manuscript submission phase.]

Nietzsche F. Der Wanderer und sein Schatten. In: Colli G, Montinari M, eds. Nietzsche Werke. Berlin: Walter de Gruyter & Co; 1880, 1967, vol. IV (3), pp. 173-342. [A collection of reflections, including many about how to write well, from one of the most brilliant writers ever.]

North American Primary Care Research Group Committee on Building Research Capacity, The Academic Family Medicine Organizations Research Subcommittee. What Does It Mean to Build Research Capacity? Fam Med. 2002; 34: 678-684. [A policy position paper from a professional society reflecting on several aspects of developing research capacity; useful background reading for anyone trying to increase the production of research.]

Not picture-perfect. Nature. 2006; 439: 891-892. [A brief editorial against editing images to idealize the data observed.]

Nuzzo R. Statistical Errors. Nature. 2014; 506: 150-152. [A science journalism article about the various problems of calculating p-values; unfortunately, this otherwise worthwhile article is sometimes muddled by Bayesian perspectives.]

Ober H, Simon SI, Elson D. Five Simple Rules to Avoid Plagiarism. Ann Biomed Eng. 2013; 41: 1-2. [This editorial with basic advice on avoiding plagiarism provides a quick and useful starting point on the subject.]

* O'Donnell M. Evidence-based illiteracy: time to rescue "the literature". Lancet. 2000; 355: 489-491. [A good essay criticizing the incomprehensible academic writing style that is pervasive in the medical literature.]

Office of Research Integrity – Office of Public Health and Science – U.S. Department of Health and Human Services. Managing Allegations of Scientific Misconduct: A Guidance Document for Editors. Rockville, MD, USA: U.S. Department of Health and Human Services; 2000. Accessed on 24 October 2017 at: https://ori.hhs.gov/images/ddblock/masm_2000.pdf [An illuminating document about what journal Editors should do in cases of allegations of scientific misconduct.]

Ohnmeiss DD. Overview of the Role of Statistic Analysis in the Design of Spine-related Studies. SAS Journal. 2009; 3: 26-29. [Although written for a readership of spine surgeons, this tutorial paper contains good beginner-level advice about statistical analysis in clinical trials, especially in regards to issues of study preparation and data collection.]

Olson KR, Shaw A. 'No fair, copycat!': what children's response to plagiarism tells us about their understanding of ideas. Dev Sci. 2011; 14: 431-439. [An experimental study showing that children develop a disapproval of plagiarism already by 6 years of age.]

Oransky I. How Publish or Perish Promotes Inaccuracy in Science—and Journalism. AMA J Ethics. 2015; 17: 1172-1175. [A magazine-tone article about the effect of publication pressure on news coverage of medical science.]

Organisation for Economic Co-Operation and Development, Global Science Forum. Best Practices for Ensuring Scientific Integrity and Preventing Misconduct. Accessed on 13 January 2018 at: www.oecd.org/science/inno/40188303.pdf [The report of an international workshop about research misconduct, focused mainly on practical administrative ways of dealing with it; instructive (but not authoritative) for medical researchers.]

* Orwell G. Politics and the English Language. In: Orwell G. Why I Write. London: Penguin; 1946, 2004, pp. 102-120. [This short essay examines how bad writing style hides dishonest thinking, and provides fundamental guidance on how to write more responsibly; essential reading for anyone striving to express themselves honestly.]

Oxford Centre for Evidence-Based Medicine, Levels of Evidence Working Group. Oxford Centre for Evidence-Based Medicine 2011 Levels of Evidence. Accessed on 18 February 2018 at: https://www.cebm.net/wp-content/uploads/2014/06/CEBM-Levels-of-Evidence-2.1.pdf [The table of the important and widely used schema of levels of evidence.]

Oxman AD, Chalmers I, Sackett DL. A practical guide to informed consent to treatment. BMJ. 2001; 323: 1464-1466. [A completely satirical suite of informed consent forms for research and routine treatment, from the godfathers of EBM.]

Oxman AD, Guyatt GH. Guidelines for reading literature reviews. CMAJ. 1988; 138: 697-703. [A useful essay about how to evaluate literature reviews.]

Oxman AD, Guyatt GH. The Science of Reviewing Research. Ann N Y Acad Sci. 1993; 703: 125-133. [An interesting historical essay about expert narrative reviews of the literature versus methodical systematic reviews of the literature.]

Oxman AD, Sackett DL, Guyatt GH; for Evidence-Based Medicine Working Group. Users' Guides to the Medical Literature, I: How to Get Started. JAMA. 1993; 270: 2093-2095. [The first in a series of articles on how to find and select journal articles to use to guide clinical care of patients; perhaps of some indirect value to people writing journal articles.]

Parker GB. On the breeding of coauthors: just call me Al. MJA. 2007; 187: 650-651. [This amusing article discusses the problem of the the the rising number of co-authors on scientific publications and proposes solutions for that.]

Pascal RP. Case Reports—Desideratum or Rubbish? Hum Pathol. 1985; 16: 759. [A somewhat useful but mostly outdated editorial about case reports.]

Pharoah P. How Not to Interpret a *P* Value? J Natl Cancer Inst. 2007; 99: 332-333. [A letter concisely summarizing the usual misguided arguments for switching to Bayesian statistics.]

Pierson DJ. How to Write an Abstract That Will Be Accepted for Presentation at a National Meeting. Respir Care. 2004; 49: 1206-1212. [This good tutorial paper provides guidance on what to write in an abstract for a scientific conference.]

Pierson DJ. The Top 10 Reasons Why Manuscripts Are Not Accepted for Publication. Respir Care. 2004; 49: 1246-1252. [This interesting paper briefly summarizes many reasons given in the literature for why manuscripts are rejected and then discusses a proposed "top 10" list of reasons more in-depth; this article is very useful for beginners, but the basic "top 10" reasons it discusses are mostly not illuminating for experienced researchers who have already published a few papers.]

Pignatelli B, Maisonneuve H, Chapuis F. Authorship ignorance: views of researchers in French clinical settings. J Med Ethics. 2005; 31: 578-581. [An interview study documenting substantial lack of awareness or disregard of authorship criteria among French Principal Investigators.]

Pitkin RM, Branagan MA. Can the accuracy of abstracts be improved by providing specific instructions? A randomized controlled trial. JAMA. 1998; 280: 267-269. [This study showed that inconsistencies in abstracts are commonplace and an intervention warning authors to avoid these specific problems was not effective.]

Pitkin RM, Branagan MA, Burmeister LF. Accuracy of Data in Abstracts of Published Research Articles. JAMA. 1999; 281: 1110-1111. [A study of papers in top-tier journals showing that the results presented in the abstracts are often inconsistent with or missing from the main body of the paper.]

Pitrou I, Boutron I, Ahmad N, Ravaud P. Reporting of Safety Results in Published Reports of Randomized Controlled Trials. Arch Intern Med. 2009; 169: 1756-1761. [This study of the literature documents substantial deficiencies in the reporting of harms.]

Plain English. J Coll Gen Pract. 1958; 1: 311-313. [A valuable editorial calling for the use of plain English and a return to well-educated writing.]

Plantin C. L'argumentation. Paris: Seuil; 1996. [A concise introductory-level book about argumentation (i.e. logic and rhetoric).]

Ploegh H. End the wasteful tyranny of reviewer experiments. Nature. 2011; 472: 391. [A viewpoint essay arguing against requests from peer reviewers for additional experiments; useful reading for all experimental researchers.]

The *PLoS Medicine* Editors. An Unbiased Scientific Record Should Be Everyone's Agenda. PLoS Med. 2009; 6: 0119-0121. [An editorial mainly about bias due to commercial and non-commercial interests, spin, and failure to publish negative findings.]

The *PLoS Medicine* Editors. Does Conflict of Interest Disclosure Worsen Bias? PLoS Med. 2012; 9: e1001210. [An editorial using the APA DSM-V as an illustration to raise the question of the ways that disclosure of financial conflicts of interest can actually worsen bias.]

The *PLoS Medicine* Editors. Getting Closer to a Fully Correctable and Connected Research Literature. PLoS Med. 2013; 10: e1001408. [A strong and original editorial about dealing with pervasive misconduct and errors in the medical literature and proposing better linkage of papers to all post-publication commentary as one solution.]

Pocock SJ, Travison TG, Wruck LM. Figures in clinical trial reports: current practice & scope for improvement. Trials. 2007; 8: 36. [A study of figures in clinical trials, along with recommendations for graphic improvements.]

Pound P, Ebrahim S, Sandercock P, Bracken MB, Roberts I; for Reviewing Animal Trials Systematically (RATS) Group. Where is the evidence that animal research benefits humans? BMJ. 2004; 328: 517-517. [A narrative review paper that, among other matters, describes deficiencies in reporting of animal studies and insufficient literature reviews before further research.]

* Primack RB, Cigliano JA, Parsons ECM. Coauthors gone bad; how to avoid publishing conflict and a proposed agreement for co-author teams. Biol Conserv. 2014; 176: 277-280. [An editorial briefly describing commonplace conflicts between co-authors at the publishing stage and proposing a partial preventive measure of a co-author agreement; recommended reading for anyone working with co-authors.]

Prinz F, Schlange T, Asadullah K. Believe it or not: how much can we rely on published data on potential drug targets? Nat Rev Drug Discov. 2011; 10: 712. [An informal but widely discussed brief report from Bayer that about two-thirds of the promising published preclinical research that they attempted to reproduce were sufficiently irreproducible that the projects were terminated; the use of three big 3D color pie-charts in their paper unintentionally confirms the hopeless depth of poor quality in medical research publications.]

Pulverer B. When things go wrong: correcting the scientific record. EMBO J. 2015; 34: 2483-2485. [A substantial and thoughtful editorial about how corrections and retractions of the literature are currently handled.]

Putnam W. Funding protected time for research: New opportunities from the Canadian Institutes of Health Research. Can Fam Physician. 2003; 49: 632-633. [This information article about grant opportunities for physicians wanting to pursue a career in research provides clear indirect evidence that it normally takes a graduate of medical school an additional 4-6 years of fellowship training to become an independent investigator.]

Qiu J. Publish or perish in China. Nature. 2010; 463: 142-143. [A news article about how rewards for publications in China drive substantial rates of scientific misconduct.]

Radford DR, Smillie L, Wilson RF, Grace AM. The criteria used by editors of scientific dental journals in the assessment of manuscripts submitted for publication. Brit Dent J. 1999; 187: 376-379. [A survey of Editors of dental journals about the criteria they use to assess manuscripts; useful reading for researchers in any medical field.]

Rawls J. A Theory of Justice. Cambridge, MA, USA: Belknap Press; 1971. [A foundational philosophy book in the branch of social ethics; of some remote relevance for understanding the ethics of scientific medical research.]

Read MEDLINE abstracts with a pinch of salt. Lancet. 2006; 368: 1394. [This brief editorial criticizes industry-sponsored journal supplements, abstracts without disclosure statements, and readers' lack of critical appraisal of full-length articles.]

Ready T. Plagiarize or perish? Nat Med. 2006; 12: 494. [A little news item about the extent of peer reviewers stealing ideas.]

Rennie D, Flanagin A, Yank V. The Contributions of Authors. JAMA. 2000; 284: 89-91. [An editorial explaining why JAMA started asking for statements of authors' contributions.]

Resnik DB, Tyler AM, Black JR, Kissling G. Authorship policies of scientific journals. J Med Ethics. 2016; 42: 199-202. [A study of the authorship policies of 600 journals across the sciences.]

Ressing M, Blettner M, Klug SJ. Systematische Übersichtsarbeiten und Metaanalysen. Dtsch Arztebl Int. 2009; 106: 456-463. [A tutorial article about various types of review papers and metaanalyses.]

Rice TW. How to Do Human-Subjects Research If You Do Not Have an Institutional Review Board. Respir Care. 2008; 53: 1362-1367. [A somewhat dull comparison of the three ways to obtain Research Ethics Committee approval if the facility where the research will be done does not have an ethics committee.]

Richardson JD. Case Reports: Boon or Bane for the Medical Editor? Am Surg. 2006; 72: 663-664. [An editorial describing a couple of scenarios that might make some surgical case reports publishable.]

Riesenberg DE. Case Reports in the Medical Literature. JAMA. 1986; 255: 2067. [An outdated editorial about what case reports should contain to be publishable.]

Riesenberg D, Lundberg GD. The Order of Authorship: Who's on First? JAMA. 1990; 264: 1857. [A very good editorial about the order of authors listed.]

Ripple AM, Mork JG, Knecht LS, Humphreys BL. A retrospective cohort study of structured abstracts in MEDLINE, 1992-2006. J Med Libr Assoc. 2011; 99: 160-163. [An information science study on the rising rate of structured abstracts on MEDLINE.]

Roberts WC. Revising Manuscripts After Studying Reviewers' Comments. Am J Cardiol. 2006; 98: 989. [An editorial advising authors to always revise their manuscripts for reviewer comments, even if they do not immediately make sense.]

Rockman HA. Great expectations. J Clin Invest. 2012; 122: 1133. [An editorial with brief comments about the history of peer review, selection of manuscripts to be sent for peer review, and a variety of brief suggestions for better reporting of data.]

Rockman HA. Waste not, want not. J Clin Invest. 2014; 124: 463. [An editorial explaining why this journal opposes calls from peer reviewers for additional experiments; highly useful for all laboratory researchers.]

Rogers LF. Salami Slicing, Shotgunning, and the Ethics of Authorship. Am J Roentgenol. 1999; 173: 265. [A short and breezy editorial about the ethical problems of "salami" publishing, plagiarism, and multiple concurrent submissions of a manuscript.]

Roman G. Read It Again: It's Good for You. JAMA. 1985; 253: 2104. [A classic, satirical editorial on the various reasons why authors should publish the same paper numerous times; worth reading.]

Roman G. Read It Again: It's Good for You. JAMA. 2009; 301: 1382. [A republication of a satirical editorial on the various reasons why authors should publish the same paper numerous times; worth rereading.]

Ronai PM. A Bad Case of Medical Jargon. AJR Am J Roentgenol. 1993; 161: 592. [An excellent little essay illustrating how and why to replace medical jargon with plain English.]

Rosenthal R. The "File Drawer Problem" and Tolerance for Null Results. Psychol Bull. 1979; 86: 638-641. [A historical attempt to quantify the effect that publication bias against studies with non-significant results would have on the overall metasynthesis of evidence on any given topic.]

Rossel M, Burnier M, Stupp R. Informed Consent: True Information or Institutional Review Board–Approved Disinformation? J Clin Oncol. 2007; 25: 5835-5836. [A substantial research letter arguing that research subjects are generally not concerned about the investigators' conflicts of interest and informed consent forms are too complex for most participants.]

Rosselot Jaramillo E, Bravo Lechat M, Kottow Lang M, Valenzuela Yuraidini C, O'Ryan Gallardo M, Thambo Becker S, Horwitz Campos N, Acevedo Pérez I, Rueda Castro L, Angélica Sotomayor M. En referencia al plagio intelectual: Documento de la Comisión de Ética de la Facultat de Medicina de le Universidad de Chile. Rev Méd Chil. 2008; 136: 653-658. [Written by the ethics committee of a medical college, this basic statement on plagiarism presents the social and moral-philosophical dimensions better than most such statements.]

Rossner M, Yamada KM. What's in a picture? The temptation of image manipulation. J Cell Biol. 2004; 166: 11-15. [A substantial editorial / tutorial paper on unacceptable editing of scientific images, specifically gels and micrographs.]

* Rothwell PM. Medical academia is failing patients and clinicians. BMJ. 2006; 332: 863-864. [A brief but very good editorial making the case that there is too little clinical research on commonplace issues that matter directly to patient care.]

Rouse A. Use short sentences. BMJ. 1997; 314: 754. [An amusing little letter criticizing long sentences.]

Royston P. Estimating Departure from Normality. Stat Med. 1991; 10: 1283-1293. [A good paper for statistical specialists presenting an approach to quantify how much a dataset departs from a Normal distribution.]

* Running the numbers. Nat Neurosci. 2005; 8: 123. [An editorial providing a quick overview of many of the commonplace errors of statistical analysis and reporting; well recommended.]

Ryder K. Guidelines for the presentation of numerical tables. Res Vet Sci. 1995; 58: 1-4. [A somewhat dated but otherwise solid tutorial paper on how to design tables.]

Sackett DL, Cook RJ. Understanding clinical trials. BMJ. 1994; 309: 755-756. [A brief tutorial paper describing various ways to present the efficacy of two treatments compared in a clinical trial.]

Sackett DL, Wennberg JE. Choosing the best research design for each question. BMJ. 1997; 315: 1636. [A brief editorial reminding readers that the best study design and research method is the one that is most appropriate for answering that particular study's research question.]

Sand-Jensen K. How to write consistently boring scientific literature. Oikos. 2007; 116: 723-727. [This sarcastic tutorial article provides 10 recommendations about how to write bad scientific literature; although amusing, if readers put in the effort to invert the sarcastic advice, only about half the recommendations are useful for writing good scientific papers, while the other half of the recommendations would actually only be useful for layperson journalistic accounts about science.]

* Saper CB. Academic Publishing, Part III: How to Write a Research Paper (So That It Will Be Accepted) in a High-Quality Journal. Ann Neurol. 2015; 77: 8-12. [Among the many tutorial papers about how to write journal papers, this is perhaps the only one with advice geared mainly toward publishing in high-impact journals; well recommended reading, especially for experienced researchers.]

Scarlat MM. Erratum, corrigenda et emendatio or "mistake, correction and amendment". Int Orthop. 2017; 41: 1071-1072. [A very clever editorial, by a French Editor, about the correction of minor errors in published papers – written with just the perfectly right amount of little errors to make his point.]

Schachman HK. From "Publish or Perish" to "Patent and Prosper". J Biol Chem. 2006; 281: 6889-6903. [A prominent life scientist's personal narrative history of research policy, funding, and ethics in America over the past half century.]

Schriger DL, Cooper RJ. Achieving Graphical Excellence: Suggestions and Methods for Creating High-Quality Visual Displays of Experimental Data. Ann Emerg Med. 2001; 37: 75-87. [This tutorial paper shows how to graph data in ways that better illuminate what the data actually shows; recommendable.]

Schriger DL, Sinha R, Schroter S, Liu PY, Altman DG. From Submission to Publication: A Retrospective Review of the Tables and Figures in a Cohort of Randomized Controlled Trials Submitted to the *British Medical Journal*. Ann Emerg Med. 2006; 48: 750-756. [An interesting study of manuscripts submitted to the BMJ, providing evidence that figures and tables in medical research are often simplistic and low-quality and are rarely improved any by peer review.]

Schroter S, Black N, Evans S, Godlee F, Osorio L, Smith R. What errors do peer reviewers detect, and does training improve their ability to detect them? J R Soc Med. 2008; 101: 507-514. [A study from a team at the BMJ showing that peer reviewers overlook most errors in manuscripts and training them has a negligible effect.]

Schulz KF, Altman DG, Moher D; for CONSORT Group. CONSORT 2010 Statement: updated guidelines for reporting parallel group randomised trials. BMJ. 2010; 340: 698-702. [Guidelines for the reporting of randomized controlled trials; essential reading for anyone writing up a randomized controlled trial, and broadly useful for reporting any other prospective clinical study too.]

Schwenzer KJ. Practical Tips for Working Effectively With Your Institutional Review Board. Respir Care. 2008; 53: 1354-1361. [A good, basic, practical review of what researchers must do (at least in the USA) to obtain approval from a Research Ethics Committee.]

* Scientific Integrity Committee of the Swiss Academies of Arts and Sciences. Authorship in scientific publications: analysis and recommendations. Swiss Med Wkly. 2015; 145: w14108. [A substantial and authoritative discussion of the determination of authorship.]

Scott T. Changing authorship system might be counterproductive. BMJ. 1997; 315: 744. [A letter of critical sociology arguing (correctly) that the people listed as authors on medical scientific papers often merely reflects the power politics of the institute behind the paper and (incorrectly) that no attempts to reform the system of authorship should be made.]

Self-plagiarism: unintentional, harmless, or fraud? Lancet. 2009; 374: 664. [A half-page editorial, conceptually muddled and lacking any references.]

* Seneca LA. Moral Essays, volume II. [Translated from the Latin by Basore JW.] Cambridge, MA, USA: Harvard University Press; (ca. 35-60), 1931, 2006. [A collection of well-written philosophical ethics essays, many of which describe the character traits and behavioral habits that are most conducive to scientific work; highly worthwhile reading.]

Seshia SS. Reproduction of Tables: Are Some Publishers Ignoring Fair Use/Dealing? Can J Neurol Sci. 2010; 37: 914-916. [A commentary on some publishers blocking fair use reproduction of tables and figures.]

Shah J, Shah A, Pietrobon R. Scientific Writing of Novice Researchers: What Difficulties and Encouragements Do They Encounter? Acad Med. 2009; 84: 511-516. [This small, poorly written, qualitative study about the difficulties novice researchers encounter when trying to write their scientific papers might be of some interest to specialists of medical education charged with teaching scientific writing to students.]

Sharp D. Kipling's Guide to Writing a Scientific Paper. Croat Med J. 2002; 43: 262-267. [Written in a vaguely quirky and eccentric tone, this informal guide to writing a scientific paper in the IMRD structure the way a journalist would is one of the most unrecommendable "expert opinion" guides to writing available in the literature.]

Shashok K. Content and communication: How can peer review provide helpful feedback about the writing. BMC Med Res Methodol. 2008; 8: 3. [A substantial discussion paper about the deficiencies of peer review feedback on composition and language aspects of manuscripts.]

Sherwin CM. Animal welfare: reporting details is good science. Nature. 2007; 448: 251. [A letter explaining why the details of animal treatment should be reported in scientific papers.]

Shih WJ. Problems in dealing with missing data and informative censoring in clinical trials. Curr Control Trials Cardiovasc Med. 2002; 3: 4. [A very useful tutorial review paper on how to deal with missing data.]

** Sigma Xi. Honor in Science. Research Triangle Park, NC, USA: Sigma Xi; 2000. [Written and published by a venerable professional society, this classic booklet about maintaining honesty in scientific research is a bit dated in style but timeless and fundamental in contents.]

Simera I, Altman DG. Writing a research article that is "fit for purpose": EQUATOR Network and reporting guidelines. Ann Intern Med. 2009; 151: JC2-2 to JC2-3. [An essay presenting the EQUATOR network and the reporting guidelines they promote.]

Simera I, Moher D, Hoey J, Schulz KF, Altman DG. A catalog of reporting guidelines for health research. Eur J Clin Invest. 2010; 40: 35-53. [This article is mostly a long list of the reporting guidelines that were available at the EQUATOR website at the time this paper was published.]

Simon SD. Understanding the Odds Ratio and the Relative Risk. J Androl. 2001; 22: 533-536. [A tutorial paper providing a thorough and comprehensible explanation of odds ratios and relative risks.]

Siontis GCM, Patsopoulos NA, Vlahos AP, Ioannidis JPA. Selection and Presentation of Imaging Figures in the Medical Literature. PLoS One. 2010; 5: e10888. [A study of the literature on the selection and presentation of medical imaging as figures, along with recommendations for improvement; useful for anyone presenting medical imaging as figures.]

Siwek J. Permission fees for reproducing tables in journal articles are exorbitant. BMJ. 2015; 351: h5128. [A letter from a journal Editor about excessive permission fees to reprint published tables.]

Slinker BK, Glantz SA. Multiple Linear Regression: Accounting for Multiple Simultaneous Determinants of a Continuous Dependent Variable. Circulation. 2008; 117: 1732-1737. [A not-so-basic introduction to multivariable linear regression.]

Smith AJ, Goodman NW. The hypertensive response to intubation. Do researchers acknowledge previous work? Can J Anaesth. 1997; 44: 9-13. [A bibliographic case study documenting how rarely researchers are aware of utterly essential literature on their own topic.]

Smith GD, Ebrahim S. Data dredging, bias, or confounding: They can all get you into the BMJ and the Friday papers. BMJ. 2002; 325: 1437-1438. [An editorial about how poor study design, data dredging, and failure to recognize confounded variables can lead to spurious research findings.]

Smith MA, Barry HC, Williamson J, Keefe CW, Anderson WA. Factors Related to Publication Success Among Faculty Development Fellowship Graduates. Fam Med. 2009; 41: 120-125. [A survey study of why many primary care faculty-development fellows never publish their research.]

Smith R. Authorship: time for a paradigm shift? BMJ. 1997; 314: 992. [An editorial describing problems with the accuracy of lists of authors and proposing solutions; though the problems are still current, this editorial's views are somewhat outdated.]

Smith R. Animal research: the need for a middle ground. BMJ. 2001; 322: 248-249. [A progressive editorial from the Editor-in-Chief of BMJ about the need to replace, reduce, and refine animal research.]

Smith R. Doctors are not scientists. BMJ. 2004; 328 (7454): 0-h. [Reflections from the Editor-in-Chief of BMJ about why physicians rarely ever read research articles in the journals they receive.]

Smith R. Letters to the editor. BMJ. 1984; 288: 1476-1477. [A brief editorial providing some insights about how to write letters about a published article.]

Smith R. Making progress with competing interests. BMJ. 2002; 325: 1375-1376. [An editorial encouraging people to openly declare their conflicts of interest.]

Smith R. The rise of medical English. BMJ. 1986. 293: 1591-1592. [An interesting editorial on the use of English as the lingua franca of medicine.]

Smith R. Time to face up to research misconduct. BMJ. 1996; 312: 789-790. [An editorial calling on the British medical profession to deal more centrally and more effectively with research misconduct.]

Smythe WR. Protected time. Surgery. 2004; 135: 232-234. [This thoughtful and well-written editorial reflects on the organizational and financial complexies of supporting the research work of clinical investigators.]

Soffer A. Can You Believe What You Read in Medical Journals? Chest. 1992; 101: 1417-1419. [A long-winded editorial about how to critically evaluate research papers.]

Sprague S, Bhandari M, Devereaux PJ, Swiontkowski MF, Tornetta P III, Cook DJ, Dirschl D, Schemitsch EH, Guyatt GH. Barriers to Full-Text Publication Following Presentation of Abstracts at Annual Orthopaedic Meetings. J Bone Joint Surg Am. 2003; 85-A: 158-163. [A survey study of why studies presented at a conference were never published in a peer-reviewed journal.]

Sprent P. Statistics in medical research. Swiss Med Wkly. 2003; 133: 522-529. [A very good introduction to basic statistical issues for clinical research, including sampling, hypothesis testing,
power, data distribution, etc.]

Spriestersbach A, Röhrig B, du Prel J-B, Gerhold-Ay A, Blettner M. Deskriptive Statistik. Dtsch
Arztebl Int. 2009; 106: 578-583. [An introductory-level tutorial article on the different types of
variables and some basic types of graphs that can be used for reporting descriptive statistics.]

Steen RG. Retractions in the scientific literature: do authors deliberately commit research fraud?
J Med Ethics. 2011; 37: 113-117. [A study of the literature comparing the characteristics of
papers retracted for fraud versus for errors.]

Sterne JAC, Smith GD. Sifting the evidence–what's wrong with significance tests? BMJ. 2001;
322: 226-231. [A thorough discussion of significance testing and p-values; occasionally con-
taminated with misguided Bayesian notions, but otherwise mostly quite good.]

Stilman A. Grammatically Correct, 2nd ed. Cincinnati, OH, USA: Writer's Digest Books; 1997,
2010. [A well-written basic guide to English punctuation, grammar, and style, with many interesting literary quotations and a high portion of medical scientific examples.]

Streiner DL. Speaking Graphically: An Introduction to Some Newer Graphing Techniques. Can J
Psychiatry. 1997; 42: 388-394. [This tutorial article about various basic data graphs is written
in a consistently silly tone and contains substantial amounts of erroneous information and bad
advice; not recommendable.]

Streit M, Gehlenborg N. Bar charts and box plots. Nat Methods. 2014; 11: 117. [A very useful
guide for constructing appropriate bar charts and box plots, yet with some minor errors of
advice and poorly referenced.]

** Strunk W Jr., White EB. The Elements of Style. Boston: Allyn & Bacon; 1959, 1979. [This
short book is the established fundamental primer of good English writing style; essential reading for anyone who wants to write anything in English.]

Sugarman J, Sulmasy DP, eds. Methods in Medical Ethics. Washington DC: Georgetown University
Press; 2001. [A book about the various scholarly approaches to the field of medical ethics; most
remote from the subject of medical scientific writing, but nonethess of some use in regards to
ethical aspects and scholarship.]

Suvarna SK, Ansary MA. Histopathology and the 'third great lie'. When is an image not a scientifically authentic image? Histopathology. 2001; 39: 441-446. [This well-written viewpoint article discusses and illustrates what is acceptable versus unacceptable digitally editing
of histopathology images, yet appears broadly applicable to all scientific photography and
imaging.]

Swinscow TVD. Statistics at Square One: V—Populations and samples. BMJ. 1976; 1 (6024):
1513-1514. [A brief but very dated introduction to this still key concept of research.]

Swinscow TVD. Statistics at Square One: VI—Variation between samples. BMJ. 1976; 1 (6025):
1585. [A very brief and useful comment on the title topic, as well as the relation between the
SD and SEM.]

Taboulet P. Advice on writing an abstract for a scientific meeting and on the evaluation of abstracts by
selection committees. Eur J Emerg Med. 2000; 7: 67-72. [This tutorial article about writing abstracts
for scientific conferences is mostly reliable and transferable to abstracts for journal papers too.]

Tallis RC. Researchers forced to do boring research... BMJ. 1994; 308: 591. [A letter on various
aspects of the occupational organization of academic research.]

Tenenbein M. Whole Bowel Irrigation and the Capsule Summary. Ann Emerg Med. 2004; 44:
666-667. [A letter criticizing inaccurate capsule summaries with unspecified authorship, with
an example.]

The cost of salami slicing. Nat Mat. 2005; 4: 1. [An editorial against salami publication; several
good points, poorly composed.]

The insider's guide to plagiarism. Nat Med. 2009; 15: 707. [A mostly narrative editorial about
plagiarism with only one reference; a rather airy account more fit for a popular magazine than
a scientific or scholarly journal.]

The long road to reproducibility. Nat Cell Biol. 2015; 17: 1513-1514. [An editorial describing some measures that the *Nature* journals took to improve the reproducibility of basic science papers.]

Thompson PJ. How To Choose the Right Journal for Your Manuscript. Chest. 2007; 132: 1073-1076. [Although a bit dated, this article contains generally good advice on selecting journals.]

Thoughts on (dis)credits. Nature. 2002; 415: 819. [A curious collection of mostly anonymous quotes about the topic of senior scientists claiming credit for work done by junior researchers.]

Tobias A. Dynamite plunger plots should not be used. Occup Environ Med. 1998; 55: 361-362. [A letter explaining why dynamite plunger graphs should be replaced with dot plots or box-and-whisker plots.]

Tramèr MR, Reynolds DJM, Moore RA, McQuay HJ. Impact of covert duplicate publication on metaanalysis: a case study. BMJ. 1997; 315: 635-640. [A well-written systematic review illustrating how duplicate publication of clinical trials distorts the overall body of evidence.]

Tscharntke T, Hochberg ME, Rand TA, Resh VH, Kraus J. Author Sequence and Credit for Contributions in Multiauthored Publications. PLoS Biol. 2007; 5: e18. [A brief discussion of various methods to allocate credit among co-authors of a paper; useful reflections on that academic squabbling.]

Tuddenham WJ. On the Art of the Abstract. Radiographics. 1989; 9: 583-584. [A brief editorial describing three inappropriate ways to compose a summary of an article.]

* Tufte ER. Envisioning Information. Cheshire, CT, USA: Graphics Press; 1990. [A beautiful and sophisticated book about how to convey information visually.]

** Tufte ER. The Visual Display of Quantitative Information, 2nd ed. Cheshire, CT, USA: Graphics Press; 1983, 2001. [A highly sophisticated, yet easily comprehensible, book about how to improve the presentation of numerical data and graphic design of figures; essential reading for anyone who makes graphs, tables, charts, etc.]

Tychinin DN, Kamnev AA. Beyond style guides: Suggestions for better scientific English. Acta Histochem. 2005; 107: 157-160. [Mostly a collection of misused English words, compiled by two Russian life scientists; well-meant and sometimes useful, but unreliable, unauthoritative, and poorly developed; not recommendable.]

* United Nations Educational, Scientific and Cultural Organization (UNESCO). Recommendation on Science and Scientific Researchers. In: United Nations Educational, Scientific and Cultural Organization (UNESCO). Report of the Social and Human Sciences Commission (SHS), 39C, 11 November 2017. Paris: UNESCO; 2017, pp. 31-47. [Although addressed to governments, these recommendations contain many enlightening descriptions of the personal qualities that scientific researchers should cultivate, as well as the humanitarian spirit required for beneficial scientific research; highly recommended reading.]

** United Nations Educational, Scientific and Cultural Organization (UNESCO). Universal Declaration on Bioethics and Human Rights. Paris: UNESCO; 2006. [A grand declaration, addressed primarily to states, on the ethical dimensions of medicine and life sciences, within a human rights framework; for individual researchers, this document is mostly useful for absorbing the general spirit of working for the betterment of humanity.]

U.S. National Library of Medicine. Samples of Formatted References for Authors of Journal Articles. Published: 09 July 2003. Updated: 02 May 2018. Accessed on 21 May 2018 at: https://www.nlm.nih.gov/bsd/uniform_requirements.html [Examples of how to format references for 44 different types of sources; authoritative.]

Van Damme H, for Editorial Board. Twelve Steps to Developing Effective Tables and Figures. Acta Chir Belg. 2007; 107: 237-238. [A brief, cursory, and basic editorial with advice for making tables and figures, most but not all of which is correct.]

Van Der Weyden MB. Managing allegations of scientific misconduct and fraud: lessons from the "Hall affair". MJA. 2004; 180: 149-151. [An illuminating scholarly editorial about how to improve the investigation of allegations of research misconduct.]

van Loon AJ. Pseudo-authorship. Nature. 1997; 389: 11. [A letter calling for an end to inflated lists of co-authors.]

van Raaij MJ. Guest authors: for contributors only. Nature. 2010; 468; 765. [A brief letter against guest authorship.]

Vandenbroucke JP, von Elm E, Altman DG, Gøtzsche PC, Mulrow CD, Pocock SJ, Poole C, Schlesselman JJ, Egger M, for STROBE Initiative. Strengthening the Reporting of Observational Studies in Epidemiology (STROBE): Explanation and Elaboration. PLoS Med. 2007; 10: e297. [Intermediate-level explanations of important guidelines for reporting observational studies; useful for the Methods and Results sections of papers, especially in regards to statistical issues, but otherwise weak with some flawed advice]

Vargas Llosa M. Cartas a un joven novelista. Madrid: Alfaguara; 2011. [An engaging book, by a Nobel Prize winner, about how to write stories; deep training for anyone wanting to write case reports or narrative accounts of medicine.]

Verhagen AP, Ostelo RWJG, Rademaker A. Is the p value really so significant? Aust J Physiother. 2004; 50: 261-262. [A translation of an unoriginal basic overview of hypothesis testing, p-values, and confidence intervals.]

Vessal K, Habibzadeh F. Rules of the game of scientific writing: fair play and plagiarism. Lancet. 2007; 369: 641. [A letter defending plagiarism of text by non-native speakers of English, on the grounds that they lack English writing expertise – elegantly written by two non-native speakers of English, thus disproving their own arguments.]

* von Elm E, Altman DG, Egger M, Pocock SJ, Gøtzsche PC, Vandenbroucke JP, for the STROBE Initiative. The Strengthening the Reporting of Observational Studies in Epidemiology (STROBE) Statement: Guidelines for Reporting Observational Studies. Ann Intern Med. 2007; 147: 573-577. [Important guidelines on what should be included in the report of observational studies, (which are the bulk of clinical studies).]

von Elm E, Costanza MC, Walder B, Tramèr MR. More insight into the fate of biomedical meeting abstracts: a systematic review. BMC Med Res Methodol. 2003; 3: 12. [A metaanalysis showing that only about one third of all abstracts submitted to conferences are ever published as full journal papers.]

Waaijers LJM. "Author pays" publishing model: Strategy is needed to get from A to B. BMJ. 2003; 327: 54. [A university librarian's insights on the costs of journals with subscription access versus open access; worth serious reflection.]

Wagena EJ. The scandal of unfair behaviour of senior faculty. J Med Ethics. 2005; 31: 308. [An ethics essay about the misappropriation by senior academics of authorship credit from junior researchers; recommended reading for anyone involved in any such intergenerational collaboration.]

Wager E. Authors, Ghosts, Damned Lies, and Statisticians. PLoS Med. 2007; 4: 0005-0006. [A commentary on the study by Gøtzsche PC, et al, 2007, listed above, which showed that statisticians are often omitted from the list of authors.]

Wager E, Williams P. "Hardly worth the effort"? Medical journals' policies and their editors' and publishers' views on trial registration and publication bias: quantitative and qualitative study. BMJ. 2013; 347: f5248. [Mostly an interesting qualitative study with a dozen or so journal Editors about the various factors influencing their decisions to accept or reject manuscripts.]

Wainer H. Depicting Error. Am Stat. 1996; 50: 101-111. [This thoughtful and well-written paper from the field of education reflects on ways to represent the uncertainty of data and results in figures and tables; recommended reading for anyone with a solid foundation in statistics and data visualization.]

Walsh M, Srinathan SK, McAuley DF, Mrkobrada M, Levine O, Ribic C, Molnar AO, Dattani ND, Burke A, Guyatt G, Thabane L, Walter SD, Pogue J, Devereaux PJ. The statistical significance of randomized controlled trial results is frequently fragile: a case for a Fragility Index. J Clin Epidemiol. 2014; 67: 622-628. [This empirical study describes and illustrates the Fragility Index – an interesting and simple statistical diagnostic tool for assessing the robustness of results; worthwhile reading for intermediate and advanced level researchers performing statistical analysis.]

Wang R, Lagakos SW, Ware JH, Huner DJ, Drazen JM. Statistics in Medicine — Reporting of Subgroup Analyses in Clinical Trials. NEJM. 2007; 357: 2189-2194. [A review of deficiencies in reporting subgroup analyses and guidelines for how they should be reported.]

Ward LG, Kendrach MG, Price SO. Accuracy of abstracts for original research articles in pharmacy journals. Ann Pharmacother. 2004; 38: 1173-1177. [A study of the literature showing that abstracts in pharmacy journals often contain information that is different from or missing in the main text.]

Watine JC. "Author pays" publishing model: Only "bad" authors should pay. BMJ. 2003; 327: 54. [A very brief letter asserting that authors should not be charged publication fees and peer reviewers should be paid for their work.]

Watson JD, Crick FHC. Molecular structure of nucleic acids: A structure for Deoxyribose Nucleic Acid. Nature. 1953; 171: 737-738. [A landmark paper cited here for the sake of example in the chapter, "Cut It Down"; not otherwise germane to the topics of this book.]

Weber EJ, Callaham ML, Wears RL, Barton C, Young G. Unpublished Research from a Medical Specialty Meeting: Why Investigators Fail to Publish. JAMA. 1998; 280: 257-259. [A survey study of why studies submitted to a conference were never published in a peer-reviewed journal.]

Weber WEJ, Merino JG, Loder E. Trial registration 10 years on: The single most valuable tool we have to ensure unbiased reporting of research studies. BMJ. 2015; 351: h3572. [A brief commentary from some Editors of this journal about the status of publications and submissions relative to the requirements for registration of trials.]

* Weissgerber TL, Milic NM, Winham SJ, Garovic VD. Beyond Bar and Line Graphs: Time for a New Data Presentation Paradigm. PLoS Biol. 2015; 13: e1002128. [A tutorial paper showing why dynamite plungers should be replaced with dot plots for the graphing of continuous variables in small samples.]

Weissmann G. Writing Science: The Abstract is Poetry, the Paper is Prose. FASEB J. 2008; 22: 2601-2604. [An editorial comparing scientific abstracts to various types of poetry; eccentric – sometimes amusing, but mostly useless.]

Welch SJ. Conflict of Interest and Financial Disclosure: Judge the Science, Not the Author. Chest. 1997; 112: 865-867. [An editorial by the Managing Editor of *Chest* about their experiences with conflict of interest disclosure policies, with a good take-home message consistent with general theories of philosophy and hermeneutics.]

West R. The end of scientific articles as we know them? J Clin Epidemiol. 2016; 70: 276. [A crackpot editorial vision about replacing scientific articles with repositories of linked datasets, metadata, and associated commentaries.]

Whalen E. An Author's Guide to the Guidelines for Authors. AJR Am J Roentgenol. 1989; 152: 195-198. [An explanation of this journal's Instructions to Authors; although some details are outdated, most of the pointers and the overall spirit of this article would help most authors prepare their manuscripts better.]

Whalen E. Why We Edit. AJR Am J Roentgenol. 1989; 152: 647-649. [This essay provides some explanation of the intended purpose of copyediting.]

Whimster WF. How I subedit. BMJ. 1976; 2 (6044): 1114-1115. [This brief editorial provides good advice and illustrations on how to edit manuscripts to eliminate excessive verbiage and other such problems of composition.]

Whitley E, Ball J. Statistic review 4: Sample size calculations. Crit Care. 2002; 6: 335-341. [A tutorial paper on calculating sample sizes for studies; more useful for understanding the issues than for actually performing the calculations, despite (or because of) extensive formulas and graphs.]

Why not to publish Case Reports? Clin Transl Oncol. 2010; 12: 157. [A brief and dull editorial about why this journal stopped publishing case reports.]

Wilcox LJ. Authorship: The Coin of the Realm, The Source of Complaints. JAMA. 1998; 280: 216-217. [An empirical study documenting and commenting on the rising rate of complaints about misallocation of authorship at one top-tier medical school.]

Wilkins RW. How to Write an Abstract. Circulation. 1958; 17: 841. [A brief editorial with good advice, mostly about how to write clearly.]

* Williams HC. How to reply to referees' comments when submitting manuscripts for publication. J Am Acad Dermatol. 2004; 51: 79-83. [This tutorial article on how to interpret jour-

nal decision letters and how to respond to peer reviewers is accurate, thorough, and useful; well-recommended.]

Winker MA. The need for concrete improvement in abstract quality. JAMA. 1999; 281: 1129-1130. [This poorly written editorial contains a useful checklist for improving the quality of abstracts.]

Woolley KL. Goodbye Ghostwriters! How to Work Ethically and Efficiently With Professional Medical Writers. Chest. 2006; 130: 921-923. [A tutorial paper about how medical researchers can work together with professional medical writers appropriately.]

Woolley KL, Barron JP. Handling Manuscript Rejection: Insights From Evidence and Experience. Chest. 2009; 135: 573-577. [A useful tutorial paper about how to determine if a paper has been completely rejected or only sent back for revision, and how to proceed in each of those scenarios; worthwhile reading.]

** World Medical Association. Declaration of Helsinki – Ethical Principles for Medical Research Involving Human Subjects. Accessed on 10 January 2018 at: https://www.wma.net/policies-post/wma-declaration-of-helsinki-ethical-principles-for-medical-research-involving-human-subjects/ [The fundamental ethical guidelines for medical research on humans; essential reading for all medical researchers, each and every time they start a new study.]

Wright DB. Making friends with your data: Improving how statistics are conducted and reported. Brit J Educ Psychol. 2003; 73: 123-136. [A substantial tutorial paper on how to improve the analysis and reporting of data, written by the Statistics Editor of a psychology journal but broadly applicable; recommendable.]

Wright JG, Swiontkowski MF, Heckman JD. Introducing Levels of Evidence to *The Journal*. J Bone Joint Surg Am. 2003; 85-A: 1-3. [A brief editorial presenting an overview of the levels of evidence system for various types of studies and an explanation of why this journal tags all articles with their level of evidence.]

Yang F, Shaw A, Garduno E, Olson KR. No one likes a copycat: A cross-cultural investigation of children's response to plagiarism. J Exp Child Psychol. 2014; 121: 111-119. [An experimental study showing that children develop a disapproval of plagiarism by 6 years of age, regardless of cultural origin from the United States, Mexico, or China.]

Yang OO. Guide to Effective Grant Writing. New York: Springer; 2005. [Although this short book is mostly about writing grant applications, and specifically NIH grant applications, some of it is useful for writing scientific reports.]

Yentis SM. Another kind of ethics: from corrections to retractions. Anaesthesia. 2010; 65: 1163-1166. [An introductory-level editorial discussing a wide range of ethical issues at the publication stage and how this journal prevents or responds to them; worthwhile reading.]

Yilmaz I. Plagiarism? No, we're just borrowing better English. Nature. 2007; 449: 658. [A letter making a (futile) attempt to defend plagiarism by scientists whose native language is not English.]

* Young J. When should you use statistics? Swiss Med Wkly. 2005; 135: 337-338. [A brief editorial from a statistician with good advice on the approach to statistical analysis for small or preliminary studies.]

Young RA, DeHaven MJ, Passmore C, Baumer JG. Research Participation, Protected Time, and Research Output by Family Physicians in Family Medicine Residencies. Fam Med. 2006; 38: 341-348. [A survey of family medicine residency programs about their research commitments and productivity; useful for understanding the time and other resources needed to conduct and report research.]

Young SN. Bias in the research literature and conflict of interest: an issue for publishers, editors, reviewers and authors, and it is not just about the money. J Psychiatry Neurosci. 2009; 34: 412-417. [A scholarly article, by the Co-Editor-in-Chief of this journal, about the wide variety of conflicts of interest that distort the scientific literature.]

Zarin DA, Tse T, Williams RJ, Rajakannan T. Update on Trial Registration 11 Years after the ICMJE Policy Was Established. NEJM. 2017; 376: 383-391. [A mixed narrative and empirical assessment of how well trial registries are fulfilling their intended goals.]

* Zinsser W. On Writing Well, 6th ed. New York: Harper Perennial; 1976, 1998. [A widely read book on the craft of writing in general; worthwhile reading for anyone who hopes to learn to write well.]

Index

The index was compiled by the author of the book, by rereading the entire text and extracting key concepts (not by merely running automatic searches for pregiven words). Page numbers in bold indicate a substantial explanation or discussion focused mainly on the index term itself; whereas, page numbers in regular font indicate that the term is used there. In many instances, occurrences of a term are not listed in the index, if they were only mentioned there fleetingly with no relevance for understanding the term, especially if the term occurs often in the book; (e.g. the index does not list every page number where the word "abstract" appears but only those page numbers where the text says something informative about abstracts). Conversely, in a few instances an index term does not appear on the page indicated, but the concept to which it refers is unmistakably discussed there in other words. Sometimes an index term is illustrated by or found in a figure, table, or example text, instead of in the main text (or additionally and separately from the main text). In such cases, an "f" after a page number indicates that the page number refers to a figure (and/or its legend) on that page; a "t" after a page number indicates that the page number refers to a table (and/or its legend) on that page; and an "e" after a page number indicates that the page number refers to an example text (and/or its integrated commentary) on that page. (Yet figures, tables, and example texts are not redundantly indicated this way, if the page numbers on which they appear are already listed in the index and the figure, table, or example text does not provide additional uses or illustrations of the index term unrelated to what is found in the main text on those pages.)

© Springer Nature Switzerland AG 2019
M. Hanna, *How to Write Better Medical Papers*,
https://doi.org/10.1007/978-3-030-02955-5

Printed in the United States
By Bookmasters